Lorraine M. Wright and Maureen Leahey

Nurses and Families

A Guide to Family Assessment and Intervention

Lorraine M. Wright, RN, PhD
International Lecturer, Blogger, Author, and Clinician
Professor Emeritus of Nursing
University of Calgary
Calgary, Alberta, Canada

Maureen Leahey, RN, PhD
Consultant, Author, Educator, and Clinician
Pugwash, Nova Scotia, Canada

EDITION 6

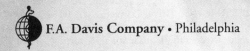

F.A. Davis Company • Philadelphia

F. A. Davis Company
1915 Arch Street
Philadelphia, PA 19103
www.fadavis.com

Printed in the United States of America

Last digit indicates print number: 10 9 8 7 6 5 4

Publisher, Nursing: Joanne Patzek DaCunha, RN, MSN
Director of Content Development: Darlene Pedersen
Project Editor: Echo Gerhart
Manager of Art and Design: Carolyn O'Brien

As new scientific information becomes available through basic and clinical research, recommended treatments and drug therapies undergo changes. The author(s) and publisher have done everything possible to make this book accurate, up to date, and in accord with accepted standards at the time of publication. The author(s), editors, and publisher are not responsible for errors or omissions or for consequences from application of the book, and make no warranty, expressed or implied, in regard to the contents of the book. Any practice described in this book should be applied by the reader in accordance with professional standards of care used in regard to the unique circumstances that may apply in each situation. The reader is advised always to check product information (package inserts) for changes and new information regarding dose and contraindications before administering any drug. Caution is especially urged when using new or infrequently ordered drugs.

Library of Congress Cataloging-in-Publication Data

Wright, Lorraine M., 1944-
  Nurses and families : a guide to family assessment and intervention / Lorraine M. Wright, Maureen Leahey. — 6th ed.
      p. ; cm.
  Includes bibliographical references and index.
  ISBN 978-0-8036-2739-0 (pbk. : alk. paper)
  I. Leahey, Maureen, 1944- II. Title.
  [DNLM: 1. Nursing Assessment. 2. Family Health. 3. Interviews as Topic—methods. WY 100.4]

  616.07'5—dc23

                                                            2012021678

After collaborating on our book *Nurses and Families* for over 30 years, we thought the time was right to dedicate this Sixth Edition to each other! Through stimulating conversations, clinical consultations, and a passionate exchange of ideas, we have experienced a constant synergy and sustained admiration for each other's knowledge and expertise. We greatly appreciate and thank one another for our deep collegiality and friendship on this incredible journey.

Lorraine M Wright
Maureen Leahey

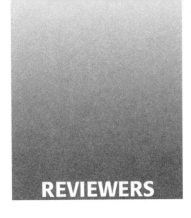

REVIEWERS

Michele D'Arcy-Evans, PhD, CNM
Professor
Lewis-Clarke State College
Lewiston, Idaho

Faith Johnson,
RN, BA, BSN, MA, CNE
Nurse Educator/Faculty
Ridgewater College
Willmar, Minnesota

Jamie Kane, MS, RN, CNE
Evening/Weekend Program Coordinator
Ellis School of Nursing
Schenectady, New York

Kara E. Keyes, MS, RNC
Instructor/Clinical Coordinator
Department of Nursing
Le Moyne College
Syracuse, New York

Stephanie Langford, RN,
BScN, MEd
Professor
University of Ottawa
Faculty of Health Sciences
School of Nursing
Ottawa, Ontario, Canada

Krista Lussier, RN, MSN
Senior Lecturer
Thompson Rivers University
Kamloops, British Columbia, Canada

M. Star Mahara, RN, BSN, MSN
Associate Professor
Thompson Rivers University
Kamloops, British Columbia, Canada

Janet McCabe, PhD, MEd, RN
Assistant Professor
University of Saskatchewan
Prince Albert, Saskatchewan, Canada

Carol Murphy Moore, MSN, CRNP
Assistant Professor of Nursing
Bloomsburg University
Bloomsburg, Pennsylvania

Judith Quaranta, MS, RN, CPN,
AE-C, Doctoral candidate
Clinical Associate Professor
Decker School of Nursing/Binghamton
University
Binghamton, New York

Helena Schaefer, RN, MN, NP
Faculty Lecturer
University of Alberta
Edmonton, Alberta, Canada

Gisele Thibodeau, BScN, RN
Faculty/Clinical Instructor
Dalhousie School of Nursing—
Yarmouth Site
Yarmouth, Nova Scotia, Canada

Sharon E. Thompson, MSN, RN
Assistant Clinical Professor
Northern Arizona University
Flagstaff, Arizona

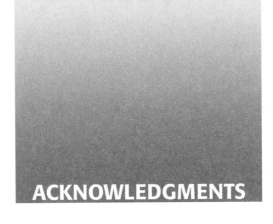

ACKNOWLEDGMENTS

We are grateful to our many colleagues, local, national, and international, for their continued support, interest, and positive comments about our book over these 30 years as we continue to evolve our ideas of how to best involve and assist families experiencing illness, loss, and/or disability. It continues to amaze and gratify us that, since 1984 when the First Edition was published, so many practicing nurses, students, and faculty have joined us in promoting family nursing worldwide.

We are especially grateful to:

- Joanne DaCunha, Publisher, Nursing Department, F.A. Davis, for her unfailing support, promptness, helpfulness, competence, and good nature as we worked on this Sixth Edition.
- Bob Martone, Publisher, Nursing Department, F.A. Davis, for his vision and support of our work, starting with the First Edition in 1984.
- Christina C. Burns, Senior Project Editor, Nursing, for her initial work on this Sixth Edition.
- Victoria White, Project Editor, Nursing, for her care in readying the manuscript for publication.
- Echo Gerhart, Project Editor, Nursing, who cheerfully walked us through the final miles of preparing the manuscript. Her attention to detail and speed in finding solutions to issues helped keep the book on track.

Finally, we are grateful to each other . . . for enduring friendship/ collegiality over some 37 years, for Caffe Beano Saturday morning conversations, fabulous restaurant experiences, and wonderful trips traveling together in Provence, Germany, Thailand, Iceland, Inle Lake, Luang Prabang, Lake O'Hara, Pugwash, Nova Scotia . . . and more adventures await!

Lorraine M. Wright
Maureen Leahey

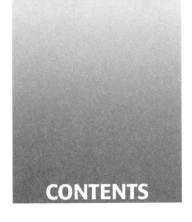

CONTENTS

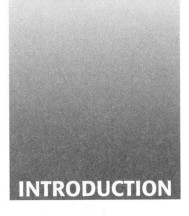

INTRODUCTION

REFLECTIONS ON THE FIRST TO SIXTH EDITIONS

We welcome you to the Sixth Edition of *Nurses and Families*. Whether you are a nursing student, practicing nurse, or nurse educator, this book is for you. We believe our book will benefit you whether you desire more relevant knowledge and essential skills for relational practice with families dealing with complex issues; information about teaching practices for family nursing; and/or the most pertinent research regarding family interaction. Our text breaches the boundaries of practice, education, and research. Research evidence and clinical narratives of families experiencing illness make it mandatory and a moral imperative for nurses to treat families with care and competence in whatever nursing context nurses find themselves. The development and evolution of family nursing have moved beyond the debate of whether families should be included in health care to a more important focus and emphasis on *how to* involve families. Therefore, the main emphasis and thrust of our Sixth Edition is to offer ideas of *how to* include families in nursing practice with the specific knowledge and skills to accomplish that. Yes, this is a "how to" book.

The First Edition of *Nurses and Families* was published in 1984, the second in 1994, the third in 2000, the fourth 2005, the fifth in 2009, and now the sixth in 2013.

Some of the changes and developments in family nursing, as well as the influence of larger societal differences in the past 30 years, are obvious and apparent to us and are discussed in our text, whereas others are more subtle and perhaps tenuous.

One example of the globalization of family nursing is our text having been translated into French, German, Icelandic, Japanese, Korean, Portuguese, Spanish, and Swedish. As well, we have developed a Web site *www.family nursingresources.com* for educational resources. We have written and produced eight educational DVDs (Wright & Leahey 2000, 2001, 2002, 2003, 2006, and 2010). See the section following the Index for additional information. These programs are also available in streaming video (.mov files and Quicktime and Windows Media Player). The programs are:

- *How to Do a 15-Minute (or Less) Family Interview* (2000)
- *Calgary Family Assessment Model: How to Apply in Clinical Practice* (2001)

- *Family Nursing Interviewing Skills: How to Engage, Assess, Intervene, and Terminate With Families* (2002)
- *How to Intervene With Families With Health Concerns* (2003)
- *How to Use Questions in Family Interviewing* (2006)
- *Common Errors in Family Interviewing: How to Avoid and Correct* (2010)
- *Tips and Microskills for Interviewing Families of the Elderly* (2010)
- *Interviewing an Individual to Gain a Family Perspective With Chronic Illness: A Clinical Demonstration* (2010)

We are delighted that these eight DVDs are being utilized by faculties, schools of nursing, and hospitals worldwide. These educational programs complement this text, *Nurses and Families*. They demonstrate family interviewing skills in action that have either been substantiated with practice-based evidence or evidence-based practice or both.

Further evidence of the expansion of family nursing assessment models worldwide is the fact that the Calgary Family Assessment Model (CFAM) continues to be widely adopted in undergraduate and graduate nursing curricula and by practicing nurses. The CFAM is utilized in nursing curricula throughout North America, Australia, Brazil, Chile, China, Denmark, England, Finland, Germany, Hong Kong, Iceland, Japan, Korea, Norway, Portugal, Qatar, Scotland, Singapore, Spain, Sweden, Switzerland, Taiwan, Thailand, and Vietnam. With this expansion, we have had to revisit and revise our thinking about the CFAM in order to acknowledge, recognize, and embrace the evolving importance of certain dimensions of family life that influence health and illness, such as class, gender, ethnicity, race, family development, and illness beliefs.

A significant amplification in our text was the development of a framework and model for interventions, namely the CFIM, which was introduced in the Second Edition. This was done in recognition of the need to give as much emphasis to intervention as there had been on assessment of families and to provide a framework within which to capture family interventions. This change was clearly influenced by the advances in family nursing research, education, and practice from a primary emphasis on assessment to an expanding and equal emphasis on intervention.

Perhaps a more subtle but equally significant development is our ever-changing and evolving relationship with the families with whom we work. This change is reflected in our choice of language to describe the nurse-family relationship that we deem most desirable. Our preferred stance/posture with families has evolved into a more collaborative, consultative, relational, and nonhierarchical relationship over the past 30 years. When we adopt this stance, we notice greater equality, respectfulness, nonjudgmentalness, and status given to the family's expertise. Therefore, the combined expertise of both the nurse and the family forms a new and effective synergy in the context of therapeutic conversations that otherwise did not and could not exist.

Another subtle development evolving throughout our six editions has been the movement toward a postmodernist worldview. We embrace the notion that there are multiple realities in and of "the world," that each family member and nurse see a world that he or she brings forth through interacting with themselves and with others through language. We encourage an openness in ourselves, our students, and the families with whom we work to the many "worlds", differences, and diversity between and among family members and health-care providers. For this reason we have included a diversity of client names representing various cultures to remind everyone of the many different "worlds" we and our clients inhabit.

We have also been influenced by dramatic restructuring in health care that has occurred over the past 20 years in Canada and the United States. With massive restructuring in health-care institutions and community clinics, budgetary constraints, and managed care, many nurses believe they cannot afford the opportunity to get involved in or attend to the needs of families in health-care settings. Nurses, particularly those in acute-care hospital settings, have expressed their frustration about the substantially reduced time to attend to families' needs and concerns because of increased caseloads, heightened acuity of patients, and short-term stays. To respect and respond to this change, we developed ideas about how to conduct a 15-minute (or less) family interview and introduced them in the Third Edition.

We have been gratified by how these ideas have been enthusiastically accepted in both our text and when presenting them at nursing workshops or conferences. More important, based on anecdotal reports, the implementation of these ideas has shown great promise. We have been encouraged by nurses' reports of softened suffering by family members and enhanced health promotion with families in their care. Equally gratifying are reports of increased job satisfaction by practicing nurses when collaborating with families, even if only for 15 minutes or less.

We consider it a privilege to collaborate and consult with families for health promotion and/or to diminish or soften emotional, physical, or spiritual suffering from illness. We are also grateful for opportunities to teach professional nurses and undergraduate and graduate nursing students about involving, caring for, and learning from families in health care. Through our own clinical practice and teaching of health professionals for over 40 years and personal family experiences with illness, we recognize the extreme importance of nurses' possessing sound family assessment and intervention knowledge, skills, and compassion in order to assist families. We also acknowledge the profound influence that families have upon our own lives and relationships.

A SNAPSHOT OF 30 YEARS OF PROGRESS AND PARADIGM EVENTS IN FAMILY NURSING

Over these 30 years since the publication of the First Edition of *Nurses and Families*, there have been paradigm events in family nursing worthy of celebration. There has been progress, and yet there are other areas where nursing still needs to put its "shoulder to the wheel." We believe one of the most far-reaching paradigm events in family nursing has been the publication of the *Journal of Family Nursing* in 1995. Since its inception, it has been under the able and competent editorship of Dr. Janice M. Bell. The establishment provided a central place, for the first time, for the uniting of family nurses and the dissemination of family nursing knowledge. Another paradigm event was the offering of the First International Family Nursing Conference in 1988, in Calgary, Canada. Without any formal organization or association, eight International Family Nursing Conferences (IFNCs) have been held in North America, South America (Chile), and (in 2007 for the first time) Asia (specifically, Bangkok, Thailand). Conferences in Chile, Iceland, Thailand, and Japan have enabled a further appreciation of family nursing's global expansion beyond the boundaries of North America. In 2009, the Ninth IFNC was held for the first time in Europe at Reykjavik, Iceland, and in 2011, the Tenth IFNC was held in Kyoto, Japan. The Eleventh IFNC returns to North America in 2013 in Minneapolis, Minnesota.

With each international family nursing conference, there is confirmation of clear, steady progress in the development and expansion of family nursing. It is evident in the presentations, workshops, and keynotes; in the advancement of knowledge in theory, research, assessment, and interventions in family work. There exists a solid commitment to focus on knowledge transfer and implementation to improve and sustain family care in actual clinical practice. The community of family nurses has expanded to be a true global force and phenomenon with enduring colleagueships and friendships.

Another momentous development occurred at the Ninth IFNC in Iceland when the International Family Nursing Association (IFNA) was created. With a formal organization, even more opportunities are now available for nurses to network and share knowledge and expertise outside of the conference format (www. internationalfamilynursing.org). One of the most exciting new developments in advancing family nursing has been the endowment of seven million dollars in 2008 to establish the Glen Taylor Nursing Institute for Family and Society (http://ahn.mnsu.edu/nursing/institute/) at the School of Nursing at Minnesota State University, Mankato. The university's vision is to create landmark innovations in the scholarship of family and society nursing practice.

The face of families has dramatically changed over the past 30 years as demographics in North America indicate an ever-increasing aging population; Baby Boomers are moving into retirement with significantly reduced numbers of Generation Xers to care for them. Marriages are being delayed or are nonexistent, as are pregnancies. Diversity in North American populations is clearly evident, demanding ever-increasing respect for a wide array of cultural, religious, and sexual orientation differences in the health-care system. Increased globalization invites the possibility for better health-care practices worldwide but also allows for the universal transmission of diseases, making it much more difficult for health-care providers to isolate, control, and segregate the origins of disease.

Amidst all the changes in demographics, technology, health-care delivery, and diversity, there are also profound changes occurring in worldviews, from modernism to postmodernism, from secularism to spiritualism. Family nursing has not been immune to these changes, nor have we.

Numerous other paradigm events have influenced families and the development of family nursing. Massive health-care restructuring and downsizing in North America, the growth of managed care in the United States, and the movements to reduce the length of stay in hospitals and to increase patient satisfaction have expanded and enlarged community-based nursing practice in the United States, Canada, and other countries. These movements have directly and indirectly placed more responsibility on families for the care of their ill members. Perhaps as a result of these dramatic changes, there is an expanded consumer movement and more collaboration with families about their health-care needs. Adding to this consumer movement is the increased technology, particularly the use of computers, personal digital assistants, instant messaging, e-mails, texting, and cellular phones. Access to the Internet and the explosion of health information through social networking such as blogs, Twitter, Facebook, Linkedin, and YouTube enable family members to be more proactive and knowledgeable about their health problems. Internet health sites and social media open doors never before possible for families to obtain current knowledge about their health problems, options for treatments, and traditional and alternative health-care resources.

THE SIXTH EDITION: WHAT IT IS, WHAT IS NEW

This revised Sixth Edition of *Nurses and Families* continues to be a "how-to" basic text for undergraduate, graduate, and practicing nurses. It is the only textbook, of which we are aware, that provides specific *how-to* guidelines for family assessment and intervention and actual skills for implementation in clinical practice with numerous clinical examples. This practical how-to guide for clinical work offers the opportunity for nursing students, practitioners, and educators to deliver better health care to families. Students and practitioners of community and public health nursing, maternal child nursing, pediatric nursing, mental health nursing, geriatric nursing, palliative care nursing, and those specializing in family systems nursing will find it most useful. Nurse educators who currently teach a family-centered approach and/or those who will be introducing the concept of the "family as the client" will find it a valuable resource. Educators involved in continuing education courses or nurse practitioner programs, especially family nurse practitioner programs, will be able to use this book to update and substantially enhance nurses' clinical knowledge and skills in family-centered care.

Our text provides specific guidelines and skills for nurses to consider when preparing for and conducting family meetings, from the first interview through to discharge or termination. Actual clinical case examples are given throughout the book. These case examples reflect ethnic, cultural, racial, and sexual orientation diversity in conjunction with various family developmental life-cycle stages and transitions. Special attention is given to the variety of family forms and structures prevalent in today's society. Issues in a variety of practice settings, including hospital, primary care, school, community, outpatient, and the home, are addressed. Innovative ideas to increase critical thinking are offered.

The clinical practice ideas are based on solid theory, research, and our own 40 years of clinical work with families. The ideas are current best practices. Due to our extensive clinical experience, both in our own practice and in the teaching and supervision of nursing and interdisciplinary students, we have been able to adapt the theoretical and clinical ideas so they can be useful. *How to Do a 15-Minute (or Shorter) Family Interview* (Chapter 9) remains one of the most popular, well-received, and useful chapters in the book as reported by numerous practicing nurses and nursing students. It assists nurses working in time-pressured environments to offer valuable assistance to families.

The major purposes of this book are to (1) provide nurses with a sound theoretical foundation for family assessment and intervention; (2) provide nurses with clear, concise, and comprehensive evidence-based family assessment and intervention models, namely the Calgary Family Assessment and Intervention Models, for current best practice; (3) provide guidelines for family interviewing skills; (4) offer detailed ideas and suggestions with clinical examples of how to prepare, conduct, use questions in, and terminate family interviews; and (5) provide nurses with an appreciation of the powerful influence of nurse-family collaboration to diminish, soften, or alleviate illness suffering.

In this Sixth Edition, the following features are new:

- A new chapter (Chapter 10) has been added: *How to Move Beyond Basic Family Nursing Skills.* We hope that this chapter will give nurses a clear idea how they can enhance their knowledge and skills, especially those nurses who have been familiar for a number of years with the skills that we discuss. This chapter offers more advanced skills in interviewing families in various settings and presents two clinical vignettes. Sample skills for interviewing families of the elderly at times of transition are highlighted as well as skills for interviewing an individual to gain a family perspective on chronic illness. Tips are offered, and microskills are delineated. Ideas for how to integrate family nursing into various practice contexts are offered.

- The Calgary Family Assessment Model (CFAM) has been thoroughly updated and expanded to include many new references to the most current research, theory, and U.S. statistics about families. These will enhance evidence-based practice. Increased attention is given to diversity issues, including ethnicity, race, culture, sexual orientation, gender, and class. CFAM is an easy-to-apply, practical, and relevant model for busy nurses working with a wide variety of complex issues and family structures and encountering various developmental stages.

- More complex genograms have been added. Recommendations for how to draw genograms for blended families with multiple parents and siblings, lesbian and gay families with children, and other family structures will enable nurses to increase their interviewing skills and take proactive steps to help families.

- The Calgary Family Intervention Model (CFIM) has been updated and revised to continue to make it more user-friendly and evidence-based. It remains, to our knowledge, the only family intervention model for nurses by nurses. It offers clear and specific family nursing interventions to assist with improving and/or sustaining family functioning and coping with illness.

- Increased complex family situations and key intervention skills will foster nurses' competence in dealing with multifaceted clinical issues, such as genetic testing, obesity, intergenerational adoption, and the impact of war and terrorism.

- Elements of the Internet, such as health networks, social networking, pornography, cybertherapy, cyberbullying, and their effects on families have been integrated into information-rich content.

- Specific suggestions for fostering collaborative nurse-family relationships are given throughout this text. Sample questions for nurses to ask themselves and the family are also offered.

- New clinical examples, vignettes, and boxes including questions used in practice are a fast and easy reference tool for busy practicing nurses.

TOUR OF THE CHAPTERS

The first five chapters provide the conceptual base for collaborating and consulting with families. To be able to interview families, identify strengths and concerns, and intervene to soften suffering, it is first necessary to have a sound conceptual framework. The specific how-to section of the book is included in Chapters 6 through 12 with numerous clinical examples in a variety of practice settings.

Chapter 1 establishes a rationale for family assessment and intervention. It describes the conceptual shift required in considering the family system, rather than the individual, as the unit of health care. It outlines the indications and contraindications for family assessment and intervention.

Chapter 2 addresses the major concepts of systems, cybernetics, communication, biology of knowing, and change theory that underpin the two models offered in this text: the CFAM and CFIM. The chapter also presents a brief description of some of the major worldviews that influence our models, such as postmodernism and gender sensitivity. Clinical examples of the application of these concepts are offered.

Chapter 3 presents the updated and revised CFAM, a comprehensive, three-pronged structural, developmental, and functional family assessment framework. This model has been thoroughly updated and expanded to reflect the current range of family forms in North American society, and it has increased emphasis on diversity issues such as ethnicity, race, culture, sexual orientation, gender, and class. Specific questions that the nurse may ask the family are provided. Two structural assessment tools—the genogram and ecomap—are described, and instructions and helpful hints are given for using them when interviewing families. Excerpts from actual family interviews are presented to illustrate how to use the model and tools in clinical practice.

Chapter 4 describes the updated and revised CFIM. The revisions enable nurses to move beyond assessment and to have available a repertoire of family interventions that will effect or sustain changes in family functioning in cognition, affect, and/or behavior. Actual clinical examples of family work are presented, and a variety of interventions are offered for consideration. Nurses traditionally have primarily focused on family assessment because there have been no family nursing intervention models within nursing to draw on.

Chapter 5 describes the family interviewing skills and competencies necessary in family-centered care. Perceptual, conceptual, and executive skills necessary for family assessment and intervention are presented. The skills are written in the form of training objectives, and clinical examples are given to help broaden the nurse's understanding of how to use these skills. Nurse educators, in particular, may find this chapter useful in focusing their evaluation of students' family interviewing skills. Ethical considerations in family interviewing are addressed.

Chapter 6 focuses on the importance of the nurse-family relationship. It presents clinical guidelines useful when preparing for family interviews. Ideas are given for developing hypotheses, choosing an appropriate interview setting, and making the first telephone contact with the family.

Chapter 7 delineates the various stages of the first interview and the remaining stages of the entire interviewing process: engagement, assessment, intervention, and termination. Actual clinical case examples in a variety of health-care settings illustrate the practice of conducting interviews.

Chapter 8 emphasizes that questions are one of the most helpful interventions nurses offer to families. Questions to engage, assess, elicit problem-solving skills, intervene, and request feedback are recommended for relational practice in various clinical settings.

Chapter 9 offers specific suggestions on how to conduct 15-minute (or less) family interviews in a manner that enhances the possibilities for healing or health promotion. These ideas respond to the realities facing many nurses in this era of managed care and health restructuring. The chapter also encourages nurses to adopt the belief that any time spent with families is better than no time.

Chapter 10 is a new chapter for this Sixth Edition and focuses on skills that are beyond the basics. Two in-depth clinical examples are given to illustrate the kind of skills that are more advanced. Ideas for how to integrate family nursing into various practice contexts are offered.

Chapter 11 offers ideas on how to avoid the three most common errors made in family nursing. Each error is defined and discussed. A clinical example is given, followed by specific ideas how each error could have been avoided. This chapter has proved useful to nurses in improving their care to families as well as enhancing their satisfaction in collaborating with families.

Chapter 12 highlights how to terminate with families in a therapeutic manner, whether after only one very short meeting, for example at the bedside, or after several meetings with a family, such as in an outpatient clinic. Ideas are given for family-initiated and nurse-initiated termination as well as for discharges determined by the health-care system.

The major difference between this book and other books on family nursing is that this book's primary emphasis is on how to meet, interview, and collaborate with families with the ultimate goal to soften suffering and/or promote health of the families in your care. We wish to emphasize, however, that this book does not offer a "cookbook" approach to family meetings and interviews. The real development of skills results from knowledge transfer to actual clinical practice and supervisory feedback.

We envision this book as a springboard for nursing students, nursing educators, nursing researchers, and practicing nurses. With a solid conceptual base and practical ideas for family assessment and intervention, we hope that more nurses will gain confidence and a commitment to engage in the nursing of families. In so doing, they will be reclaiming some aspects of nursing that have been directly or inadvertently given to other health professionals. In the process, nurses will continue to regain an important and expected dimension of nursing practice and be instrumental in the health promotion and healing of families with whom they care for and collaborate. We appreciate and are grateful for your interest and support of the ideas we offer in our book.

References

Wright, L.M., & Leahey, M. (Producers). (2000). *How to do a 15-minute (or less) family interview.* [DVD]. Calgary, Canada: www.familynursingresources.com.

Wright, L.M., & Leahey, M. (Producers). (2001). *Calgary Family Assessment Model: How to apply in clinical practice.* [DVD]. Calgary, Canada: www.familynursing resources.com.

Wright, L.M., & Leahey, M. (Producers). (2002). *Family nursing interviewing skills: How to engage, assess, intervene, and terminate with families.* [DVD]. Calgary, Canada: www.familynursingresources.com.

Wright, L.M., & Leahey, M. (Producers). (2003). *How to intervene with families with health concerns.* [DVD]. Calgary, Canada: www.familynursingresources.com.

Wright, L.M., & Leahey, M. (Producer). (2006). *How to use questions in family interviewing.* [DVD]. Calgary, Canada: www.familynursingresources.com.

Wright, L.M & Leahey, M. (Producers). (2010). Common Errors in Family Interviewing: How to Avoid & Correct. [DVD]. Calgary, Canada: www.FamilyNursingResources.com

Wright, L.M & Leahey, M. (Producers). (2010). Tips and Microskills for Interviewing Families of the Elderly. [DVD]. Calgary, Canada: www.FamilyNursingResources.com

Wright, L.M & Leahey, M. (Producers). (2010). Interviewing an Individual to Gain a Family Perspective with Chronic Illness: A Clinical Demonstration. [DVD]. Calgary, Canada: www.FamilyNursingResources.com

Chapter

Family Assessment and Intervention: An Overview

Nurses have an ethical and moral obligation to involve families in their health-care practice. This bold statement is due to evidence that the family has a significant impact on the health and well-being of individual members. Family-centered care is achieved responsibly and respectfully by relational practices consisting of collaborative nurse-family relationships together with sound family assessment and intervention knowledge and skills.

A rich tradition of nursing literature about the involvement of families in nursing care has been evolving over the past 35 years. Some of the classic and more recent texts on family nursing have enabled a new language to emerge through naming, describing, and communicating about the involvement of families in health care. Terms such as *family interviewing* (Wright & Leahey, 2013), *family health promotion nursing* (Bomar, 2004), *family health care nursing* (Hanson, 2001; Hanson & Boyd, 1996; Kaakinen, Gedaly-Duff, Coehlo, & Hanson, 2010), *family nursing* (Bell, Watson, & Wright, 1990; Broome, et al, 1998; Friedman, Bowden, & Jones, 2003; Gilliss, 1991; Gilliss, et al, 1989; Svavarsdottir & Jonsdottir, 2011; Wegner & Alexander, 1993; Wright & Leahey, 1990), *family nursing practice* and *family systems nursing* (Bell, 2009; Wright & Leahey, 1990; Wright, Watson, & Bell, 1990), *nursing of families* (Feetham, et al, 1993), and *family nursing as relational inquiry* (Doane & Varcoe, 2005) have all helped to bring forth a vital aspect of nursing practice heretofore overlooked, neglected, or minimized.

Perhaps the most significant, but not necessarily well-known, publication about family nursing is the monograph published by the International Council of Nurses titled *The Family Nurse: Frameworks for Practice* developed by Madrean Schober and Fadwa Affara (2001). It is a convincing validation for an emerging new role and specialty that the influential International Council of Nurses identifies the "family nurse" and "family nursing" as two of the important new and ongoing movements in nursing.

As nurses theorize about, conduct research on, and involve families more in health care, they modify their usual patterns of clinical practice. The implication for this change in practice is that nurses must become competent in assessing and intervening with families through collaborative nurse-family relationships. Nurses who embrace the belief that illness needs to be treated as a family affair can more efficiently learn the knowledge and clinical skills required to conduct family interviews (Wright & Bell, 2009). This belief invites nurses to think interactionally, or reciprocally, about families. The dominant focus of family nursing assessment and intervention must be the reciprocity between health and illness and the family.

It is most helpful and enlightening for nurses to assess the impact of illness on the family and the influence of family interaction on the cause, course, and cure of illness. Additionally, the reciprocal relationship between nurses and families is also a significant component of both softening suffering and enhancing healing.

EVOLUTION OF THE NURSING OF FAMILIES

Throughout nursing's history, family involvement has always been part of health-care, but it has not always been labeled as such. Because nursing originated in patients' homes, family involvement and family-centered care were natural occurrences. With the transition of nursing practice from homes to hospitals during the Great Depression and World War II, families became excluded not only from involvement in caring for ill members but also from major family events such as birth and death. After having undergone all these developmental changes, the practice of nursing has now come full circle, with an obligation to invite families once again to participate in their own health care. However, this invitation is being made with much more knowledge, research evidence, respect, and collaboration than at any other time in nursing history.

The history, evolution, and theory development of the nursing of families in North America have been discussed in depth in the literature (Anderson, 2000; Doane, 2003; Feetham, et al, 1993; Ford-Gilboe, 2002; Friedman, Bowden, & Jones, 2003; Gilliss, 1991; Gilliss, et al, 1989; Hartrick, 2000; Kaakinen, Gedaly-Duff, Coehlo, et al, 2010). These authors have made significant contributions to the advancement of family nursing knowledge.

The evolution, development, and practice of family nursing are well established and are being documented in many countries outside North America, such as Brazil (Angelo, 2008), Finland (Astedt-Kurki, 2010; Astedt-Kurki & Kaunonen, 2011), Iceland (Svavarsdottir, 2008; Svavarsdottir & Sigurdardottir, 2011), Hong Kong (Simpson, et al, 2006), Japan (Bell, 1999; Moriyama, 2008; Sugishita, 1999), Nordic countries (Svavarsdottir, 2006), Nigeria (Irinoye, Ogunfowokan, & Olaogun, 2006), Scotland (O'Sullivan Buchard, et al, 2004), Sweden (Saveman, 2010; Saveman & Benzein, 2001), and Thailand (Wacharasin & Theinpichet, 2008), to name a few.

Perhaps the boldest and most ambitious global effort to enhance care to families by implementing and improving the education and practice of nurses is the World Health Organization (WHO) Family Health Nurse Multinational Study (World Health Organization, 2006). Eighteen European countries were involved in this multinational study whose aim was to implement and evaluate the concept of family health nurse (FHN) within their various health and educational systems. The inclusion of countries such as Slovenia, Kyrgyzstan, Tajikistan, Republic of Moldova, and Lithuania indicates the continued global expansion of family nursing. An FHN was defined as a skilled generalist family/community nurse who combined illness prevention and management and other duties determined by family/community needs.

In 2006, there was a final meeting in Berlin, Germany, 6 years after the start of the study. At this meeting, the conclusion was that "the project was very much an action research and action learning process. Participants showed great enthusiasm and commitment to the research aims. Implementing a new nursing service is a change management process and in-country change cycles at the time of the multinational study were diverse. Some had developed a fully functional FHN programme and had advanced into a second phase. Some countries had not yet implemented the FHN programme whilst others were in the process of their implementation" (p. 10). One example of a country that published an impressive report upon completion of the Family Health Nurse Project initiated by WHO was Scotland, at the University of Stirling (Murray, 2008).

The evolution of family nursing is most evident in the textbooks utilized in the field. Five major textbooks on family health nursing in North America referenced throughout this text are now in their second to sixth editions. Providing nurses with a framework for family assessment and the interventions for treating families can facilitate the transition from thinking in an individualistic manner toward thinking interactionally and, thus, thinking "family."

FAMILY ASSESSMENT

Numerous disciplines have attempted to define and conceptualize the concept of *family*. Each discipline has its own point of view or frame of reference for viewing the family, and all have an ever-increasing appreciation of diversity issues. Economists, for example, have been concerned with how the family works together to meet material needs. Sociologists are concerned with the family as a specific group in society. Mischke-Berkey, Warner, and Hanson (1989); Hanson and Boyd (1996); and Tarko and Reed (2002) have identified and described several family assessment models and instruments developed by nurses and non-nurses. It is helpful for nurses to be aware of the many models offered by various disciplines and the distinct variables emphasized in each model because no one assessment model explains all family phenomena.

In any clinical practice setting, nurses benefit from adopting a clear conceptual framework, or map, of the family. This framework encourages the synthesis of data so that family strengths and problems can be identified and a useful nursing plan devised. When no conceptual framework exists, it is extremely difficult for the nurse to group disparate data or to examine the relationships among the multiple variables that affect the family. Use of a family assessment framework helps to organize this massive amount of seemingly different information. It also provides a focus for intervention.

CALGARY FAMILY ASSESSMENT MODEL: AN INTEGRATED FRAMEWORK

The Calgary Family Assessment Model (CFAM) was one of the four models identified in *The Family Nurse: Frameworks for Practice* monograph by the International Council of Nurses (Schober & Affara, 2001). The CFAM is a multidimensional framework consisting of three major categories: structural, developmental, and functional (see Chapter 3). The model is based on a theory foundation involving systems, cybernetics, communication, and change. It was adapted from Tomm and Sanders' (1983) family assessment model and has been substantially embellished since the first edition of this textbook in 1984. The model is also embedded within larger worldviews of postmodernism, feminism, and biology of cognition. Diversity issues are also emphasized and appreciated within this model.

Of course, any model is useful only if it can be comprehended by nurses and then transferred into their generalist practice with families. One encouraging study to substantiate that CFAM is an easily comprehensible model was conducted at the University of Hong Kong with senior baccalaureate nursing students. Following the teaching of CFAM, there was a significant increase in the perceived understanding of all subcategories in CFAM compared with the control group of baccalaureate nursing students who completed an elective nursing course in women's health (Lee, Leung, Chan, et al, 2010).

An advancement in research has been the psychometric development of the Iceland-Family Perceived Support Questionnaire (ICE-FPSQ) and the Iceland-Expressive Family Functioning Questionnaire (ICE-EFFQ), based on the CFAM and CFIM (Sveinbjarnardottir, Svavarsdottir, & Hrafnkelsson, in press; Sveinbjarnardottir, Svavarsdottir, & Hrafnkelsson, in press). These questionnaires will provide further credence and validity to the usefulness of the CFAM and CFIM. See Chapter 3 for a detailed description of CFAM and Chapter 4 for CFIM.

INDICATIONS AND CONTRAINDICATIONS FOR A FAMILY ASSESSMENT

It is important to identify guidelines for determining which families will automatically be considered for family assessment. Because families now tend to have increased health-care awareness and knowledge, nurses are encountering families who present themselves as a unit for assistance with family health and illness issues. Frequently, however, families believe the illness involves only one family member. Therefore, with each illness situation, a judgment must be made about whether that particular illness or problem should be approached within a family context.

Here are some examples of indications for a family assessment:

- A family is experiencing emotional, physical, or spiritual suffering or disruption caused by a family crisis (e.g., acute or chronic illness, injury, or death).

- A family is experiencing emotional, physical, or spiritual suffering or disruption caused by a developmental milestone (e.g., birth, marriage, youngest child leaving home).

- A family defines an illness or problem as a family issue, and a motivation for family assessment is present.

- A child or adolescent is identified by the family as having difficulties (e.g., cyberbullying, fear of cancer treatment).

- The family is experiencing issues that jeopardize family relationships (e.g., end-of-life illness, addictions).

- A family member is being admitted to the hospital for psychiatric or mental health treatment.

- A child is being admitted to the hospital.

Conducting and completing a family assessment does not absolve nurses from assessing serious risks, such as suicide and homicide, or serious illnesses in individual family members. Family assessment is neither a panacea nor a substitute for an individual assessment. In advanced nursing practice, particularly family systems nursing, assessment of individuals and of the family system occur simultaneously (Wright & Leahey, 1990).

Some situations contraindicate family assessment:

- Family assessment compromises the individuation of a family member (e.g., if a young adult has recently left home, a family interview may not be desirable).

- The context of a family situation permits little or no leverage (e.g., the family might have a constraining belief that the nurse is working as an agent of some other institution, such as the court).

During the engagement process, nurses must explicitly present the rationale for a family assessment. (Suggestions for how to do this are given in Chapters 6 and 7.) A nurse's decision to conduct a family assessment should be guided by sound clinical principles and judgment. The nurse can take advantage of opportunities to consult with peers and supervisors if questions exist about the suitability of such an assessment.

After the nurse has completed the family assessment, he or she must decide whether to intervene with the family. In the next section, general ideas about intervention are discussed. Specific ideas for nurses to consider when making clinical decisions about interventions with particular families are presented in Chapters 4, 8, and 9. The three most common errors in working with families are discussed in Chapter 11.

NURSING INTERVENTIONS: A GENERIC DISCUSSION

Numerous terms are used to distinguish and label the treatment portion of nursing practice, including *intervention, treatment, therapeutics, action, activity, moves,* and *micromoves* (Bulechek & McCloskey, 1992, 1999; Wright & Bell, 2009). This textbook prefers the designation *intervention.* The most rigorous effort to standardize the language for nursing interventions is the work of Bulechek and McCloskey (1992, 1999) and their colleagues at the University of Iowa. More recently, these authors have worked to build taxonomies such as the Nursing Interventions Classification, which is based on nurses' reports of their practice (Bulechek, Butcher, & McCloskey Dochterman, 2008).

Our practice differs in that after assessing a family, we prefer to generate a list of strengths and problems rather than diagnoses. We conceptualize the list as one observer's perspective, not as the "truth" about a family. The list presents problems or concerns that nurses can address. It has been our experience that nursing diagnoses have become too rigid and do not include enough consideration of ethnic and cultural issues. We prefer to identify the strengths of a family and list them alongside the problems. The advantage of this type of listing is that it gives a balanced view of a family. It also asks nurses not to be blinded by a family's problems or diagnosis but to realize that every family has strengths and resources, even in the face of potential or actual health problems.

Definition of a Nursing Intervention

Bulechek and McCloskey (1999) define nursing interventions as "any treatment based upon clinical judgment that a nurse performs to enhance patient/client outcomes. Nursing interventions include both direct and indirect care; those aimed at individuals, families, and the community; including nurse-initiated, physician-initiated treatments and other provider-initiated treatment" (p. xix). Wright and Bell (2009) offer an alternate definition: "any action or response of the clinician, which includes the clinician's overt therapeutic actions and internal cognitive-affective responses, that occurs in the context of a clinician-client relationship offered to effect individual, family, or community functioning for which the clinician is accountable." Wright and Bell (2009) expand on their definition of intervention by suggesting that an intervention "usually implies a one-time act with clear boundaries, frequently offering something or doing something to someone else." Interventions are normally purposeful and conscious and usually involve observable behaviors of the nurse.

Context of a Nursing Intervention

Nursing interventions should focus on the nurse's behavior and the family's response followed by the nurse's response to the family and so forth. We believe that nurse behaviors and client behaviors are contextualized in the nurse-client relationship and are therefore interactional. This differs from nursing diagnoses and nursing outcomes, which focus on client behavior (Bulechek & McCloskey, 1999) and are not usually interactional in nature. An interactional phenomenon occurs whereby the responses of a nurse (interventions) are invited by the responses of clients/family members (outcome) that are, in turn, invited by the responses of a nurse. To focus on only client behaviors or nurse behaviors does not take into account the relationship between nurses and clients. All of our nursing interventions are interactional—that is, not doing to or for the patient but *with* the patient. Nursing interventions are actualized only in a relationship.

However, some nurses do find the classification of nursing interventions to be helpful in providing a language to describe and conceptualize specific treatment efforts (Bulechek, Butcher, & McCloskey Dochterman, 2008).

Intent of Nursing Interventions

The intent or aim of any nursing intervention is to effect change, whether to decrease a high temperature of a patient or improve family functioning when caring for a young boy with chronic illness and his family. Therefore, effective nursing interventions are those to which clients and families respond because of the "fit," or meshing between the intervention offered by the nurse and the biopsychosocial-spiritual structure of family members. In relational practice with families, there is no predetermined, standardized intervention to use across a number of families. Rather, the nurse, in collaboration with a specific family, determines what interventions are most useful for a family experiencing a particular illness.

NURSING INTERVENTIONS FOR FAMILIES: A SPECIFIC DISCUSSION

Nurses can intervene with families in numerous ways, depending on the compassion, competence, skills, and even imagination of each nurse and, most importantly, depending on the nurse's relationship with each family (Bell, 2011). This next section discusses some specific aspects of family interventions. It also presents indications for and contraindications to family interventions.

Conceptualization of Interventions With Families

Notions about reality gleaned from postmodernism and social constructionism are helpful when conceptualizing ideas about interventions. It is unwise to attempt to ascertain what is "really" going on with a particular family or what the "real" problem or suffering is. Rather, nurses should recognize that what is "real" to them as nurses is always a consequence of the nurse's construction of the world. Maturana (1988) presents an intriguing notion of reality by submitting that individuals (living systems) bring forth reality—they do not construct it, and it does not exist independent of them. This concept has implications for nurses' clinical work with families—specifically, what nurses perceive about particular situations with families is influenced by how nurses behave (i.e., their interventions), and how they behave depends on what they perceive. (Refer to Chapter 2 for more understanding of Maturana's biology of cognition.)

Therefore, one way to change the "reality" that family members have constructed is to assist them with developing new ways of interacting in the family. The interventions that we use in this endeavor focus on changing cognitive, affective, or behavioral domains of family functioning. As family members' perceptions or beliefs about each other and the illness in their family change, so do their behaviors.

The effectiveness of family interventions in the treatment of physical illness has been examined in two integrative reviews conducted by Campbell and Patterson (1995) and Campbell (2003). These reviews included only studies that used a control group. Support was found for the effectiveness of interventions directed to the family rather than just the individual diagnosed with the illness.

Another important study to examine if family interventions improve health in persons with chronic illness and their family members across the life span was conducted by Chesla (2010). Her results were encouraging in that the review of family intervention studies with adults indicated there were beneficial effects for family member health and for patient mental health. There was also reasonable evidence that a family-centered approach for children with type 1 diabetes was helpful. Nurses were involved in one quarter to one third of the research studies that were reviewed.

Weihs and colleagues (2002) reported the efforts of a multidisciplinary group that reviewed and collated existing literature about family interventions in chronic illness. Three general goals for family-focused interventions were identified: helping families cope with the challenges of chronic illness management, mobilizing family support, and reducing intrafamilial hostility and suffering.

Evidence has been found for a significant reduction in the use of healthcare services following individual, marital, and family therapy (Crane & Payne, 2011; Law, Crane, & Berge, 2003). These studies substantiate the need for more family intervention research in nursing.

There are now a few studies that have begun to uncover family interventions with families experiencing physical illness, particularly about the usefulness of family interventions that target family interactions and examine the influence of each family member's illness experiences on other family members (Duhamel & Dupuis, 2004; Duhamel & Talbot, 2004; Noiseux & Duhamel, 2003; O'Farrell, Murray, & Hotz, 2000). Konradsdottir and Svavarsdottir (2011) conducted a quasi-experimental study of families with adolescents who had diabetes. Following their educational and support intervention with these families utilizing CFAM and CFIM, there was a significant positive difference between parents' coping patterns than before the intervention.

Documentation of clinical experience indicates that interventions normally directed at challenging the meanings or constraining beliefs about suffering tend to have the most sustaining changes (Bell, Moules, & Wright, 2009; Bell & Wright, 2011; Bohn, Wright, & Moules, 2003; Duhamel & Talbot, 2004; Houger Limacher & Wright, 2003, 2006; Moules, 2002, 2009; Moules, et al, 2007; Moules, Thirsk, & Bell, 2006; Wright & Bell, 2009).

Efforts to develop and identify intervention strategies for family health promotion are also being made, although little documentation of their effectiveness is evident (Loveland-Cherry & Bomar, 2004). Family health promotion is an area of family nursing in which there are tremendous opportunities for the development and testing of family interventions. An example of nurses taking the initiative to promote family health, in this case children with attention deficit hyperactivity disorder (ADHD), is an in-home intervention called Parents and Children Together (PACT) (Kendall & Tabacco, 2011). Recognizing that families with children with ADHD have more interpersonal conflict and negativity in their family and social life, Kendall and Tabacco designed a program to provide both assessment and resources. This is an impressive effort to empower families, particularly mothers, in their daily management of these children.

Another innovative intervention program promoting family health is a Web-based asthma education project (Garwick, Seppelt, & Belew, 2011). This program addressed the cultural and literacy backgrounds of families and involved family members in the actual needs assessment and in the development of the Web site.

Nurses need to keep the element of time in mind with regard to interventions. Interventions are an integral part of family interviewing, spanning engagement to termination. Normally, interventions used during family interviewing are based on the nurse's and family's influence on the experience of suffering, a problem, or an illness. If engagement and assessment have been adequate, the interventions are generally more effective. For example, if a nurse working with a Latino family perpetually addresses family members other than the father first, the family may disengage. The opportunity to further intervene will be eliminated. In this example, the nurse must possess family interviewing skills and must be sensitive to ethnic issues before embarking on specific goal-oriented interventions.

Family nurse clinicians are grounded in the everyday complexities and uniqueness of each family they serve. Although clinicians may benefit from the research literature that offers a description of family responses in health and illness, they are intimately involved in *doing* intervention and consequently find themselves wanting to know about the specific practice offered to families. We have found it heartening to learn about the increased examples of intervention programs to assist families.

Indications and Contraindications for Family Interventions

After a family assessment, a nurse must decide whether to intervene with a family. The nurse should consider the family's level of functioning, his or her own skill level, and the resources available. We recommend intervention in the following circumstances:

- **A family member presents with an illness that has an obvious detrimental impact on other family members.** For instance, a grandfather's Alzheimer's disease may cause his grandchildren to be afraid of him, or a young child's cyberbullying behavior may be related to his mother's deterioration from multiple sclerosis.

- **A family member contributes to another family member's symptoms or problems.** For example, lack of visitation from adult children exacerbates physical or psychological symptoms in an elderly parent.

- **One family member's improvement leads to symptoms or deterioration in another family member.** For example, decreased asthma symptoms in one child correlate with increased abdominal pain in a sibling.

- **A child or an adolescent develops an emotional, behavioral, or physical problem in the context of a family member's illness.** For example, an adolescent with diabetes suddenly requests that his mother administer his daily insulin injections even though he has been injecting himself for the past 6 months.

- **Illness is first diagnosed in a family member.** If family members have no previous knowledge of or experience with a particular illness, they require information and may also require reassurance and support.

- **A family member's condition deteriorates markedly.** Whenever deterioration occurs, family patterns may need restructuring, and intervention is indicated.

- **A chronically ill family member moves from a hospital or rehabilitation center back into the community.** For example, a young adult returns home after being hospitalized for 6 months at a drug rehabilitation center.

- **An important individual or family developmental milestone is missed or delayed.** For example, an adolescent is unable to move out of the home at the anticipated time.

- **A chronically ill patient dies.** Although the patient's death may be a relief, the family might feel a tremendous void when the caregiving role is lost.

After the nurse and family have decided that intervention is indicated, they must then collaboratively decide on the duration and intensity of the family sessions. If sessions occur too frequently, the family may have insufficient time to recalibrate and process the change. The optimal number of days, weeks, or months between sessions is difficult to state categorically. We recommend that nurses ask family members when they would like to have another meeting, particularly if the family meetings are occurring on an outpatient basis. Families are much better judges than nurses of how frequently they need to be seen to resolve a particular problem.

Furthermore, nurses should be aware that the duration and intensity of sessions depend on the context in which the family is seen. For example, if a hospital nurse is working with a family, he or she may have the opportunity for only one or two meetings before discharge, whereas a community health nurse may be able to schedule a series of meetings. The context in which the nurse encounters families commonly dictates the frequency and number of family meetings. Whether a nurse has one or ten meetings with a family for assessment or intervention, there are important considerations for terminating with families. Additional information on termination is discussed in Chapter 12.

Family intervention is not always required, and contraindications for family intervention exist, including:

- All family members state that they do not wish to pursue family meetings or treatment even though it is recommended.

- Family members state that they agree with the recommendation for family meetings or treatment but would prefer to work with another professional.

These contraindications are generally evident to the nurse immediately after the family assessment. Sometimes during the course of intervention, however, families indicate a desire to stop treatment. This situation will be discussed more fully in Chapter 12.

Nurses working with patients and families in a variety of health-care settings need to have a good understanding of when family involvement is indicated and when it is contraindicated. Not only for their own benefit but also for each family's benefit, nurses should distinguish between family assessment and family intervention. Families are often willing to come for an assessment when they can see the nurse face-to-face and make their own assessment of the nurse's competence. When a nurse does a careful, credible assessment, he or she has an easier time initiating family interventions.

DEVELOPMENT, IDENTIFICATION, AND IMPLEMENTATION OF NURSING INTERVENTIONS WITH FAMILIES

The slower pace of developing nursing interventions with families has been due in part to the lack of appreciation for the interactional aspect of families and illness. The lack of specific interventions with families has been caused by the lack of nurse educators who are also skilled family clinicians. Lack of administrative support for implementation of family nursing and the lack of ongoing educational support of family interventions in clinical settings have negatively influenced the adoption of family nursing (Leahey & Harper-Jaques, 2010). However, since the fifth edition of *Nurses and Families* (2009), significant strides have been made in all of these areas.

Because interventions related to the family are independent nursing actions for which nurses are accountable, nurse-educators and researchers need to name, specify, explore, understand, and test interventions related to the family. Very few nursing interventions with families have been tested. This fact is not surprising given that the nursing profession is still at a very early stage in simply identifying and describing family interventions. However, there are encouraging signs with more publications in the *Journal of Family Nursing* and presentations at the International Family Nursing Conferences discussing family interventions. More nurses are committed to increasing knowledge of family nursing interventions through describing and examining their effectiveness in actual clinical practice and through quantitative and qualitative studies. We believe these trends will continue with even more rigor and dedication over the next few years.

In a thoughtful editorial about evidence-based nursing, interventions, and family nursing, Hallberg (2003) offers specific recommendations for nursing interventions with individuals and families. Specifically, the author recommends that nurses develop and examine "interventions that acknowledge family members as experts and that acknowledge their role as primary caregivers; interventions directed at older people, especially those between 80 and 100 years and those dependent on others as opposed to independent older people; and interventions that elaborate on ways in which professionals can cooperate with families caring for older people in their homes and that apply a perspective of family caregiving as more complex than only a burden or a strain" (p. 21). Hallberg strongly emphasizes the belief that interventions with older people and their families are the most urgent need of the three. Therefore, nurse educators, researchers, and practicing nurses in the area of geriatric nursing have an urgent call for more knowledge about how to best assist and intervene with elderly families and their caregivers.

One program of research has responded to this call and is reported by Ducharme (2011) and her team, who have developed an in-home psycho-educational intervention program for family caregivers of seniors. Although they acknowledge that this program does not address the family from a systemic perspective, their program does respond to the family's needs and offers important education to the primary family caregiver of the senior. The family caregiver is often the member suffering the most under the burden and strain of caring for a loved one.

Nurses in direct clinical contact with families perceive family interventions differently from nurses who predominantly conduct research or engage in theory development. Nurse educators and researchers need to understand more about the challenges, successes, and difficulties of implementing family nursing in practice settings. One such clinical project shed some light on nurses' primary needs and concerns in their work with families (Duhamel, Dupuis, & Wright, 2009). Nurses were found to have difficulty integrating the theoretical aspects of family systems nursing into their practice and therefore desired to acquire additional clinical skills. Specifically, the nurses stated their most pressing need was to develop their abilities to deal with relational issues such as conflict between families and health professionals and family-communication problems. However, they frequently labeled families as "demanding" or "complaining," which was perceived as separate from the relational aspect of care.

In this project, one of the conclusions was that nurses' beliefs about families often led them to label families' responses to illness as being "dysfunctional" or members being in "denial" rather than more benevolent responses such as family members suffering, being under stress, or experiencing anxiety. This project led these nursing educators to further study three methods of training in FSN for successful knowledge transfer into practice (Duhamel, et al, 2009). This study called attention to the need for more educational support in the clinical setting to promote utilization of FSN knowledge in addition to the provision of administrative support. Through these various studies, it becomes evident that a circular, interactional process between education, research, and practice needs to be adhered to and respected (Duhamel & Dupuis, 2011).

FAMILY RESPONSES TO INTERVENTIONS

The previous discussion of interventions in family nursing practice primarily focused on the nurse's behaviors. However, interventions are actualized only in a relationship. Therefore, it is equally important to ascertain the responses of family members to interventions that are offered. Since the last edition of this text, more intervention studies have been conducted. These studies increase nurses' understanding of what is helpful to families and what is not. Bell and Wright (2007) challenge the predominant belief within "good science" that before intervention research can be designed and conducted, there first must be a thorough understanding of the phenomena (i.e., an in-depth knowledge of what the variables are that mediate families' response to health and illness). They offer an alternate view that in daily nursing practice, nurses encounter families suffering in a variety of clinical settings that require immediate care and intervention. Therefore, family nursing practice as it occurs in the daily life of nurses needs to be described, explored, and evaluated to gain an understanding of what is working in the moment. What are nurses actually doing and saying that is helpful to families in their experience of illness?

A seminal study by Robinson and Wright (1995), which is also one of the top ten cited articles in the *Journal of Family Nursing*, identified what nurses do that makes a positive difference to families. They found that families who experienced difficulty managing a member's chronic condition and sought assistance in an outpatient nursing clinic could readily identify interventions that alleviated or softened their suffering. The nursing interventions that made a difference for these families fell within two stages of the therapeutic change process:

- Bringing the family together to engage in new and different conversations (this fell within the stage of "creating the circumstances for change").
- Establishing a therapeutic relationship between the nurse and family, particularly in the areas of providing comfort and demonstrating trust (within the stage of "creating the circumstances for change").

Within the stage of "moving beyond and overcoming problems," families identified four interventions that promoted healing:

- Inviting meaningful conversation
- Noticing and distinguishing family and individual strengths and resources
- Paying careful attention to and exploring concerns
- Putting illness problems in their place

Recent studies indicate that nurses are eager to learn more about the usefulness of family interventions that target family interactions and examine the influence of each family member's illness experiences on other family members (O'Farrell, Murray, & Hotz, 2000).

A few additional qualitative studies have also been useful in examining particular family interventions. Studies such as unpacking the interventions of commendations (Houger Limacher & Wright, 2003, 2006), spiritual care practices (McLeod, 2003), and therapeutic letters (Moules, 2002, 2003) have enhanced our understanding of how, when, and why these interventions are healing for families. Other intervention studies have focused on what is significant for therapeutic change to occur (Bell & Wright, 2011; Duhamel & Talbot, 2004; Wright & Bell, 2009), while still others examined particular populations experiencing illness: interventions for parents with children undergoing bone marrow transplants (Noiseux & Duhamel, 2003), interventions in perinatal family care (Goudreau & Duhamel, 2003), interventions for families experiencing chronic illness (Robinson, 1998; Robinson & Wright, 1995), interventions for families experiencing heart disease (Tapp, 2001), interventions for families experiencing childhood cancer (West, 2011), interventions for grieving families (Thirsk, 2009), and interventions for families experiencing HIV/AIDS (Wacharasin, 2010).

Duhamel and Talbot (2004) conducted an ambitious, labor-intensive study to evaluate the usefulness of a family systems nursing approach utilizing the CFAM and CFIM with families experiencing cardiovascular and cerebrovascular diseases. Because interventions are actualized only within the context of a relationship between the nurse and the family, it is important to study the process itself rather than simply the results. The Duhamel and Talbot (2004) study was extremely beneficial because it was based on a participatory research design that allowed for continuous feedback and improvement of the interventions throughout the study.

In such a study, the participants are all concerned with the problem: nurses, patients, their spouses, and caregivers. Family members described the "humanistic attitude of the nurse, constructing a genogram, interventive questioning, offering educational information, normalization, and exploring the illness experience in the presence of other family members" (Duhamel & Talbot, 2004, p. 21) as the most useful interventions. Although all of these interventions are part of CFAM and CFIM, Duhamel and Talbot's 2004 study results provide interesting insights to substantiate their usefulness.

The study also had a positive impact on the nurses involved as co-investigators—a revealing finding. For example, the nurses indicated that they gained a better understanding of the illness's impact on the family members' relationships, acquired an appreciation of the importance of active listening and a humanistic and personalized approach, centered on family members' specific concerns to reduce their anxiety, and integrated new family systems nursing interventions into their practice.

The identification of these interventions offers incredibly useful ideas for improving the care of families experiencing illness. However, many more studies are needed to ascertain families' responses to the interventions offered.

CALGARY FAMILY INTERVENTION MODEL: AN ORGANIZING FRAMEWORK

The CFIM is an organizing framework for conceptualizing the relationship between families and nurses that helps change to occur and healing to begin. Specifically, the model highlights the family–nurse relationship by focusing on the intersection between family member functioning and interventions offered by nurses (see Chapter 4). It is at this intersection that healing can take place. The CFIM is a resilience and strength-based, collaborative, nonhierarchical model that recognizes the expertise of family members experiencing illness and the expertise of nurses in managing illness and promoting health. The model is rooted in notions from postmodernism and the biology of cognition. It can be applied and used with patients and families from diverse cultures because it emphasizes fit of particular interventions from a particular cultural viewpoint. To the best of our knowledge, it remains the only family nursing intervention model that is currently documented.

NURSING PRACTICE LEVELS WITH FAMILIES: GENERALIST AND SPECIALIST

Schober and Affara (2001) emphasize that nursing practice with families is directed by whether the concept of the family is defined as *family as context* or *family as client*. One way to alleviate potential confusion of practice levels is to clearly distinguish two levels of expertise in nursing with regard to clinical work with families: generalists and specialists. Typically, generalists are nurses at the baccalaureate level who predominantly use the concept of the family as context (Wright & Leahey, 1990), although upper-level baccalaureate students begin to conceptualize the family as the unit of care. Specialists, on the other hand, are nurses at the graduate (master's or doctoral) level who predominantly use the concept of family as the unit of care. This requires specialization in family systems nursing (Wright & Leahey, 1990). Family systems nursing specialization requires that "the focus is always on interaction and reciprocity. It is not 'either/or' but rather 'both/and'" (Wright & Leahey, 1990, p. 149).

Family systems nursing integrates nursing, systems, cybernetics, change, and family therapy theories (Bell, 2009; Wright & Leahey, 1990). It requires familiarity with an extensive body of knowledge: family dynamics, family systems theory, family assessment, family intervention, and family research. It also requires accompanying competence in family interviewing skills. Family systems nursing focuses simultaneously on the family and individual systems (Bell, 2009; Wright & Leahey, 1990). All nurses should be knowledgeable about and competent in involving families in health care across all domains of nursing practice. Consequently, the emphasis in the practice of family nursing at the generalist level is on the family as context.

In contrast, the practice of family systems nursing at the specialist level emphasizes the family as the unit of care. However, these boundaries can become blurred, with upper-level baccalaureate students recognizing the importance of focusing on interaction and reciprocity. These students often develop nursing competence and are able to deal with individual and family systems simultaneously. At Brandon University, a Family Case Model was developed within the curriculum that embedded family nursing across five courses in an undergraduate curriculum (Fast Braun, Hyndman, & Foster, 2010). This method of teaching family nursing to undergraduate students invited a focus on the reciprocity between illness, family members, and the nurse across courses.

CONCLUSIONS

We consider it a great privilege to work with families experiencing illness and/or suffering, loss, and disability. We are also grateful for opportunities to teach professional nurses and nursing students how to involve families in health care. Through this process, we recognize the extreme importance of nurses having sound family assessment and intervention knowledge, skills, and compassion. The remainder of this textbook is our effort to help nursing students, practicing nurses, and nurse educators learn new ways to heal families with our offering of specific knowledge and skills for maximizing family collaboration and healing.

References
Anderson, K.H. (2000). The family health system approach to family systems nursing. *Journal of Family Nursing, 6,* 103–119.

Angelo, M. (2008). The emergence of family nursing in Brazil. *Journal of Family Nursing, 14*(4), 436–441.

Astedt-Kurki, P. (2010). Family nursing research for practice: The Finnish perspective. *Journal of Family Nursing, 16*(3), 256–268.

Astedt-Kurki, P., & Kaunonen, M. (2011). Family nursing interventions in Finland: Benefits for families. In E. Svavarsdottir & H. Jonsdottir (Eds.): *Family Nursing in Action.* Reykjavik, Iceland: University of Iceland Press, pp. 115–129.

Bell, J.M. (1999). Family nursing network: Family nursing in Japan—A firsthand glimpse. *Journal of Family Nursing, 5*(2), 236–238.

Bell, J.M. (2009). Family systems nursing: Re-examined. *Journal of Family Nursing, 15*(2), 123–129.

Bell, J.M. (2011). Relationships: The heart of the matter in family nursing. *Journal of Family Nursing, 17*(1), 3–10.

Bell, J.M., Moules, N.J., & Wright, L.M. (2009). Therapeutic letters and the Family Nursing Unit: A legacy of advanced nursing practice. *Journal of Family Nursing, 15*(1), 6–30.

Bell, J.M., Watson, W.L., & Wright, L.M. (Eds.) (1990). *The Cutting Edge of Family Nursing.* Calgary, Alberta: Family Nursing Unit Publications.

Bell, J.M., & Wright, L.M. (2007). La recherche sur la pratique des soins infirmiers a la famille. In F. Duhamel (Ed.): *La Sante et la Famille: Une Approache Systemique en Soins Infirmieres* (2nd ed.). Montreal, Quebec, Canada: Gaetan Morin editeru, Cheneliere Education.

Bell, J.M., & Wright, L.M. (2011). Creating practice knowledge for families experiencing illness suffering: The Illness Beliefs Model. In E. Svavarsdottir & H. Jonsdottir (Eds.): *Family Nursing in Action.* Reykjavik, Iceland: University of Iceland Press, pp. 15–51.

Bohn, U., Wright, L.M., & Moules, N.J. (2003). A family systems nursing interview following a myocardial infarction: The power of commendations. *Journal of Family Nursing, 9*(2), 151–165.

Bomar, P.J. (Ed.). (2004). *Promoting health in families: Applying family research and theory to nursing practice* (3rd ed.). Philadelphia: W.B. Saunders.

Bulechek, G.M., Butcher, H., & McCloskey Dochterman, J. (2008). *Nursing Interventions Classification (NIC)* (5th ed.). New York: Elsevier.

Bulechek, G.M., & McCloskey, J.C. (Eds.). (1992). Defining and validating nursing interventions. *Nursing Clinics of North America, 27*(2), 289–299.

Bulechek, G.M., & McCloskey, J.C. (Eds.). (1999). *Nursing Interventions: Effective Nursing Treatments* (3rd ed.). Philadelphia: W.B. Saunders Company.

Campbell, T.L. (2003). The effectiveness of family interventions for physical disorders. *Journal of Marital and Family Therapy, 29*(2), 545–583.

Campbell, T.L., & Patterson, J.M. (1995). The effectiveness of family interventions in the treatment of physical illness. *Journal of Marital and Family Therapy, 21*(4), 545–583.

Chesla, C.A. (2010). Do family interventions improve health? *Journal of Family Nursing, 16*(4), 355–377.

Cousins, N. (1979). *Anatomy of an Illness As Perceived by the Patient: Reflections on Healing and Regeneration.* New York: Bantam Books.

Crane, D.R., & Payne, S.H. (2011). Individual versus family psychotherapy in managed care: Comparing the costs of treatment by the mental health professions. *Journal of Marital and Family Therapy, 37*(3), 273–289.

Doane, G.H. (2003). Through pragmatic eyes: Philosophy and the re-sourcing of family nursing. *Nursing Philosophy, 4*(1), 25–33.

Doane, G.H., & Varcoe, C. (2005). *Family Nursing as Relational Inquiry*. Philadelphia: Lippincott Williams & Wilkins.

Ducharme, F. (2011). A research program on nursing interventions for family caregivers of seniors: Development and evaluation of psycho-educational interventions. In E. Svavarsdottir & H. Jonsdottir (Eds.): *Family Nursing in Action*. Reykjavik, Iceland: University of Iceland Press, pp. 233–250.

Duhamel, F., & Dupuis, F. (2004). Guaranteed returns: Investing in conversations with families of cancer patients. *Clinical Journal of Oncology Nursing, 8*(1), 68–71.

Duhamel, F., & Dupuis, F. (2011). Towards a Triology Model of family systems nursing knowledge utilization: Fostering circularity between practice, education, and research. In E. Svavarsdottir & H. Jonsdottir (Eds.): *Family nursing in Action*. Reykjavik, Iceland: University of Iceland Press, pp. 53–68.

Duhamel, F., Dupuis, F., Goudreau, J., et al. (2009). Implementing family systems nursing in clinical practice: An insight on the process of knowledge utilization. Presentation at the 9th International Family Nursing Conference, Reykjavik, Iceland.

Duhamel, F., Dupuis, F., & Wright, L.M. (2009). Families' and nurses' responses to the "one question question": Reflections for clinical practice, education, and research in family nursing. *Journal of Family Nursing, 15*(4), 461–485.

Duhamel, F., & Talbot, L.R. (2004). A constructivist evaluation of family systems nursing interventions with families experiencing cardiovascular and cerebrovascular illness. *Journal of Family Nursing, 10*(1), 12–32.

Fast Braun, V., Hyndman, K., & Foster, C. (2010). Family nursing for undergraduate nursing students: The Brandon University family case model approach. *Journal of Family Nursing, 16*(2), 161–176.

Feetham, S.L., et al. (1993). *The Nursing of Families: Theory, Research, Education, and Practice*. Newbury Park, CA: Sage Publications.

Ford-Gilboe, M. (2002). Developing knowledge about family health promotion by testing the developmental model of health and nursing. *Journal of Family Nursing, 8*(2), 140–156.

Friedman, M.M., Bowden, V.R., & Jones, E.G. (2003). *Family Nursing: Research, Theory and Practice* (5th ed.). Upper Saddle River, NJ: Prentice Hall.

Garwick, A., Seppelt, A., & Belew, J.L. (2011). Addressing family health literacy to create a family-centered, culturally relevant web-based asthma education project. In E. Svavarsdottir & H. Jonsdottir (Eds.): *Family nursing in action*. Reykjavik, Iceland: University of Iceland Press, pp. 251–266.

Gilliss, C.L. (1991). Family nursing research, theory and practice. *Image: Journal of Nursing Scholarship, 23*(1), 19–22.

Gilliss, C.L., et al. (Eds.). (1989). *Toward a Science of Family Nursing*. Menlo Park, CA: Addison-Wesley.

Goudreau, J., & Duhamel, F. (2003). Interventions in perinatal family care: A participatory study. *Families, Systems, & Health, 21*(2), 165–180.

Hallberg, I.R. (2003). Evidence-based nursing, interventions, and family nursing: Methodological obstacles and possibilities. *Journal of Family Nursing, 9*(3), 3–22.

Hanson, S.M.H. (2001). *Family Health Care Nursing: Theory, Practice, and Research* (2nd ed.). Philadelphia: F. A. Davis.

Hanson, S.M.H., & Boyd, S.T. (1996). *Family health care nursing: Theory, practice, and research*. Philadelphia: F. A. Davis.

Hartrick, G. (2000). Developing health promoting practice with families: One pedagogical experience. *Journal of Advanced Nursing, 31*(1), 27–34.

Houger Limacher, L., & Wright, L.M. (2003). Commendations: Listening to the silent side of a family intervention. *Journal of Family Nursing, 9*(2), 130–135.

Houger Limacher, L., & Wright, L.M. (2006). Exploring the therapeutic family intervention of commendations: Insights from research. *Journal of Family Nursing, 12,* 307–331.

Irinoye, O., Ogunfowokan, A., & Olaogun, A. (2006). Family nursing education and family nursing practice in Nigeria. *Journal of Family Nursing, 12*(11), 442–447.

Kaakinen, J.R., Gedaly-Duff, V., Coehlo, D., et al. (Eds.). (2010). *Family Health Care Nursing: Theory, Practice, and Research* (4th ed.). Philadelphia: F. A. Davis.

Kendall, J., & Tabacco, A. (2011). Parents and children together: In-home intervention for families and children with children with attention-deficit/hyperactivity disorder. In E. Svavarsdottir & H. Jonsdottir (Eds.): *Family Nursing in Action.* Reykjavik, Iceland: University of Iceland Press, pp. 185–216.

Konradsdottir, E., & Svavarsdottir, E.K. (2011). How effective is a short-term educational and support intervention for families of an adolescent with type 1 diabetes? *Journal for Specialists in Pediatric Nursing, 16,* 295–304.

Law, D.D., Crane, D.R., & Berge, J.M. (2003). The influence of individual, marital, and family therapy on high utilizers of health care. *Journal of Marital and Family Therapy, 29*(3), 353–363.

Leahey, M., & Harper-Jaques, S. (2010). Integrating family nursing into a mental health urgent care practice framework: Ladders for learning. *Journal of Family Nursing, 16*(2), 196–212.

Lee, A.C.K., Leung, S.O., Chan, P.S.I., et al. (2010). Perceived level of knowledge and difficulty in applying family assessment among senior undergraduate nursing students. *Journal of Family Nursing, 16*(2), 177–195.

Loveland-Cherry, C.J., & Bomar, P.J. (2004). Family health promotion and health protection. In P.J. Bomar (Ed.): *Promoting Health in Families: Applying Family Research and Theory to Nursing Practice* (3rd ed.). Philadelphia: Saunders.

Maturana, H. (1988). Reality: The search for objectivity or the quest for a compelling argument. *Irish Journal of Psychology, 6*(1), 25–83.

McLeod, D.L. (2003). Opening space for the spiritual: Therapeutic conversations with families living with serious illness. Unpublished doctoral thesis, University of Calgary, Alberta, Canada.

Mischke-Berkey, K., Warner, P., & Hanson, S. (1989). Family health assessment and intervention. In P.J. Bomar (Ed.): *Nurses and Family Health Promotion: Concepts, Assessment, and Interventions.* Baltimore: Williams & Wilkins.

Moriyama, M. (2008). Family nursing practice and education: What is happening in Japan? *Journal of Family Nursing, 14*(4), 442–455.

Moules, N.J. (2002). Nursing on paper: Therapeutic letters in nursing practice. *Nursing Inquiry, 9*(2), 104–113.

Moules, N.J. (2003). Therapy on paper: Therapeutic letters and the tone of relationship. *Journal of Systemic Inquiries, 22*(1), 33–49.

Moules, N.J., et al. (2007). The soul of sorrow work: Grief and therapeutic interventions with families. *Journal of Family Nursing, 13*(2), 117–141.

Moules, N.J. (2009). Therapeutic letters in nursing: Examining the character and influence of the written word in clinical work with families experiencing illness. *Journal of Family Nursing, 15*(1), 31–49.

Moules, N.J., Thirsk, L.M., & Bell, J.M. (2006). A Christmas without memories: Beliefs about grief and mothering—A clinical case analysis. *Journal of Family Nursing, 12*(11), 426–441.

Murray, I. (2008). Family health nurse project—An education program of the World Health Organization: The University of Stirling experience. *Journal of Family Nursing, 14*(4), 469–485.

Noiseux, S., & Duhamel, F. (2003). La greffe de moelle osseuse chez l'enfant. Evaluation constructiviste de l'intervention aupres des parents. [Bone marrow transplantation in children. Constructive evaluation of an intervention for parents]. *Perspective Infirmiere, 1*(1), 12–24.

O'Farrell, P., Murray, J., & Hotz, S.B. (2000). Psychological distress among spouses of patients undergoing cardiac rehabilitation. *Heart and Lung, 29*(2), 97–104.

O'Sullivan Burchard, D.J.H., Claveirole, A., Mitchell, R., et al. (2004). Family nursing in Scotland. *Journal of Family Nursing, 10*(3), 323–337.

Psychometric Development of the Iceland-Expressive Family Functioning Questionnaire (ICE-EFFQ). *Journal of Family Nursing.*

Psychometric Development of the Iceland-Family Perceived Support Questionnaire (ICE-FPSQ). *Journal of Family Nursing.*

Robinson, C.A. (1998). Women, families, chronic illness, and nursing interventions: From burden to balance. *Journal of Family Nursing, 4*(3), 271–290.

Robinson, C.A., & Wright, L.M. (1995). Family nursing interventions: What families say makes a difference. *Journal of Family Nursing, 1*(3), 327–345.

Saveman, B. (2010). Family nursing research for practice: The Swedish perspective. *Journal of Family Nursing, 16*(1), 26–44.

Saveman, B., & Benzein, E. (2001). Here come the Swedes! A report on the dramatic and rapid evolution of family-focused nursing in Sweden. *Journal of Family Nursing, 7*(3), 303–310.

Schober, M., & Affara, F. (2001). *The Family Nurse: Frameworks for Practice.* Geneva: International Council of Nurses.

Simpson, P., et al. (2006). Family systems nursing: A guide to mental health care in Hong Kong. *Journal of Family Nursing, 12*(8), 276–291.

Sugishita, C. (1999). Development of family nursing in Japan—Present and future perspectives. *Journal of Family Nursing, 5*(2), 239–244.

Svavarsdottir, E.K. (2006). Listening to the family's voice: Nordic nurses' movement toward family centered care. *Journal of Family Nursing, 12*(4), 346–367.

Svavarsdottir, E.K. (2008). Excellence in nursing: A model for implementing family systems nursing in nursing practice at an institutional level in Iceland. *Journal of Family Nursing, 14*(4), 456–468.

Svavarsdottir, E.K., & Jonsdottir, H. (2011). *Family Nursing in Action.* Reykjavik, Iceland: University of Iceland Press.

Svavarsdottir, E.K., & Sigurdardottir, A.O. (2011). Implementing family nursing in general pediatric nursing practice: The circularity between knowledge translation and clinical practice. In E.K. Svavarsdottir & H. Jonsdottir (Eds.): *Family Nursing in Action.* Reykjavik, Iceland: University of Iceland Press, pp. 161–184.

Sveinbjarnardottir, E.K., Svavarsdottir, E.K., & Hrafnkelsson, B. (In press).

Tapp, D.M. (2001). Conserving the vitality of suffering: Addressing family constraints to illness conversations. *Nursing Inquiry, 8*(4), 254–263.

Tarko, M.A., & Reed, K. (2002). Taxonomy of family nursing diagnosis based upon the Neuman systems model of nursing. Unpublished manuscript. New Westminster, British Columbia, Canada: Douglas College.

Thirsk, L.M. (2009). Understanding the nature of nursing practice and interventions with grieving families. Unpublished doctoral thesis, University of Calgary, Alberta, Canada.

Tomm, K., & Sanders, G. (1983). Family assessment in a problem oriented record. In J.C. Hansen & B.F. Keeney (Eds.): *Diagnosis and Assessment in Family Therapy.* London: Aspen Systems Corporation, pp. 101–102.

Wacharasin, C. (2010). Families suffering with HIV/AIDS: What family nursing interventions are useful to promote healing? *Journal of Family Nursing, 16*(3), 302–321.

Wacharasin, C. & Theinpichet, S. (2008). Family nursing practice, education, and research: What is happening in Thailand? *Journal of Family Nursing, 14*(4), 429-435.

Wegner, G.D., & Alexander, R.J. (Eds.). (1993). *Readings in Family Nursing.* Philadelphia: J.B. Lippincott Company.

Weihs, K., Fisher, L., & Baird, M. (2002). Families, health, and behavior. *Families, Systems, & Health, 20*(1), 7–46.

West, C.H. (2011). Addressing illness suffering in childhood cancer: Exploring the beliefs of family members in therapeutic nursing conversations. Unpublished doctoral thesis. Alberta, Canada: University of Calgary.

World Health Organization. (2006). *Fifth workshop on the WHO Family Health Nurse Multinational Study: Evaluation Six Years After the Munich Declaration.* Copenhagen, Denmark: World Health Regional Office for Europe, Author.

Wright, L.M., & Bell, J.M. (2009). *Beliefs and Illness: A Model for Healing.* Calgary, AB: 4th Floor Press.

Wright, L.M., & Leahey, M. (1990). Trends in nursing of families. *Journal of Advanced Nursing, 15*(2), 148–154.

Wright, L.M., & Leahey, M. (2009). *Nurses and Families: A Guide to Family Assessment and Intervention* (5th ed.). Philadelphia: F.A. Davis.

Wright, L.M., & Leahey, M. (2013). *Nurses and Families: A Guide to Family Assessment and Intervention* (6th ed.). Philadelphia: F.A. Davis.

Wright, L.M., Watson, W.L., & Bell, J.M. (1990). The family nursing unit: A unique integration of research, education, and clinical practice. In J.M. Bell, W.L. Watson, & L.M. Wright (Eds.): *The Cutting Edge of Family Nursing.* Calgary, Alberta: Family Nursing Unit Publications, pp. 95–109.

2

Theoretical Foundations of the Calgary Family Assessment and Intervention Models

Models are useful ways to bring clusters of ideas, notions, and concepts into awareness. However, models cannot stand alone. For example, nursing practice models are built on a foundation of many worldviews, theories, beliefs, premises, and assumptions. These models are more comprehensible and meaningful if the underlying theories, assumptions, and premises are explained. Therefore, to comprehend and use the Calgary Family Assessment Model (CFAM; see Chapter 3) and the Calgary Family Intervention Model (CFIM; see Chapter 4) in nursing practice with individuals, couples, and families, nurses must understand the theoretical assumptions underlying these models.

We believe no one overall model or theory of family nursing exists. "No one theoretical or conceptual framework adequately describes the complex relationships of family structure, function, and process. No single theoretical perspective gives nurses a sufficiently broad base of knowledge and understanding for use as a guide to family assessment and interventions with families. Thus there is no single theoretical basis that guides nursing care of families. Rather, nurses must draw on multiple theories and frameworks to guide their work with families and take an integrated approach to practice, research, and education in family nursing" (Kaakinen & Hanson, 2004, p. 111). We concur with Kaakinen and Hanson on this.

The six theoretical foundations and worldviews that inform the CFAM and CFIM (and the family nursing practice guidelines presented in the rest of this textbook) are postmodernism, systems theory, cybernetics, communication theory, change theory, and biology of cognition. Each theory or worldview and some of its distinguishing concepts are presented and related to clinical practice with individuals, couples, and families.

POSTMODERNISM

Humans seem to delight in rethinking, reexamining, reconstructing, and deconstructing their history and culture. One popular way to do this is through the lens of postmodernism. Anything before the present "enlightened" worldview is considered modernist and therefore less desirable to those who rigidly hold postmodernist beliefs. Consequently, the influence of the ideas, conditions, and beliefs of postmodernism have been demonstrated in art, literature, architecture, science, culture, religion, philosophy, and, more recently, in family therapy and nursing, particularly family nursing (Becvar & Becvar, 2003; Glazer, 2001; Kermode & Brown, 1996; Moules, 2000; Tapp & Wright, 1996; Watson, 1999). The popularity and increasing acceptance of postmodern ideas in nursing are even making their way into propositions of spiritual care and postmodernism coexisting, although this is an unlikely connection (Salladay, 2011).

We, too, have been influenced by and have embraced many of the notions of postmodernism. These ideas have proved useful in our clinical nursing practice with families. However, we do not wish to imply that we have been able to successfully distance ourselves from all modernist ideas, nor would we want to. We concur with Glazer (2001), who criticizes the postmodern movement for abandoning the biological underpinnings of nursing. We cannot deny our history and culture and how they have influenced who we were and are. Therefore, we acknowledge the previous and continuing influences of both modernist and postmodernist paradigms on our lives and our practice of relational family nursing.

CONCEPT 1

Pluralism is a key focus of postmodernism.

Postmodernism offers the end of a single worldview and a resistance to single explanations and offers a respect for difference. One of the major notions of postmodern thinking is the idea of pluralism, or a belief in multiplicity—there are as many ways to understand and experience the world as there are people who experience it (Moules, 2000; Watson, 1999; Wright & Bell, 2009). In family nursing practice, this idea becomes operational by recognizing that there are as many ways to understand and experience illness as there are families experiencing it. In an ethical and relational family nursing practice, it becomes operational by acknowledging the multiplicity of cultural, ethnic, and religious beliefs and their influence on various complex family structures.

CONCEPT 2

Postmodernism is a debate about knowledge.

Postmodernism is partly a reaction to the modernist claim that knowledge emerges primarily from science and technology (Glazer, 2001). The belief that progressive technology necessarily leads to a better world has become open to reexamination, questioning, and doubt (Tapp & Wright, 1996). Therefore, an intense critique is being made of the grand belief systems that have formed the foundation of many scientific, religious, and political movements and institutions. As they are questioned, opportunities arise to deconstruct or uncover certain beliefs and practices that are taken for granted, to hear voices of marginal groups, and to value knowledge from a variety of domains heretofore not legitimized (Tapp & Wright, 1996; Watson, 1999).

In encounters with families experiencing illness, much more emphasis is now given to the illness narratives and experiences of family members within their particular cultural context not just to medical narratives. Honoring the voices of families about their illness narratives has profound implications for nursing practice with families. It invites collaboration and consultation between nurses and families to honor the knowledge and expertise of both nurses and family members. These practices are the cornerstone of relational nursing. Inviting the illness narratives of families also enhances the possibilities for healing as their stories are heard, understood, and witnessed.

Some offshoots of postmodernism include constructivism, social constructionism, and biology of cognition (also called *"bring forthism"*; Bell & Wright, 2011; Maturana & Varela, 1992; Moules, 2000; Wright & Bell, 2009). Biology of cognition is the offshoot we have found most useful in our clinical work and we discuss it in more detail later in this chapter.

The postmodernist movement has been strongly critiqued by feminists, who claim that women's voices continue to be diminished or ignored because of patriarchy and oppression (Kermode & Brown, 1996). This has not been our experience in working with families. Evidence for the importance of acknowledging women's voices and their illness burden in family systems nursing practice can be found in Robinson's 1998 study. She discovered that women in families experiencing chronic illness are vulnerable to the demands of illness's responsibility, work, and problems. As a more equitable balance of illness demands was sought by the nurse and family members, the women in this study found better lives for themselves and were able to live beyond illness and the problems they experienced. They also took on new views of their situations and thus behaved differently. This study's recognition of women's voices as distinct and different from a collective "family voice" seems in keeping with the best that the postmodernist movement has to offer.

SYSTEMS THEORY

For a number of years, health professionals have applied general systems theory, introduced in 1936 by von Bertalanffy, to the understanding of families. In addition to the original writings on systems theory by von Bertalanffy (1968, 1972, 1974), numerous articles and chapters in books have been written on this subject and its concepts. This proliferation of systems information is also evident within nursing literature. We agree with Kaakinen and Hanson (2010) in their belief that "family systems theory has been the most influential of all the family social science frameworks" (p. 73).

One of the most useful analogies that highlights systems concepts as applied to families is offered by Allmond, Buckman, and Gofman (1979). They suggest that, when thinking of the family as a system, it is useful to compare it to a mobile:

> Visualize a mobile with four or five pieces suspended from the ceiling, gently moving in the air. The whole is in balance, steady yet moving. Some pieces are moving rapidly; others are almost stationary. Some are heavier and appear to carry more weight in the ultimate direction of the mobile's movement; others seem to go along for the ride. A breeze catching only one segment of the mobile immediately influences movement of every piece, some more than others, and the pace picks up with some pieces unbalancing themselves and moving chaotically about for a time. Gradually the whole exerts its influence in the errant part(s) and balance is reestablished but not before a decided change in direction of the whole may have taken place. You will also notice the changeability regarding closeness and distance among pieces, the impact of actual contact one with another, and the importance of vertical hierarchy. Coalitions of movement may be observed between two pieces. Or one piece may persistently appear isolated from the others; yet its position of isolation is essential to the balancing of the entire system (p. 16).

Keeping the analogy of the mobile in mind, some of the most useful concepts of systems theory, which have frequent application in clinical practice with families, are highlighted in the following paragraphs. These systems concepts provide a theoretical foundation for understanding the family as a system. A *system* can be defined as a complex of elements in mutual interaction. When this definition is applied to families, it allows us to view the family as a unit and thus focus on observing the interaction among family members and between the family and the illness or problem rather than studying family members individually. However, remember that each family member is both a subsystem and a system in his or her own right. An individual system is both a part and a whole, as is a family.

CONCEPT 1

A family system is part of a larger suprasystem and is composed of many subsystems.

The concept of hierarchy of systems is very useful when applied to families. It is especially helpful for nurses struggling with how to conceptualize complex family situations. A family is composed of many subsystems, such as parent-child, marital, and sibling subsystems. These subsystems are also composed of subsystems of individuals. Individuals are extremely complex systems composed of various subsystems, some of which are physical (e.g., the cardiovascular and reproductive systems) or psychological (e.g., cognitive, affective, and behavioral systems). At the same time, the family is just one unit nested in larger suprasystems, such as neighborhoods, organizations, or church communities. Drawing a large circle and placing elements, parts, or variables inside the circle can be a helpful way to visualize a system. Inside the circle, lines can be drawn among the component parts to represent relationships between elements. Outside the circle is the larger context, where all other factors impinging on the system can be placed. Thus, a nurse can draw a circle to visualize a family and then place the individual family members within it (Fig. 2–1).

Systems are arbitrarily defined by their boundaries, which aid in specifying what is inside or outside the system. Normally, boundaries associated with living systems are physical in nature, such as the number of people in a family.

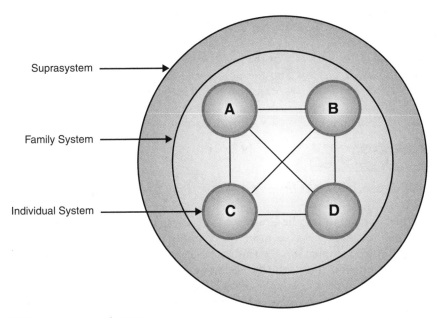

FIGURE 2-1: Family system.

It is also possible to construct a boundary and therefore create a system around ideas, beliefs, expectations, or roles. For example, a person may have a system of multiple roles, such as daughter, partner, colleague, wife, sister, nurse, mother, and grandmother. However, from time to time, it may be useful to draw an imaginary boundary and create, for example, a system of parental beliefs about the use of nonmedical drugs by their children.

When working with families, nurses should initially consider:

- Who is in this family system?
- What are some of the important subsystems?
- What are some of the significant suprasystems to which the family belongs?

In addition, within family systems and their subsystems, nurses should assess the permeability of the boundaries (see Chapter 3 for further understanding about boundaries when conducting a family assessment). In family systems, the boundaries must be both permeable and limiting. If the family boundary is too permeable, the system loses identity and integrity (e.g., members may be too open to input from the outside environment, such as extended family, friends, or health professionals) and therefore does not allow the family to use its own resources in decision-making. However, if the boundary is too closed or impermeable, necessary interaction with the larger world is shut off (e.g., an immigrant family from Afghanistan that relocates to Pennsylvania may inadvertently remain closed initially because of great differences in language and culture). With increased use of cellular phones; the Internet; personal digital assistants; e-mail; e-Books; blogs; Skype; chat rooms; and social networking sites such as Facebook, Twitter, and YouTube, the permeability of boundaries has changed dramatically in the last decade.

Hierarchy of systems and the boundaries that create systems are useful concepts to apply when working with and attempting to conceptualize the uniqueness of each particular family. Among certain ethnic groups—for example, Iranian families—honoring hierarchies and boundaries is essential.

CONCEPT 2

The family as a whole is greater than the sum of its parts.

When applied to families, this concept of systems theory emphasizes that the family's "wholeness" is more than simply the addition of each family member. It also emphasizes that individuals are best understood within their larger context, which is normally the family. To study individual family members separately does not equate to studying the family as a unit. By studying the whole family, it is possible to observe interaction among family members, which often more fully explains individual family member functioning. Consider this clinical scenario: A young Filipino mother whose 3-year-old child has temper tantrums that she cannot control asks a community health nurse (CHN) for guidance. The CHN could intervene in a variety of ways:

- See the mother individually and discuss some behavioral methods that could be used to assist in controlling her child's temper tantrums.
- See the child individually and do an individual assessment.
- See the whole family (mother, father, and child) and perform a child-and-family assessment (see Chapter 3) in order to understand the child, the child's behavior in the family context, and the Filipino family's beliefs about discipline.

Because the CHN understood the importance of Concept 2, she chose to see the whole family. During the first session with the family, the child was well behaved for the first half hour of the interview. Then the child had a temper tantrum, in response to which the mother became annoyed and the father withdrew. The CHN was astute enough to observe the sequence of interaction before the temper tantrum. When the child had the temper tantrum, the parents were in a heated argument about their parenting styles. Once the tantrum started, the parents stopped arguing and focused on the child. This child might have been responding to the tension between the parents and using the temper tantrums to stop the parents' conflict. Thus, the temper tantrums were understood quite differently in the context of the family than they would have been if the child had been assessed in isolation. In this example, the family is the client, but an individual family member is the reason for initiating care (Schober & Affara, 2001). Any time a family seeks assistance because of a concern or problem with an individual family member, the nurse can initiate family nursing with the entire family unit.

Therefore, when possible, nurses should see whole families and observe family interaction to more fully understand family member functioning. This type of observation enables assessment of the relationships among family members and individual family member functioning. You cannot understand the parts of a body, a family, or a theory unless you understand how the whole works, for the parts can be understood only in relation to the whole. Conversely, you cannot grasp how the whole works unless you have an understanding of its parts. However, family nursing is not about how many family members are present in the room with the nurse but rather how the nurse conceptualizes the interaction between illness and family dynamics. (See Chapter 10 for a clinical example of interviewing an individual to obtain a family perspective with chronic illness.)

CONCEPT 3

A change in one family member affects all family members.

This concept aids the recognition that any significant event or change in one family member affects all family members to varying degrees as was illustrated in the analogy of the mobile. It can be most useful to nurses considering the impact of illness on families. For example, the father of a Somali family experienced a myocardial infarction. This event affected all family members and various family relationships. The father and mother were unable to continue their joint participation in sports, and the mother increased her employment from part-time to full-time to supplement the substantially reduced income during the father's convalescence. The eldest daughter, who had been isolated from the family since her marriage, began visiting her father more often. The youngest daughter provided emotional support and so became closer to her mother. Thus, all family members were affected, and the organization and functioning of the family changed.

This concept can also be used to understand how a nurse can change the family system by implementing family interventions—that is, if one family member changes, other family members cannot respond as they previously did because the individual family member now behaves differently.

CONCEPT 4

The family is able to create a balance between change and stability.

Over the past few years, there has been a shift away from the belief that families tend toward maintaining equilibrium. Instead, the popular belief now is that families are really in constant states of flux and are always changing. The pendulum has now swung to the other end of the continuum. However, von Bertalanffy (1968) warned many years ago to avoid this polarized view of families. He suggested that systems, in this case family systems, can achieve balance among the forces operating within them and on them and that change and stability can coexist in living systems (see the "Change Theory" section later in this chapter).

However, when change occurs in a family, the disturbance can cause a shift to a new position of balance. The family reorganizes in a way that is different from any previous organization. For example, if a family member is diagnosed with a long-term chronic illness, such as multiple sclerosis, the entire family must reorganize itself in ways that are totally different from the ways it was organized before the diagnosis. The balance between change and stability constantly shifts during periods of remission and exacerbation; however, a balance between change and stability is most common.

The concept of change and stability coexisting is perhaps one of the most difficult concepts of systems theory for nurses to understand. This is partly because, in actual clinical practice, families frequently present themselves as being either in rigid equilibrium or in constant change rather than manifesting an observable balance between the two. However, the more experienced one becomes in family nursing, the greater appreciation one has for the complexity of families. In many cases, when families are "stuck" or experiencing severe difficulties, they are polarized in maintaining rigid equilibrium or are in a phase of too much change. Eventually, the family needs to find ways to obtain a more equal balance between the phenomena of stability and change. In our own practice over the last several years, we have noticed how military families and other families directly affected by terrorism and war have developed creative solutions to cope with the fluctuations of stability and change.

CONCEPT 5

Family members' behaviors are best understood from a view of circular rather than linear causality.

One method of dealing with the massive amounts of data presented in a family interview is to observe for patterns. Tomm (1981) offers a useful discussion of the differences between linear and circular patterns:

> One major difference between linear and circular patterns lies in the overall structure of the connections between elements of the pattern. Linear patterns are limited to sequences (e.g., A → B → C) whereas circular patterns form a closed loop and are recursive (e.g., A → B → C → A → ... or A → B, B → C, C → A). A less obvious but more significant difference lies in the relative importance usually given to time and meaning when making the connections or links in the pattern. Linearity is heavily rooted in a framework of a continuous progression of time....Circularity...is more heavily dependent on a framework of reciprocal relationships based on meaning (p. 85).

Linear causality, defined as a relationship in which one event causes another, can serve as a useful and helpful function for individuals and families. For example, when the clock strikes 6:00 PM, a family routinely eats supper. This is an example of linear causality because event A (the clock striking 6:00 PM) is seen as the cause of event B (the eating of supper), or A → B, whereas event B does not affect event A.

However, circular causality occurs when event B does affect event A. For example, if a husband takes an interest in his wife's ostomy care (event A) and the wife responds by explaining the daily procedures (event B), then it is likely to result in the husband continuing to take an interest and offer support regarding his wife's ostomy care and his wife continuing to feel supported; thus, the cycle continues (A → B → A). Each individual's behavior has an effect on and influences the other individual's behavior. A method for diagramming these very useful circular interactional patterns is discussed in Chapter 3.

The application of these concepts in clinical practice affects the nurse's style of questioning during a family interview. Linear questions tend to explore descriptive characteristics (e.g., "Is the father fearful of another heart attack?"), whereas circular questions tend to explore interactional characteristics. Types of circular questions include difference questions (e.g., "Who is most worried about Sunil having another heart attack?"), behavioral effect questions (e.g., "What do you do, Amal, when your wife's pain becomes unbearable for you?"), hypothetical or future-oriented questions (e.g., "What might you do in the future to prevent your elderly father from falling?"), and triadic questions (e.g., "When your dad shows support to your sister Manisha, how does your mom feel?") (Loos & Bell, 1990; Selvini-Palazzoli, et al, 1978; Tomm, 1984, 1985, 1987a, 1987b, 1988; Wright & Bell, 2009). Bateson (1979) offers the idea that "information consists of differences that make a difference" (p. 99). Tomm (1981) connects the idea of "differences" to relationships:

> Differences between perceptions, objects, events, ideas, etc. are regarded as the basic source of all information and consequent knowledge. On closer examination, one can see that such relationships are always reciprocal or circular. If she is shorter than he, then he is taller than she. If she is dominant, then he is submissive. If one member of the family is defined as being bad, then the others are being defined as being good. Even at a very simple level, a circular orientation allows implicit information to become more explicit and offers alternative points of view. A linear orientation on the other hand is narrow and restrictive and tends to mask important data (p. 93).

Various types of assessment and interventive questions that could be asked during a family interview are highlighted in Chapters 3, 4, and 6 through 10.

With regard to family member interaction, the assumption is made that each person contributes to adaptive and maladaptive interaction. For example, in geriatric health-care facilities, it is common for elderly parents to complain that their adult children do not visit enough and therefore withdraw; on the other hand, the adult children complain that their elderly parents constantly nag them when they visit (see Chapter 10 for a clinical example). Each family member is "correct" in the perception of the other, but neither recognizes how his or her own behavior influences the behavior of the other family member.

Normally, families and their individual members need help to move from a linear perspective of their situation to a more interactional, reciprocal, and systemic view. This shift is possible only if the nurse avoids linear thinking when attempting to understand family dynamics.

The five concepts previously listed are by no means inclusive of all systems concepts, but they reflect those that are deemed most significant and important to the theoretical foundation for working with families.

CYBERNETICS

Cybernetics is the science of communication and control theory. The term *cybernetics* was originally coined by the mathematician Norbert Weiner. It is important to differentiate between general systems theory and cybernetics. We do not use the terms synonymously although some people regard each as a branch of the other. Systems theory is primarily concerned with changing the conceptual focus from parts to wholes, whereas cybernetics is concerned with changing focus from substance to form.

CONCEPT 1

Family systems possess self-regulating ability.

Interpersonal systems, particularly family systems, "may be viewed as feedback loops, since the behavior of each person affects and is affected by the behavior of each other person" (Watzlawick, Beavin, & Jackson, 1967, p. 31). We have found this idea to be very useful in family work because recognizing that each family member's behavior affects other family members and, in turn, that person is affected by other family members' behavior removes any tendency or impulse a nurse may have to blame one person in a family for the difficulties that an entire family is facing. For any substantial change to occur in a relationship, the regulatory limits must be adjusted so that a new range of behaviors is possible or an entirely new pattern can emerge (transformation). Tomm (1980) offers a useful method of applying cybernetic regulatory concepts to actual clinical interviewing. His method of diagramming circular patterns of communication is discussed in Chapter 3.

CONCEPT 2

Feedback processes can simultaneously occur at several systems levels with families.

Initially, the application of cybernetic concepts in family work began by observations of simple phenomena (e.g., a wife criticizes, the husband withdraws); this is generally referred to as *simple cybernetics*. However, as cyberneticians began examining more complex orders of phenomena, they recognized different orders of feedback (such as feedback of feedback and change of change). Maturana and Varela (1980) suggest a higher-order cybernetics that links the organization of living process and cognition.

Therefore, the simple feedback phenomenon observed in the interactional pattern of criticizing wife—withdrawing husband may also be understood to be part of a larger feedback loop involving the couple's relationship to their families of origin, which may recalibrate the lower-order loop of the couple's interaction. This concept can be especially helpful to nurses working with complex family situations. Thus, cybernetics of cybernetics moves into a larger context that includes both the observer and the observed.

COMMUNICATION THEORY

The study of communication focuses on how individuals interact with one another. Within families, the function of communication is to assist family members in clarifying family rules regarding behavior, to help them learn about their environment, to explicate how conflict is resolved, to nurture and develop self-esteem for all members, and to model expressions of feeling states constructively within the family as a unit. One of the most significant contributions to the understanding of interpersonal processes is the classic book *Pragmatics of Human Communication* (1967) by Watzlawick, Beavin, and Jackson. The concepts presented here are primarily drawn from this important book on communication and have been updated by the research studies of Dr. Janet Beavin Bavelas in 1992.

CONCEPT 1

All nonverbal communication is meaningful.

This concept helps us to realize that there is no such thing as not communicating because all nonverbal communication by a person carries a message in the presence of another (Watzlawick, Beavin, & Jackson, 1967). In personal communications and in her 1992 publication, Dr. Beavin Bavelas states that she now distinguishes between nonverbal behavior (NVB) and nonverbal communication (NVC). NVC is viewed as a subset of NVB. NVB involves an "inference-making observer," whereas NVC involves a "communicating person" (encoder). In the original text by Watzlawick, Beavin, and Jackson, the concept was presented that all NVB is meaningful.

A significant component of this concept is context. Behavior is relevant and meaningful only when the immediate context is considered. For example, if a mother complains to a CHN that she has been experiencing insomnia for 2 months and finds herself irritable because of the prolonged sleep deprivation, the mother's behavior must be understood in her immediate context. On further exploration, the nurse discovers that this mother has a child on an apnea monitor and that the father sleeps soundly. Also, the family apartment is close to a subway. With this additional context information, the mother's insomnia can be more fully understood and treated by the CHN.

CONCEPT 2

All communication has two major channels for transmission: digital and analog.

Digital communication is commonly referred to as *verbal communication*. It consists of the actual content of the message, or the brute facts. For example, a man might proudly say, "I lost 15 pounds this past month," or a 10-year-old girl might say, "I can now give myself my own insulin." However, when the analogical communication is also taken into account, the meaning of these statements may change dramatically.

Analogical communication consists not only of the usual types of NVC, such as body posture, facial expression, and tone, but also of music, poetry, and painting. For example, a man who is obese and proudly states that he lost 15 pounds in a month sends a more positive message, both digitally and analogically, than a man who is emaciated and states that he lost 15 pounds.

When discrepancies exist between analogical and digital communication, then the analogical message is considered more pertinent to the nurse's observing eye. For example, a teenager who has been placed in a cumbersome cast for a fractured femur might state, "It doesn't bother me," but her eyes are filled with tears. In this situation, the nurse must recognize the importance of the analogical message. To the teenager's boyfriend, the digital communication may be the most relevant. He may not perceive the significance of the analogical communication. More suggestions for operationalizing this concept are included in the CFAM in Chapter 3.

CONCEPT 3

A dyadic relationship has varying degrees of symmetry and complementarity.

The terms *symmetry* and *complementarity* are useful in identifying typical family interaction patterns. Jackson (1973) defined these terms:

> A complementary relationship consists of one individual giving and the other receiving. In a complementary relationship, the two people are of unequal status in the sense that one appears to be in the superior position, meaning that he initiates action and the other appears to follow that action. Thus the two individuals fit together or complement each other. The most obvious and basic complementary relationship would be the mother and infant. A symmetrical relationship is one between two people who behave as if they have equal status. Each person exhibits the rights to initiate action, criticize the other, offer advice and so on. This type of relationship tends to become competitive; if one person mentions that he has succeeded in some endeavor, the other person mentions that he has succeeded in an equally important endeavor. The individuals in such a relationship emphasize their equality or their symmetry with each other. The most obvious symmetrical relationship is a pre-adolescent peer relationship (p. 189).

Both complementary and symmetrical relationships are appropriate and healthy in certain situations. For example, a staff nurse must take a "one-down" position to her nurse manager most of the time. If the staff nurse cannot do this, conflict could result and the relationship could become predominantly symmetrical. This symmetrical escalation could result in the nurse manager filing incident reports about the staff nurse or the staff nurse quitting on unpleasant terms. An example of a healthy symmetrical relationship is one between spouses, who may, for instance, debate where to spend their next vacation.

In family relationships, predominance of either complementary or symmetrical behavior usually results in problems. However, some cultural groups may prefer one style over another. Couples need to balance symmetry and complementarity in their various experiences. Parent-child relationships, however, typically gradually shift from a predominantly complementary relationship to a more symmetrical, egalitarian relationship as the child moves into the teenage and young adult years.

CONCEPT 4

All communication has two levels: content and relationship.

Communication consists of what is being said (content) and information that defines the nature of the relationship between those interacting. For example, a father might say to his son, "Come over here, son. I want to tell you something," or he might say, "Get over here. I've got something to tell you!" These statements are similar in content, but each implies a very different relationship. The first statement could be viewed as part of a loving relationship, whereas the second statement implies a conflictual relationship. In this instance, it is the tone of the content that gives evidence to a particular kind of relationship. Therefore, "family communication not only reveals a message about 'who is saying what and when,' it also conveys a message about the structure and functions of family relationships in relation to the power base, decision-making processes, affection, trust, and coalitions" (Crawford & Tarko, 2004, p. 162).

CHANGE THEORY

The process of change is a fascinating phenomenon, and researchers and clinicians have a variety of ideas about how and what constitutes change in family systems. In the discussion of change theory that follows, the most profound and salient points from an extensive review of the literature are synthesized and presented along with our own beliefs about change and the conditions that affect the change process.

Systems of relationships appear to possess a tendency toward progressive change. However, a French proverb states, "the more something changes, the more it remains the same." This paradox beautifully highlights the dilemma frequently faced in working with families. The nurse must learn to accept the challenge of the paradoxical relationship between persistence (stability) and change. Maturana (1978) explains the recursiveness of change and stability in this way: Change is an alteration in the family's structure that occurs as compensation for perturbations and has the purpose of maintaining structure and stability. Change itself is experienced as a perturbation to the system, so change generates further change and stability. A change in state is exhibited as behavior; therefore, differences in family interactional patterns must be explored. Changes in behavior may or may not be accompanied by insight. However, "the most profound and sustaining change will be that which occurs within the family's belief system (cognition)" (Bell & Wright, 2011; Wright & Bell, 2009).

Watzlawick, Weakland, and Fisch (1974) were the first to suggest that persistence and change must be considered together despite their opposing natures. These researchers offer a widely accepted notion of change and suggest that two different types or levels of change exist. They refer to one type as change occurring within a given system that remains unchanged itself. In other words, the system itself remains unchanged, but its elements or parts undergo some type of change. This type of change is referred to as *first-order change*. It is a change in quantity, not quality. First-order change involves using the same problem-solving strategies over and over again. Each new problem is approached mechanically. If a solution to the problem is difficult to find, more old strategies are used and are usually more vigorously applied. An example of first-order change is the learning of a new behavioral strategy to deal with a child's excessive computer use. A parent who formerly disciplined his child by restricting the child's access to the computer is said to have undergone first-order change when he then limits the child's spending money.

The second type of change, referred to as *second-order change*, is one that changes the system. Second-order change is thus a "change of change." It appears that the French proverb is applicable only to first-order change. For second-order change to occur, actual changes in the rules governing the system must occur, and therefore the system is structurally transformed. It is important to note that second-order change is often in the nature of a discontinuity or jump and can be sudden and radical. Other times, second-order change occurs in a logical sequence with the person almost seemingly unaware of the change until it is noted by others.

This type of change represents a quantum jump in the system to a different level of functioning. Second-order change can be said to occur, for example, when a family now spends more time together and is able to raise conflictual issues with one another as a result of resolving their teenager's refusal to eat with the family.

Watzlawick, Weakland, and Fisch (1974) also refer to the most obvious type of change, spontaneous change. In spontaneous change, problem resolution occurs in daily living without the input of professionals or sophisticated theories. For example, an anorexic young woman suddenly and apparently spontaneously begins to eat regularly after 2 years of not doing so, or a man suffering from shingles (herpes zoster) reports that his chronic pain disappeared overnight.

Bateson (1979) offers a most thought-provoking statement with regard to change when he proposes that people are almost always unaware of changes. He suggests that changes in social interactions and in the environment are dramatically and constantly occurring but that people become accustomed to the "new state of affairs before our senses can tell us that it is new" (p. 98). Bateson also offers the idea that, with regard to the perception of change, the mind can receive only news of difference. Therefore, as Bateson states, change can be observed as "difference which occurs across time" (p. 452). These ideas concur with those of Maturana and Varela (1992), who offer the idea that change occurs in humans from moment to moment. This change is either triggered by interactions or perturbations from the environment in which the system (family member) exists or is a result of the system's (family member's) own internal dynamics.

Our own view of change in family work draws from the above authors and from our clinical experience in working with families. Change is constantly evolving in families, and people are frequently unaware of it. This type of continuous or spontaneous change occurs with everyday living and progression through individual and family stages of development. These changes may or may not occur with professional input.

Major transformations of an entire family system can occur and can be precipitated by major life events—such as serious illness; disability; divorce; unemployment; addictions; terrorism; displacement from home as a result of terrorism, war, floods, hurricanes, or tsunamis; or death of a family member—or through interventions offered by nurses. Change within a family can occur within the cognitive, affective, or behavioral domains, but change in any one domain impacts the other domains. Therefore, family-nursing interventions can be aimed at any domain or all three domains. Interventions are discussed further in Chapter 4, in which the CFIM is presented. We believe that directly correlating interventions with resulting changes is impossible; therefore, predicting outcomes or the types of change that will occur within families is also impossible.

An important role for nurses (operating from a systems perspective) is to carefully observe the connections between systems. To effect change within the original system (the individual), it is necessary to intervene at a higher systems level or at the metalevel (the family system [see Fig. 2–1]). In other words, if nurses wish to effect change within family systems, they need to be able to maintain a metaposition to each family. They must simultaneously conceptualize both the family system interactions and their own interactions with the family. However, if a problem arises between the nurse and the family, this problem must be resolved at a higher level than the nurse-family system, preferably by a supervisor, who can examine the problem from a higher metaposition.

CONCEPT 1

Change is dependent on the perception of the problem.

In a now-famous statement, Alfred Korzybski proclaimed that "the map is not the territory." In other words, the name is different from the thing named and the description is different from what is described. In applying this concept to family interviewing, the "mapping" of a particular situation or a nurse's perception of a problem follows from how that nurse chooses to see it. How a nurse perceives a particular problem has profound implications for how the nurse will intervene and therefore how change will occur and whether it will be effective.

One of the most common traps for nurses working with families is acceptance of one family member's perception or perspective as the "truth" about the family. There is no one "truth" or "reality" about family functioning, or perhaps it is more accurate to say that there are as many "truths" or "realities" as there are members of the family (Maturana & Varela, 1992). The error of taking sides in relational family nursing is discussed in Chapter 11. The important task for the nurse is to accept all family members' perceptions, perspectives, and beliefs and offer the family another view of their health concerns, illness, or problems. Individual family members construct their own realities of a situation based on their history of interactions with people throughout their lives and their genetic history (Maturana & Varela, 1992). Maturana, in an interview with Simon (1985), offers an even more radical idea with regard to different family members' perceptions:

> Systems theory first enabled us to recognize that all the different views presented by the different members of a family had some validity. But, systems theory implied that these were different views of the same system. What I am saying is different. I am not saying that the different descriptions that the members of a family make are different views of the same system. I am saying that there is no one way which the system is; that there is no absolute, objective family. I am saying that for each member there is a different family; and that each of these is absolutely valid (p. 36).

Maturana and Varela (1992) emphasize that human systems "bring forth" reality, in language and living with others. Problems can be perceived in very different, yet valid, ways. However, nurses are part of a larger societal system and thus are bound by moral, legal, cultural, and societal norms that require them to act in accordance with these norms regarding illegal or dangerous behaviors (Wright & Bell, 2009).

If a nurse does not conceptualize human problems from a systems or cybernetics perspective, the nurse's perceptions of the family and their illness, problems, and concerns will be based on a completely different conception of "reality" based on different theoretical assumptions. This text emphasizes different theoretical assumptions as opposed to more correct or "right" views of problems.

CONCEPT 2

Change is determined by structure.

Changes that occur in living systems (i.e., human systems) are governed by the present structure of that system. The concept of structural determinism (Maturana & Varela, 1992) offers the notion that each individual's biopsychosocial-spiritual structure is unique and is a product of that person's genetic history (phylogeny) and his or her history of interactions over time (ontogeny).

The implication for nursing practice is that an individual's present structure determines the interpersonal, intrapersonal, and environmental influences that are experienced as perturbations (i.e., that trigger structural changes). Therefore, we cannot say beforehand which family nursing interventions will be useful in promoting change for this particular family member at this time and which will not. Consequently, individuals are selectively perturbed by the interventions that are offered by nurses according to what does or does not "fit" their unique biopsychosocial-spiritual structures. We cannot predict which family nursing interventions will fit for a particular person and which will disturb that person's structure. This theoretical assumption is why we prefer that interventions be tailored to each family rather than standardized interventions for particular kinds of problems.

A deep respect and awe for and curiosity about family members develop in nurses who are cognizant of the notion of structural determinism. When structural determinism is applied to clinical work with families, Wright and Levac (1992) suggest that the description of families as noncompliant, resistant, or unmotivated is not only "an epistemological error but a biological impossibility" (p. 913). This concept has made a dramatic difference in the way in which we think about families and the interventions that we offer.

CONCEPT 3

Change is dependent on context.

Efforts to promote change in a family system must always take into account the important variable of context. Interventions must be planned with sufficient knowledge of the contextual constraints and resources. This is particularly important considering the emphasis in the health-care industry on accountability, cost-effectiveness, efficiency, and time-effective intervention. Nurses need to be aware of their position in the health-care delivery system vis-à-vis the family. For example, are other professionals involved with the family, and if so, what are their roles with the family? How do these roles differ from the nurse's role? How are the nurse and family influenced by and influential on the context in which they find themselves, be it a hospital, a primary care clinic, or an extended-care facility? It is particularly useful to underscore the positive contributions each health-care stakeholder can make to the family's care rather than attributing or assuming self-serving motives to stakeholders who have different vested interests in family care (such as limiting costs).

Larger systems (e.g., schools, mental health agencies, hospitals, public service delivery systems) frequently impose certain "rules" on families that ultimately serve to maintain the larger system's stability and impede change (Imber-Black, 1991; Imber Coppersmith, 1983). One example is the rule of *linear blame*—that is, institutions tend to blame families for difficulties (e.g., lack of motivation) and tend to make referrals for family treatment in order to "cure" or "fix" the family. This process is similar to the one that families use to refer another family member to be "cured."

Because members of some larger systems, particularly nursing staff, become intensely involved in a patient's or family member's life, they commonly tend to go beyond the immediate concerns. The end result is that patients in hospitals and their families find themselves inundated with services that commonly usurp the family's own resources. This then places the family in a "one-down" position in terms of articulating what they perceive their present needs to be. When a nurse is asked to complete a family assessment, he or she may become one more irritant in the family's life and can be hamstrung before even beginning because of the number of professionals involved. This is another reason why nurses should carefully assess the larger context in which the family and the staff find themselves. In some cases, the more serious problem is at the interface of the family with other professionals rather than within the family itself. Thus, interventions aimed at the family–professional system would need to occur before addressing problems at the family system level.

Another situation that can arise is unclear expertise and leadership. Families may find themselves in a larger system, such as an outpatient drug assessment and treatment clinic. They may receive different ideas on how to deal with a particular problem (e.g., cocaine addiction), depending on whether they are seen at the clinic, at home, or in a class. This usually occurs because no one clinic or educational program offered within a hospital setting has more decision-making power than another regarding a particular family's treatment plan.

Conflicts can also occur between larger systems or between families and larger systems. Unacknowledged or unresolved conflicts commonly result in triads, which inhibit healthy behavior. For example, if parents wish to send their adolescent son to a drug rehabilitation center but the nurse and rehabilitation director have been in conflict over rehabilitation policies, the family is placed in a situation in which pressure from the larger system (nurse–rehabilitation director system) leads them to align or take sides with either the nurse or the rehabilitation director.

How the family is being influenced by and is exerting influence on their involvement with these suprasystems is important information. Change within a family can be thwarted, sabotaged, or impossible if the issue of context is not addressed.

CONCEPT 4

Change is dependent on co-evolving goals for treatment.

Change requires that goals between nurses and families co-evolve within a realistic time frame. In many cases, the main reason for failure in working with families is either the nurse or family setting unrealistic or inappropriate goals. Frank and open discussions with family members regarding treatment goals can help avoid misunderstandings and disappointments on both sides.

Because one of the primary goals of family intervention is to alter the family's views or beliefs of the problem or illness and alleviate suffering (Wright & Bell, 2009), nurses should help family members to search for alternative behavioral, cognitive, and affective responses to problems. Therefore, one of the nurse's goals is to help the family discover or reclaim its own solutions to problems.

The task of setting specific goals for treatment is accomplished in collaboration with the family. Part of the assessment process is to identify the current suffering or problems with which the family is most concerned and the changes they would like to see. This provides a baseline for the goals of family interviews and becomes the therapeutic contract.

Contracts with families can be either verbal or written. In our clinical practice and in the practice of our nursing students, we typically make verbal contracts with families that state which problems will be tackled during what specified period of time or number of sessions. At the end of that period, progress is evaluated and either contact with the family is terminated or a new contract is made if further therapeutic work is required.

In most instances, clear goals (in the form of a contract) can be set with families with verbal commitments by family members to work on the problems outlined. On conclusion of the contract, evaluation should consist of assessing changes in the family system and in the identified patient.

In summary, family assessment and intervention are often more effective and successful if they are based on clear therapeutic goals. However, families rarely come to family interviews with the understanding or desire that family change is required. Therefore, in addition to goal setting, the nurse must help the family to obtain a different view of their problems. First, the nurse needs to engage the family; this can most easily be accomplished by first focusing on understanding and exploring their current suffering, the presenting problems and concerns, and the changes the family desires in relation to them. More detailed information about goal setting, contracts, and termination is given in Chapters 7, 10, and 12.

CONCEPT 5

Understanding alone does not lead to change.

Changes in family work rarely occur by increasing a family's understanding of problems but rather through effecting changes in their beliefs and/or behavior. Too often, health professionals engaged in family work assume that understanding a problem brings about a solution by the family. From a systems perspective, however, solutions to problems occur as beliefs about health and illness, problems, and patterns change, regardless of whether this is accompanied by insight (Wright & Bell, 2009).

There has been a tendency in nursing to believe that one must understand "why" in order to solve a problem. Thus, nurses with good intentions spend many hours attempting to obtain masses of data (usually historical) in order to understand the "why" of a problem. In many cases, patients and families encourage the nurse in this quest and participate in it. For example, a patient might ask, "Why did I have my heart attack?" "Why won't my son give up crack?" or "Why did my wife have to die so young?" We strongly discourage searching for the answers, because we do not believe this is a precondition for change; rather, it steers one away from effective efforts at change. The prerequisite or precondition for change is not understanding the "why" of a situation but rather understanding the "what." Therefore, we recommend that nurses ask, "What is the effect of the father's heart attack on him and his family?" and "What are the implications of the father's heart attack on his employment?" These questions serve a much more useful purpose in paving the way for possible interventions than do those focusing on the "why" of the situation.

"Why" questions seem to be entrenched in psychoanalytic roots that bring forth psychopathologies. These perspectives are not congruent with a systems or cybernetic foundation of understanding family dynamics that focuses on human problems such as the experience of illness, loss, or disability as interpersonal crises or dilemmas. Even if the "why" of a problem is occasionally understood, it rarely contributes to a solution. Therefore, it is more useful to explore what is being done in the here and now that perpetuates the problem and what can be done in the here and now to effect a change. The search for causes should be avoided because it inadvertently can invite family members to view problems from a linear rather than a systemic or interactional perspective. In other words, we prefer to believe that most problems reside between persons rather than within persons—that is, they are relational.

CONCEPT 6

Change does not necessarily occur equally in all family members.

Recall the analogy of the mobile previously presented in this chapter. Imagine the mobile after a wind has passed it. Some pieces turn or react more rapidly or energetically than do others. This is similar to change in family systems in that one family member may begin to respond or change more rapidly than others and, by this very process, set up an opportunity for change throughout the rest of the family. This occurs because other family members cannot respond in the same way to the family member who is changing, so a ripple effect of change occurs through the system. We have observed this phenomenon in practice with military families when a spouse returns home from a war or a peacekeeping mission. The desire for family members to "return to normal" (i.e., their pre-posting functioning) often conflicts with the returning member's experience of change. This event typically precipitates a time of intense adjustment for all family members.

Robinson's (1998) research also highlighted the concept that when families experience chronic illness, all family members are affected but not necessarily equally. In her study, women suffered more emotionally than other family members whether the illness was their own, their spouse's, or their child's.

Change depends on the recursive (cybernetic) nature of a family system. Therefore, a small intervention can lead to a variety of reactions, with some family members changing more dramatically or quickly than others.

CONCEPT 7

Facilitating change is the nurse's responsibility.

We believe that it is the nurse's responsibility to facilitate change in collaboration with each family. Facilitating change does not imply that a nurse can predict the outcome, and a nurse should not be invested in a particular outcome. However, there is a distinct difference between facilitating change, directing change, being an expert in resolving family problems, or assuming what must change. We believe families possess expertise about their experiences of their health, illness, and disabilities, whereas nurses have expertise in ideas about health promotion and management of serious illness and disability. It is also crucial for nurses to avoid making value judgments about how families should function. Otherwise, the changes or outcomes in a family system may not be satisfying to the nurse if they are incongruent with how the nurse perceives a family should function. It is more important that the family be satisfied with their new level of functioning than that the nurse be satisfied.

From time to time, nurses must evaluate the level or degree of responsibility they feel for treatment. The level of responsibility is out of proportion if a nurse feels more concerned, worried, or responsible for family problems than the families feel themselves. In the opposite response, sometimes nurses experience a detachment or a lack of concern, compassion, or responsibility for facilitating change within families. Both of these extreme responses indicate the need to obtain clinical supervision.

How much change nurses should expect to facilitate in family work depends on their own competence, their capacity for compassion, the context of family treatment, and the family's response. Nurses need to be cognizant that they are not change agents; they cannot and do not change anyone (Bell & Wright, 2011; Wright & Bell, 2009; Wright & Levac, 1992). For some nurses, not being a change agent is counterintuitive to their desire and manner of being helpful. But when nurses can let go of the notion of being a change agent and instead become a facilitator of change, they can move into a truly relational and collaborative relationship with families entrusted in their care.

Ultimate and sustained changes in family members are determined by each member's biopsychosocial-spiritual structures, not by the nurse (Maturana & Varela, 1992). Therefore, it is the nurse's responsibility to facilitate a context for change. Paying attention to windows of opportunity for facilitating change is one idea put forth by Robinson, Bottorff, and Torchalla (2011). Their findings support the idea that at the time of a diagnosis of lung cancer, families may be more open to addressing smoking-cessation strategies.

CONCEPT 8

Change occurs by means of a "fit" or meshing between the therapeutic offerings (interventions) of the nurse and the biopsychosocial-spiritual structures of family members.

The concept of "fit" or "meshing" arises from the notion of structural determinism (Maturana & Varela, 1992). That is, the family member's structure, not the nurse's therapeutic offering, determines whether the intervention is experienced as a perturbation that triggers, facilitates, or stimulates change. This concept is aligned with the guiding principle that the nurse is not a change agent (Wright & Levac, 1992) but rather one who, among other things, creates a context for change (Bell & Wright, 2011; Wright & Bell, 2009). In our clinical experience, family members who respond to particular therapeutic offerings do so because of a fit, or meshing, between their current biopsychosocial-spiritual structures and the family nursing intervention offered. (For more information on this, see Chapter 4 and the discussion of the CFIM.) This includes nurse sensitivity to the family's race, ethnicity, sexual orientation, and social class.

The concept of "fit" allows nurses to be nonblaming of patients and themselves when nonfit—and consequently nonadherence and non-follow-through—occurs (Bell & Wright, 2011; Wright & Bell, 2009; Wright & Levac, 1992). Nurses operating from a therapeutic stance who appreciate fit can be highly curious about ways to increase the suitability of interventions for particular family members at a specific time. When the concept of fit is over-looked, neglected, or not appreciated, nurses operate with more lecturing, prescribing behaviors, and often labeling family members as noncompliant, not ready for change, or defiant of the professional system.

CONCEPT 9

Change can be the result of a myriad of causes or reasons.

Change is influenced by so many different variables that, in most cases, knowing specifically what precipitated, stimulated, or triggered the change is difficult. Change is not always a result of well-thought-out intervention. Commonly, it can be the result of a collaborative relationship between the nurse and family and/or the method of inquiry into family problems. Asking interventive questions (see Chapter 4 for an in-depth discussion about the nurse–family relationship and questions within the CFIM, and see Chapters 8 and 9 for how to use questions in family interviewing) may in and of itself promote change. It is more important for nurses to attribute change to families than to concern themselves with what they did to create change (see Chapter 12 for more information on concluding meetings with families). To search for or take undue credit for change is inappropriate at this stage of our knowledge of the change process in families.

BIOLOGY OF COGNITION

The biology of cognition has been described and articulated by two neurobi-ologists, Maturana and Varela (1992), in their landmark publication *The Tree of Knowledge: The Biological Roots of Human Understanding*. They offer the idea that humans bring forth different views to their understanding of events and experiences in their lives. This idea is not new, but Maturana and Varela's perspective on how humans make and claim observations is much more radical: It is based on biology and physiology, not philosophy (Bell & Wright, 2011; Wright & Bell, 2009; Wright & Levac, 1992). If a nurse adopts a particular view of reality, it then follows that he or she now encompasses a particular view of people and their functioning, relationships, and illnesses.

CONCEPT 1

Two possible avenues for explaining our world are objectiv-ity and objectivity-in-parentheses (Maturana & Varela, 1992; Wright & Bell, 2009; Wright & Levac, 1992; Wright, Watson, & Bell, 1990).

The view of objectivity assumes that one ultimate domain of reference ex-ists for explaining the world. Within this domain, entities are assumed to exist independent of the observer. Such entities are as numerous and broad as imagination might allow and may be explicitly or implicitly identified as mind, knowledge, truth, and so on. Within this avenue of explanation, people come to believe they have access to a true and correct view of the world and its events, an objective reality. From this "objectivist" view, "a system and its components have a constancy and a stability that is independent of the observer that brings them forth" (Mendez, Coddou, & Maturana, 1988, p. 154). Nursing diagnoses, emotional conflict, pride, and politics are all products of an "objective" view of reality.

When objectivity is "placed in parentheses," people recognize that objects do exist but that they are not independent of the living system that brings them forth. The only "truths" that exist are those brought forth by observers, such as nurses and family members. Each person's view is not a distortion of some presumably correct interpretation. Instead of one objective universe waiting to be discovered or correctly described, Maturana has proposed a "multiverse," where many observer "verses" coexist, each valid in its own right. To increase options and possibilities for families to cope with illness using a variety of strategies or to improve their well-being, nurses need to help family members drift toward objectivity-in-parentheses. When nurses are able to maintain an objective stance, they are increasingly able to invite family members to resist the "sin of certainty"—that is, to resist the notion that there is only one true or correct way to manage health or illness, loss, or disability.

CONCEPT 2

We bring forth our realities through interacting with the world, ourselves, and others through language.

We propose that reality does not reside "out there" to be absorbed; rather, people exist in many domains of the realities that they bring forth to explain their experiences (Maturana & Varela, 1992). The ability to bring forth personal meaning and to respond to and interact with the world and with each other, but always with reference to a set of internal coherences, can be seen as the essential quality of living. Maturana and Varela (1980) assert that this statement applies to all organisms, with or without a nervous system. They further suggest that it is best to think of cognition as a continual inter-action between what people expect to see (owing to unconscious premises or beliefs) and what they bring forth. In a telephone interview, Maturana (1988) embellished this notion of reality as follows:

> We exist in many domains of realities that we bring forth . . . What I'm saying in the long-run is that there is no possibility of saying ab-solutely anything about anything independent from us. So whatever we do is always our total responsibility in the sense that it depends completely on us, and all domains of reality that we bring forth are

> equally legitimate although they are not equally desirable or pleasant to live in. But they are always brought forth by us, in our coexistence with other human beings. So if we bring forth a community in which there is misery, well, this is it. If we bring forth a community in which there is well-being, this is it. But it is us always in coexistence with others that . . . are bringing forth reality. Reality is indeed an explanation of the world that we live [in] with others.

In sum, the world everyone sees is not the world but a world that they bring forth with others (Maturana & Varela, 1992). When nurses adopt this particular ethical stance, they find themselves more curious about the world each family member brings forth and how this world influences the person's ability or inability to cope with or manage his or her illness.

CONCLUSIONS

Nursing is striving to articulate and describe more clearly the theories that inform clinical practice models. In an important and useful review of family studies and interventions, Hallberg (2003) found "a lack of congruence between the theoretical framework, the intervention, and the outcome measure" (p. 9). This chapter has attempted to provide insight about the theories or worldviews that provide the foundations of the CFAM and CFIM. This was done to clarify the connection between our theoretical frameworks and our family assessment and intervention models. Nurses need to continue to conduct research-based practice and practice-based research that enhance our understanding of which theories are most significant to inform practice, especially the offering of interventions.

References
Allmond, B.W., Buckman, W., & Gofman, H.F. (1979). *The Family Is the Patient: An Approach to Behavioral Pediatrics for the Clinician.* St. Louis: Mosby.

Bateson, G. (1979). *Mind and Nature.* New York: E.P. Dutton.

Bavelas, J.B. (1992). Research into the pragmatics of human communication. *Journal of Strategic and Systemic Therapies, 11(2),* 15–29.

Becvar, D.S., & Becvar, R.J. (2003). *Family Therapy: A Systemic Integration (5th ed.).* Boston: Allyn and Bacon.

Bell, J.M., & Wright, L.M. (2011). Creating practice knowledge for families experiencing illness suffering: The Illness Beliefs Model. In E. Svavarsdottir & H. Jonsdottir (Eds.): *Family Nursing in Action.* Reykjavik, Iceland: University of Iceland Press, pp. 15–52.

Crawford, J.A., & Tarko, M.A. (2004). Family communication. In P.J. Bomar (Ed.): *Promoting Health in Families: Applying Family Research and Theory to Nursing Practice* (3rd ed.). Philadelphia: Saunders.

Glazer, S. (2001). Therapeutic touch and postmodernism in nursing. *Nursing Philosophy, 2(3),* 196–230.

Hallberg, I.R. (2003). Evidence-based nursing, interventions, and family nursing: Methodological obstacles and possibilities. *Journal of Family Nursing, 9(3),* 3–22.

Imber-Black, E. (1991). The family-larger-system perspective. *Family Systems Medicine, 9(4),* 371–396.

Imber Coppersmith, E. (1983). The place of family therapy in the homeostasis of larger systems. In M. Aronson & R. Wolberg (Eds.): *Group and Family Therapy: An Overview*. New York: Brunner/Mazel, pp. 216–227.

Jackson, D.D. (1973). Family interaction, family homeostasis and some implications for conjoint family psychotherapy. In D.D. Jackson (Ed.): *Therapy, Communication and Change* (4th ed.). Palo Alto, CA: Science & Behavior Books, pp. 185–203.

Kaakinen, J.R., & Hanson, S.M.H. (2010). Theoretical foundations for the nursing of families. In J.R. Kaakinen, V. Gedaly-Duff, D.P. Coehlo, & S.M.H. Hanson (Eds.): *Family Health Care Nursing: Theory, Practice and Research* (4th ed.). Philadelphia, PA: F.A. Davis, pp. 63–102.

Kermode, S., & Brown, C. (1996). The postmodernist hoax and its effects on nursing. *International Journal of Nursing Studies, 33(4)*, 375–384.

Loos, F., & Bell, J.M. (1990). Circular questions: A family interviewing strategy. *Dimensions in Critical Care Nursing, 9(1)*, 46–53.

Maturana, H. (1978). Biology of language: The epistemology of reality. In G.A. Miller & E. Lenneberg (Eds.): *Psychology and Biology of Language and Thought*. New York: Academic Press, pp. 27–63.

Maturana, H.R. (1988). Telephone conversation: Calgary/Chile coupling [Telephone transcript]. Calgary, Canada: University of Calgary.

Maturana, H.R., & Varela, F.J. (1980). *Autopoiesis and Cognition: The Realization of the Living*. Dordrecht, Holland: D. Reidl Pub.

Maturana, H.R., & Varela, F. (1992). *The Tree of Knowledge: The Biological Roots of Human Understanding*. Boston: Shambhala Publications.

Mendez, C.L., Coddou, F., & Maturana, H.R. (1998). The bringing forth of pathology. *Irish Journal of Psychology, 9(1)*, 144–172.

Moules, N.J. (2000). Postmodernism and the sacred: Reclaiming connection in our greater-than-human worlds. *Journal of Marital and Family Therapy, 26(2)*, 229–240.

Robinson, C.A. (1998). Women, families, chronic illness, and nursing interventions: From burden to balance. *Journal of Family Nursing, 4(3)*, 271–290.

Robinson, C.A., Bottorff, J.L., & Torchalla, I. (2011). Exploring family relationships: Directions for smoking cessation. In E.K. Svavarsdottir & H. Jonsdottir (Eds.): *Family Nursing in Action*. Reykjavik, Iceland, University of Iceland Press, pp. 137–160.

Salladay, S.A. (2011). Confident spiritual care in a postmodern world. *Journal of Christian Nursing, 28(2)*, 102–108.

Schober, M., & Affara, F. (2001). *The Family Nurse: Frameworks for Practice*. Geneva: International Council of Nurses.

Selvini-Palazzoli, M., et al. (1978). A ritualized prescription in family therapy: Odd days and even days. *Journal of Marriage and Family Counseling, 4(3)*, 3–9.

Simon, R. (1985). Structure is destiny: An interview with Huberto Maturana. *Family Therapy*, May–June, 32–43.

Tapp, D.M., & Wright, L.M. (1996). Live supervision and family systems nursing: Postmodern influences and dilemmas. *Journal of Psychiatric and Mental Health Nursing, 3(4)*, 225–233.

Tomm, K. (1980). Towards a cybernetic-systems approach to family therapy at the University of Calgary. In D.S. Freeman (Ed.): *Perspectives on Family Therapy*. Toronto: Butterworths, pp. 3–18.

Tomm, K. (1981). Circularity: A preferred orientation for family assessment. In A.S. Gurman (Ed.): *Questions and Answers in the Practice of Family Therapy* (vol. 1). New York: Brunner/Mazel, pp. 874–887.

Tomm, K. (1984). One perspective on the Milan systemic approach: Part II. Description of session format, interviewing style and interventions. *Journal of Marital and Family Therapy, 10(3),* 253–271.

Tomm, K. (1985). Circular interviewing: A multifaceted clinical tool. In D. Campbell & R. Draper (Eds.): *Applications of Systemic Family Therapy: The Milan Approach.* London: Grune & Stratton, pp. 33–45.

Tomm, K. (1987a). Interventive interviewing: Part I. Strategizing as a fourth guideline for the therapist. *Family Process, 26(1),* 3–13.

Tomm, K. (1987b). Interventive interviewing: Part II. Reflexive questioning as a means to enable self-healing. *Family Process, 26(6),* 167–183.

Tomm, K. (1988). Interventive interviewing: Part III. Intending to ask lineal, circular, strategic, or reflexive questions? *Family Process, 27(1),* 1–15.

Varela, F.J. (1979). *Principles of Biological Autonomy.* New York: Elsevier North Holland.

von Bertalanffy, L. (1968). *General Systems Theory: Foundations, Development, Applications.* New York: George Braziller.

von Bertalanffy, L. (1972). The history and status of general systems theory. In G.J. Klir (Ed.): *Trends in General Systems Theory.* New York: Wiley-Interscience.

von Bertalanffy, L. (1974). General systems theory and psychiatry. In S. Arieti (Ed.): *American Handbook of Psychiatry.* New York: Basic Books, pp. 1095–1117.

von Glaserfeld, E. (1984). An introduction to radical constructivism. In P. Watzlawick (Ed.): *The Invented Reality: Contributions to Constructivism.* New York: Norton, pp. 17–40.

Watson, J. (1999). *Postmodern Nursing and Beyond.* Philadelphia: Churchill Livingstone.

Watzlawick, P. (Ed.). (1984). *The Invented Reality: Contributions to Constructivism.* New York: Norton.

Watzlawick, P., Beavin, J.H., & Jackson, D.D. (1967). *Pragmatics of Human Communication: A Study of Interactional Patterns, Pathologies, and Paradoxes.* New York: Norton.

Watzlawick, P., Weakland, J.H., & Fisch, R. (1974). *Change: Principles of Problem Formulation and Problem Resolution.* New York: Norton.

Wright, L.M., & Bell, J.M. (2009). *Beliefs and Illness: A Model for Healing.* Calgary, AB: 4th Floor Press.

Wright, L.M., & Levac, A.M. (1992). The non-existence of non-compliant families: The influence of Humberto Maturana. *Journal of Advanced Nursing, 17(8),* 913–917.

Wright, L.M., & Watson, W.L. (1988). Systemic family therapy and family development. In C.J. Falicov (Ed.): *Family Transitions: Continuity and Change Over the Life Cycle.* New York: Guilford Press, pp. 407–430.

Wright, L.M., Watson, W.L., & Bell, J.M. (1990). The family nursing unit: A unique integration of research, education, and clinical practice. In J.M. Bell, W.L. Watson, & Wright, L.M. (Eds.): *The Cutting Edge of Family Nursing.* Calgary, Alberta: Family Nursing Unit Publications, pp. 95–109.

Chapter **3**

The Calgary Family Assessment Model

The Calgary Family Assessment Model (CFAM) is an integrated, multidimensional framework based on the foundations of systems, cybernetics, communication, and change theory and is influenced by postmodernism and biology of cognition. This text discusses the distinction between using CFAM to assess a family and using it as an organizing framework, or template, for helping families to resolve issues.

CFAM has received wide recognition since the first edition of this book in 1984. Our model has been adopted by many faculties and schools of nursing and hospital settings in some 26 countries: Australia, Great Britain, Brazil, Hong Kong, Canada, Chile, China, Denmark, Japan, Finland, Sweden, Korea, Taiwan, Portugal, Singapore, Spain, Iceland, New Zealand, Norway, Qatar, Germany, Scotland, Switzerland, United States, Vietnam, and Thailand. It has also been referenced frequently in the literature, especially in the *Journal of Family Nursing*. In addition, the International Council of Nurses has recognized it as one of the four leading family assessment models in the world (Schober & Affara, 2001). Originally adapted from a family assessment framework developed by Tomm and Sanders (1983), CFAM was substantially revised in 1994, 2000, 2005, and 2009, and it is now even more developed in this Sixth Edition.

CFAM consists of three major categories:

1. Structural
2. Developmental
3. Functional

Each category contains several subcategories. It is important for *each* nurse to decide which subcategories are relevant and appropriate to explore and assess with *each* family at *each* point in time—that is, not all subcategories need to be assessed at a first meeting with a family, and some subcategories need never be assessed. If the nurse uses too many subcategories, he or she may become overwhelmed by all the data. If the nurse and the family discuss too few subcategories, each may have a distorted view of the family's strengths or problems and the family situation.

It is useful to conceptualize these three assessment categories and their many subcategories as a branching diagram (Fig. 3–1). As nurses use the subcategories on the right of the branching diagram, they collect more and more microscopic data. It is important for nurses to be able to move back and forth on the diagram to draw together all of the relevant information into an integrated assessment. This process of synthesizing data helps nurses working with complex family situations.

It is also important for a nurse to recognize that a family assessment is based on the nurse's personal and professional life experiences and beliefs and his or her relationships with those being interviewed. It should not be considered as "the truth" about the family, but rather one perspective at a particular point in time.

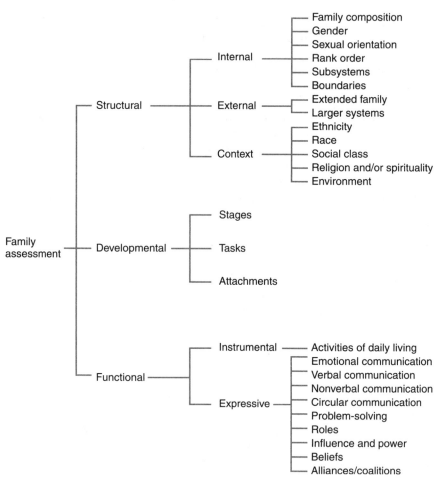

FIGURE 3-1: Branching diagram of CFAM.

We believe it is useful for nurses to determine whether they are using CFAM as a model to assess a family or as an organizing framework for clinical work to help a specific family address their health issue. When learning CFAM, students and practicing nurses new to family work will likely find the model helpful for directly assessing families. Similarly, researchers seeking to assess families will also find the model useful. This use of the model involves asking family members questions about themselves for the purpose of gaining a snapshot of the family's structure, development, and functioning at a particular point in time.

In our own work, we have used CFAM in a clinical rather than a research manner. Once a nurse becomes experienced with the categories and subcategories of CFAM, he or she can use CFAM as a clinical organizing framework to help families solve problems or issues. For example, a single-parent family in the developmental stage of families with adolescents will have many positive experiences from earlier developmental stages to draw from in coping with their teenager's unexpected illness. The nurse, being reminded of family developmental stages by using CFAM, will draw forth those resiliencies. She will ask questions and collaboratively develop interventions with the family to enhance their functioning during this health-care episode.

Families do not generally present to health-care professionals to be "assessed." Rather, they present themselves or are encountered by nurses while coping or suffering with an illness, loss, and/or disability or are seeking assistance to improve their quality of life. CFAM helps guide nurses in helping families.

In this chapter, each assessment category is discussed separately. Terms are defined, and sample questions relevant to each CFAM category are proposed for the nurse to ask family members. It is important that nurses do not ask these questions in a routine or disembodied manner. Real-life clinical examples are provided in Chapters 4, 7, 8, 9, and 10 so that readers can see how to use the sample questions and apply CFAM.

To assist in understanding further how to implement the CFAM in clinical practice, we have produced the educational DVD *Calgary Family Assessment Model: How to Apply in Clinical Practice* (Wright & Leahey, 2001) (www. familynursingresources.com). The use of assessment and interventive questions will be discussed in Chapter 4. Again, we wish to emphasize that not all questions about various subcategories of the model need to be asked at the first interview, and questions about each subcategory are not appropriate for every family. Families are obviously composed of individuals, but the focus of a family assessment is less on the individual and more on the interaction *among* all of the individuals within the family.

STRUCTURAL ASSESSMENT

In assessing a family, the nurse needs to examine its structure—that is, who is in the family, what is the connection among family members vis-à-vis those outside the family, and what is the family's context. Three aspects of family structure can most readily be examined: internal structure, external structure, and context. Each of these dimensions of family structural assessment is addressed separately.

Internal Structure

Internal structure includes six subcategories:

1. Family composition
2. Gender
3. Sexual orientation
4. Rank order
5. Subsystems
6. Boundaries

Family Composition

The subcategory "family composition" has several meanings because of the many definitions given to family. Wright and Bell (2009) define family as a group of individuals who are bound by strong emotional ties, a sense of belonging, and a passion for being involved in one another's lives. There are five critical attributes to the concept of family:

1. The family is a system or unit.
2. Its members may or may not be related and may or may not live together.
3. The unit may or may not contain children.
4. There is commitment and attachment among unit members that include future obligation.
5. The unit's caregiving functions consist of protection, nourishment, and socialization of its members.

Using these ideas, the nurse can include the various family forms that are prevalent in society today, such as the biological family of procreation; the nuclear family (family of origin); the sole-parent family; the stepfamily; the communal family; the child-free by choice family; and the lesbian, gay, bisexual, queer, intersexed, transgendered, or twin-spirited (LGBQITT) couple or family. Designating a group of people with terms such as *couple, nuclear family, multinuclear family,* or *single-parent family* specifies attributes of membership, but these distinctions of grouping are not more or less "families" by reason of labeling. Rather, attributes of affection, strong emotional ties, a sense of belonging, and durability of membership determine family composition.

Nurses need to find a definition of family that moves beyond the traditional boundaries that limit membership using the criteria of blood, adoption, and marriage. We have found the following definition of family to be most useful in our clinical work: *The family is who they say they are.* With this definition, nurses can honor individual family members' ideas about which relationships are significant to them and their experience of health and illness. For example, does the family include the surrogate mother and the commissioning couple?

Although we recognize the dominant North American type of separately housed nuclear families, our definition allows us to address the emotional past, present, and anticipated future relationships within the family system. For example, we support the American Academy of Pediatrics (2002) policy advocating that children who are born or adopted by one member of a same-sex couple deserve the security of two legally defined parents. We know that gays and lesbians often refer to their friendship network as "family" and that for many gays and lesbians, this family is often as crucial and influential as their family of origin and at times even more so.

Other family configurations include grandparents as primary caregivers for their grandchildren. In the United States, 1 child in 10 lives with a grandparent, and according to the Pew Research analysis of census data, there has been a sharp increase in 2007–2008 along with the recession (Livingston & Parker, 2010). Approximately 41% of those children are being raised by their grandparent.

Some authors, such as Penn (2007), have questioned the commonly held belief that all couples want to live together. He discusses "commuter couples," an alternate form of relationship in which each partner retains his or her own separate living quarters while remaining in a committed, monogamous, loving relationship. A rhythm that ensures both solitude and passionate connection is highly valued by these couples. Dual-dwelling duos (DDDs) and other new alternative pair-bonding structures, such as cohabitation and nonmarital coparenting, have also emerged. Our definition of family is based on the family's conception of family rather than on who lives in the household.

Changes in family composition are important to note. These changes could be permanent, such as the loss of a family member or the addition of a new person such as a new baby, an elderly parent, a nanny, or a boarder. Changes in family composition can also be transient. For example, stepfamilies commonly have different family compositions on weekends or during vacation periods when children from previous relationships cohabit. Families with a child in placement or those experiencing homelessness often live temporarily with other relatives and then move on. In New York City in 2002, more than 13,000 children spent their nights shuttling between shelters and other living accommodations (Egan, 2002).

Losses tend to be more severe depending on how recently they have occurred, the younger some of the family members are when loss occurs, the smaller the family, the greater the numerical imbalance between male and female members of the family resulting from the loss, the greater the number of losses, and the greater the number of prior losses. The circumstances surrounding the loss may be of exquisite concern for the nurse. For example, some parents of severely mentally ill children have reported that they were encouraged to give up custody of their children to foster care as a way of securing intense health-care treatment for them.

Serious illness or death of a family member, especially by violence or war, can lead to profound disruption in the family. The simultaneous deaths of both parents by car or plane crash, murder/suicide, natural disasters such as earthquakes and tsunamis, wars, terrorist acts such as September 11, domestic terrorism such as the Virginia Tech killings, or the absence of one parent in jail and the death of the other parent can result in aunts and uncles raising nieces and nephews or grandparents raising grandchildren, an often undernoticed family structural arrangement. Other family arrangements can occur when one parent is in a rehab facility owing to military injuries.

The extent of a death's impact on the family depends on the social and ethnic meaning of death, the history of previous losses, the timing of the death in the life cycle, and the nature of the death (Becvar, 2001, 2003). Research by Bowse and colleagues (2003) indicates that the extent of HIV risk-taking in adulthood is positively related to unexpected deaths experienced early in life and related inadequate mourning. We agree with these authors' recommendation that prevention efforts need to be more family-based and family-focused.

Our own reflections in the aftermath of September 11 and those of the families we work with have only increased our sensitivity to loss, its meaning in our culture, and its very specific meaning for each family in terms of how they cope and deal with uncertainty. Every family touched by tragedy faces the task of making sense of what happened, why it happened, and how to adjust to the changed landscape. Families can find inspiration from many sources to cope with unprecedented tragedy.

The position and function of the person who died in the family system and the openness of the family system must also be considered. We have found it useful to note the family's losses and deaths during the structural assessment process but do not immediately assume that these losses are of major significance to the family. By taking this stance, we disagree with the position taken by some clinicians who assert that it is important to track patterns of adaptation to loss as a routine part of family assessment even when it is not initially presented as relevant to chief complaints.

In our clinical practice with families, we have found it useful to ask ourselves these questions to determine the composition of families: Who is in *this* family? Who does *this* family consider to be "family"?

Questions to Ask the Family. Could you tell me who is in your family? Does anyone else live with you—for example, grandparents, boarders? So, your family consists of you and Faris, your 35-year-old son who just returned from Afghanistan. Anyone else? Has anyone recently moved out? Is there anyone else you think of as family who does not live with you? Anyone not related biologically?

Gender

The subcategory of gender is a basic construct, a fundamental organizing principle. We believe in the constructivist "both/and" position—that is, we view gender as both a universal "reality" operational in hierarchy and power and as a reality constructed by ourselves from our particular frame of reference. We recognize gender as a fundamental basis for all human beings and as an individual premise. Gender is important for nurses to consider because the difference in how men and women experience the world is at the heart of the therapeutic conversation. We can help families by assuming that differences between women and men can be changed, discarding unhelpful cultural scripts for women and men, and recognizing and attending to hidden power and influence issues. We think it is also important to consider friendship networks in our discussions with men and women. McGoldrick (2011b) asserts that for women, "close female friendships appear second only to good health in importance for satisfaction throughout the life cycle" (p. 56). Mock (2011) believes men seek companionship and comfort in closeness through shared activities with other men rather than through communication at a deep emotional level or through intimacy. In addition, friendships can be an important source of support for families dealing with illness.

In couple relationships, the problems described by men and women commonly include unspoken conflicts between their perceptions of gender—that is, how their family and society or culture tell them that men and women should feel, think, or behave—and their own experiences.

Gender is, in our view, a set of beliefs about or expectations of male and female behaviors and experiences. These beliefs have been developed by cultural, religious, and familial influences and by class and sexual orientation. They are in some ways more important than anatomic differences, although persons with ambiguous genitalia are often referred to as having an intersex orientation.

Gender plays an important role in family health care, especially child health care. Differences in parental roles in caring for an ill child may be significant sources of family stress. For example, when a child is ill, the majority of help-seeking is initiated by the mother. Robinson (1998) found role strain among families in which chronic illness became an unwelcome, dominant, powerful burden: "It became clear that the women—the wives and mothers in these families—were responsible for day-to-day, 24-hour, day-in, day-out protection" (p. 277). The women carried both the burden of responsibility and the majority of the workload.

In 2009, Neufeld and Kushner reported on men's experiences as family caregivers and what the men found as nonsupportive interactions, such as a lack of orientation to the caregiving situation, an unsatisfactory linkage to support sources, insufficient support, and hurtful interactions. We have found that men and women report more similar than dissimilar challenges in caregiving.

Levac, Wright, and Leahey (2002) recommend that assessment of the gender's influence is especially important when societal, cultural, or family beliefs about male and female roles are creating family tension. In this situation, couples may desire to establish more equal relationships, with characteristics such as:

- Partners hold equal status (e.g., equal entitlement to personal goals, needs, and wishes).

- Accommodation in the relationship is mutual (e.g., schedules are organized equally around each partner's needs).

- Attention to the other in the relationship is mutual (e.g., equal displays of interest in the other's needs and desires by both partners).

- Enhancement of the well-being of each partner is mutual (e.g., the relationship supports the psychological health of each equally).

In our clinical supervision with nurses doing relational family practice, we have found it useful to have them consider their own ideas about male, female, intersexed, and transgendered persons. Examples of questions we ask them to consider include the following: As a woman, how do you believe you should behave toward men? How do you expect them to behave toward you? How do you believe men should behave toward ill family members? What ways have you noticed that men express emotion? What are your thoughts about couples who choose a child's sex? Whose work do you express more interest in: husband's or wife's? Who do you feel more comfortable inviting to an interview: husband or wife? If a father answers the phone, who do you ask to set the appointment with: father, mother, or both?

Questions to Ask the Family. Sabeen, what effect did your parents' ideas have on your own ideas of masculinity and femininity? If your arguments with your male children were about how to stay connected rather than how to separate, would your arguments then be different? If you would show the feelings you keep hidden, Hashim, would your wife think more or less of you? How did it come to be that Mom assumes more responsibility for the dialysis than Dad does?

Sexual Orientation

The subcategory of sexual orientation includes sexual majority and sexual minority populations. *Heterosexism,* the preference of heterosexual orientation over other sexual orientations, is a form of multicultural bias that has the potential to harm both families and health-care providers. Sexual minority populations include LGBQITT persons. This acronym attempts to be inclusive but is not definitive. *Queer* refers to individuals whose gender identity does not strictly conform with societal norms traditionally ascribed to either male or female and who define themselves outside of these definitions. The premise is that sexual identity is socially constructed. Although the term *queer* previously was used in a negative manner, now it has a more positive connotation. *Intersexed* describes someone with ambiguous genitalia or chromosomal abnormalities. *Two-spirited* denotes an individual in the Aboriginal culture with close ties to the spirit world and who may or may not identify as being lesbian, gay, bisexual, or transgender. Overall, it indicates a duality existent in a person.

Discrimination, lack of knowledge, stereotyping, and insensitivity about sexual orientation are being addressed in North American society. However, discussions about gay marriage have at times clouded the issue of equal treatment. Despite the fact that approximately 1% of all U.S. households are identified as consisting of same-sex couples (*USA Today,* 2003), the topic of sexual orientation is one that nurses approach with varying levels of acceptance, comfort, and knowledge. For example, nurses' first encounters with transgendered persons often pose unfamiliar challenges. Weber (2010) points out that "families headed by parents who are sexual orientation or gender minorities may require special guidance for navigating an unusually complicated terrain related to parenting and family life" (p. 379). We agree with him. Lesbians, gay men, queers, and heterosexual women and men live in partially overlapping but partially separate cultures, and their gender role development often follows distinctive trajectories leading to different outcomes. In addition, immigrants may have also been exposed to varying beliefs about gay culture. Samir (2002) states that "there's absolutely no gay culture in Iraq. Not a hint of it. The only Arab country establishing a gay culture is Lebanon ... Homosexuality in most Arab countries is frowned upon and in some it is a crime punishable by extreme sentences" (p. 98).

In our clinical supervision of relational family nursing, we have found it useful to reflect critically on attitudes about sexual orientation. When comparing lesbian couples with heterosexual couples, we use parallel terms as opposed to comparing them to "normal" couples—that is, we do not say that lesbian couples as compared to "normal" couples have more coping skills. Rather, we say that lesbian couples believe this and heterosexual couples believe that. We do not assume that what applies to gay relationships can be applied to lesbian relationships or that a patient is heterosexual if the patient says that he or she is dating. We know there are mixed orientation marriages in which gay, bisexual, and lesbian spouses manage homoerotic feelings or activities while maintaining their marital relationship and being sensitive to the needs of their partner (Hernandez, Schwenke, & Wilson, 2011). We believe that nurses should be able to support a patient along whatever sexual orientation path he or she takes and that the patient's sense of integrity and interpersonal relatedness are the most important goals of all. If a nurse is not able to support a patient's explorations or decision to live openly or not as a heterosexual, homosexual, bisexual, queer, intersexed, or transgendered person, the nurse should excuse himself or herself from treating such patients.

We have found the sample questions exploring heteronormative assumptions posed by McGeorge and Carlson (2011) useful for self-reflection. We ask ourselves, What did my family of origin teach me about sexual orientation, bisexuality, and same-sex relationships? What are my beliefs about how a person "becomes" gay, lesbian, or bisexual? What is my initial reaction when I see a gay or lesbian couple expressing physical affection? What do the religious or spiritual texts of my particular faith teach me about sexual orientation?

Questions to Ask the Family. Elsbeth, at what age did you first engage in sexual activity (rather than asking, At what age did you first have intercourse)? When LaCheir first told your mom that she was lesbian, what effect did it have on your mom's caregiving with her? When your brother, LeeArius, announced that he was gay and leaving his marriage, how did your parents respond? What did your parents tell you, Lilah, about your ambiguous genitals?

Rank Order

The subcategory "rank order" refers to the position of the children in the family with respect to age and gender. Birth order, gender, and distance in age between siblings are important factors to consider when doing an assessment, because sibling relationships can be significant across the family developmental life cycle. Siblings tend to spend the most time with each other as youngsters; in later life, with parents living longer, the siblings' relationship is often intensified as brothers and sisters have to work out long-term caregiving arrangements.

Toman (1993) has been a major contributor to research about sibling configuration. In his main thesis, the duplication theorem, he asserts that the more new social relationships resemble earlier intrafamilial social relationships, the more enduring and successful they are. For example, the marriage between an older brother (of a younger sister) and a younger sister (of an older brother) has good potential for success because the relationships are complementary. If the marriage is between two firstborns, a symmetrical competitive relationship might exist, with each one vying for the position of leadership.

The following factors also influence sibling constellation: the timing of each sibling's birth in the family history, the child's characteristics, the family's idealized "program" for the child, and the parental attitudes and biases regarding sex differences. For example, we have found that siblings of children with attention deficit hyperactivity disorder (ADHD) frequently felt victimized by their ADHD sibling and that their experiences were often minimized or overlooked in the family. Bellin, Bentley, and Sawin (2009) argue for multilevel interventions to support siblings based on their study of siblings of youths with spina bifida.

Although we believe that sibling patterns are important to note, we urge nurses to remember that different child-rearing patterns have also emerged as a result of increased use of birth control, the women's movement, the large number of women in the workforce, and the great variety of family configurations. Newman (2011) notes that in the last 20 years, the number of families with just one child in the United States has more than doubled to between 20% and 30%. In Spain and Portugal, 30% of families have one child and in England it's up to 46% while in Canada it is approximately 40%.

We hold the view that sibling position is an organizing influence on the personality, but it is not a fixed influence. Each new period of life brings a reevaluation of these influences. An individual transfers or generalizes familial experiences to social settings outside the family, such as kindergarten, schools, and clubs. Given the availability and powerful influence of the Internet, the universe of available relationships and experiences is greatly expanded. As an individual is influenced by the environment, his or her relationships with colleagues, friends, and spouses are also generally affected. With time, multiple influences in addition to sibling constellation can affect personality organization.

Prior to meeting with a family, we encourage nurses to hypothesize about the potential influence of rank order on the reason for the family interview. For example, nurses could ask themselves, If this child is the youngest in the family, could this be influencing the parents' reluctance to allow him to give his own insulin injection? The nurse could also consider the influence of birth order on motivation, achievement, and vocational choice. For example, is the firstborn child under pressure to achieve academically? If the youngest child is starting school, what influence might this have on the couple's persistent attempts with in vitro fertilization? We urge clinicians not only to consider rank order when children are young but also its relevance when working with siblings in later life. Overlooking the fact that individuals may be influenced by old or ongoing conflicts may lead to missed opportunities for healing.

Questions to Ask the Family. How many children do you have, Amber? Who is the eldest? How old is he or she? Who comes next in line? Have there been any miscarriages or abortions? If your older sister, Gerda, showed more softness and were less controlling of your mom, might you be willing to talk more with your mom? Would you be willing to talk about difficult issues such as her giving up driving because of her macular degeneration?

Subsystems

Subsystems is a term used to discuss or mark the family system's level of differentiation; a family carries out its functions through its subsystems. Dyads, such as husband–wife or mother–child, can be seen as subsystems. Subsystems can be delineated by generation, sex, interest, function, or history.

Each person in the family is a member of several different subsystems. In each, that person has a different level of power and uses different skills. A 65-year-old woman can be a grandmother, mother, wife, and daughter within the same family. An eldest boy is a member of the sibling subsystem, the male subsystem, and the parent–child subsystem. In each of the subsystems, he behaves according to his position. He has to concede the power that he exerts over his younger brother in the sibling subsystem when he interacts with his stepmother in the parent–child subsystem. An only girl living in a single-parent household has different subsystem challenges when she lives on alternate weekends with her father, his new wife, and their two daughters. The ability to adapt to the demands of different subsystem levels is a necessary skill for each family member. It is also an important factor for nurses to consider in working with families. For example, children are often affected by a parent's mental (Beardslee, 2002) or physical illness. The nurse could inquire if the parent is worried about the children. The response to this question might shed light not only on the parental subsystem but also on the sibling subsystem.

In our clinical practice, we have found it useful to consider whether clear generational boundaries are present in the family. If they exist, does the family find them helpful or not? For example, we ask ourselves whether one child behaves like a parent or husband surrogate. Is the child a child, or is there a surrogate–spouse subsystem? By generating these hypotheses before and during the family meeting, we are able to connect isolated bits of data to either confirm or negate a hypothesis.

Questions to Ask the Family. Some families have special subgroups; for example, the women do certain things while the men do other things. Do different subgroups exist in your family? If so, what effect does this have on your family's stress level? If you were to look at your family as being made up of two teams, who would be on each team? When Mom and your sister, DeRong, stay up at night and talk about Dad's use of crack, what do the boys do? Which subgroup in the family is most affected by Cleve's crack problem and how? Who gets together in the family to talk about Shabana's self-mutilating behaviors?

When asking questions pertaining to subsytems, nurses can focus on particular ones such as parent-child, marital, or sibling.

Parent–child: How has your relationship with Bamboo changed since her diagnosis with severe acute respiratory syndrome?

Marital: How much couple time can you and Gbope carve out each month without talking about the children?

Sibling: On a scale of 1 to 10, with 10 being the most, how scared were you when AhPoh developed congestive heart failure?

Boundaries

The subcategory "boundaries" refers to the rule "defining who participates and how" (Minuchin, 1974, p. 53). Family systems and subsystems have boundaries, the function of which is to define or protect the differentiation of the system or subsystem. For example, the boundary of a family system is defined when a father tells his teenage daughter that her boyfriend cannot move into the household. A parent–child subsystem boundary is made explicit when a mother tells her daughter, "You are not your brother's parent. If he is not taking his medication, I will discuss it with him."

Boundaries can be diffuse, rigid, or permeable. As boundaries become diffuse, the differentiation of the family system decreases. For example, family members may become emotionally close and richly cross-joined. These family members can have a heightened sense of belonging to the family and less individual autonomy. A diffuse subsystem boundary is evident when a child is "parentified," or given adult responsibilities and power in decision making.

When rigid boundaries are present, the subsystems tend to become disengaged. A husband who rigidly believes that only wives should visit the elderly and whose wife agrees with him can become disengaged from or peripheral to the senior adult–child subsystem. Clear, permeable boundaries, on the other hand, allow appropriate flexibility. Under these conditions, the rules can be modified. We do not support the pathologizing of coalitions or subsystems just because they exist. In working with families from different cultures, races, and social classes or those from rural settings, we have found that fostering other central ties may be most beneficial for the family.

Boundaries tend to change over time and can become ambiguous during the process of reorganization after acquisition or loss of a member. This is particularly evident with families experiencing separation or divorce. As couples make the transition to parenthood, they may experience the desired child as a family member who is psychologically present but physically absent. This is particularly relevant if there is a surrogate mother or a known sperm donor involved during the pregnancy. Families caring for a member with Alzheimer's disease may experience the opposite phenomenon: The member is physically present but may often be psychologically absent.

Other variations include the ambiguity experienced by some families when a family member is in prison and then returns home. With approximately 650,000 ex-convicts leaving state or federal American prisons in 2006 (Penn, 2007), the impact on families is significant. Family boundaries can also be challenged when family members, especially young parents, are soldiers at war or live in a rehab hospital following a tour of duty. The concept of ambiguous boundaries was quite evident in the days shortly following 9/11 or Hurricane Katrina, when people were missing. Boss (2002) named the situation "ambiguous loss" and further described it as the most difficult loss there is, because families and friends feel helpless and the cultural tendency in the United States is to seek closure. During the early days post September 11, 2001, there was little closure for families who had missing relatives. Many Arab Americans and other immigrant groups experienced flashbacks of terror and connected to a history of oppression in the Middle East.

Boundary styles can facilitate or constrain family functioning. For example, an immigrant family that moves into a new culture may be very protective of its members until it gradually adapts to the cultural milieu. Its boundaries vis-à-vis outside systems may be quite firm and rigid but may gradually become more flexible. For example, some Muslim families' preference for greater connectedness, more hierarchical family structure, traditional dress, and an implicit communication style can be a challenge for their teens adjusting to a North American urban lifestyle.

The closeness-caregiving dimension of boundaries is another aspect for nurses to consider. The relative sharing of territory can be assessed along aspects of contact time (time together), personal space (physical nearness, touching), emotional space (sharing of affects), information space (information known about each other), shared private conversations separate from others, and decision space (extent to which decisions are localized within various individuals or subsystems). The closeness-caregiving dimension of a boundary may be very significant for nurses to assess when dealing with older people with chronic illnesses and their adult children.

In our clinical supervision with nurses, we encourage them to consider how each family differentiates itself from other families in the neighborhood and in the city. The nurse considers whether there is a parental subsystem, a marital subsystem, a sibling subsystem, and so forth. Are the boundaries clear, rigid, or diffuse? Does the boundary style facilitate or constrain the family? If there are multiple stepfamilies, which boundary predominates?

Questions to Ask the Family. The nurse can infer the boundaries, for example, by asking a husband if there is anyone with whom he can talk when he feels stressed by his upcoming retirement. The nurse can ask the wife the same question. To whom would you go if you felt happy? If you felt sad? Would there be anyone in your family opposed to your talking with that person? Who would be most in favor of your talking with that person? What impact might it have on your mom's ability to deal with your dad's illness if she had more support from your grandparents?

External Structure

External structure includes two subcategories:

1. Extended family
2. Larger systems

Extended Family

The subcategory of extended family includes the family of origin and the family of procreation as well as the present generation and stepfamily members. Multiple loyalty ties to extended family members can be invisible but may be very influential forces in the family structure. Special relationships and support can exist at great geographical distances. Also, conflictual and painful relationships can seem fresh and close at hand despite the extended family living far away or not in frequent contact. How each member sees himself or herself as a separate individual yet part of the "family ego mass" (Bowen, 1978) is a critical structural area for assessment.

We recommend assessment of the quantity and type of contact with extended family to provide information about the quality and quantity of support. For example, the importance of social media connections cannot be overemphasized. A young man paralyzed following a sports injury need not be isolated. Contact through Facebook, Twitter, Pinterest, and blogs is a helpful way for the family, friends, and colleagues to link to the patient and to each other. Such connective interaction "does hope," a notion we support and find healing.

In our clinical work, we consider whether there are many references to the extended family. How significant is the extended family to the functioning of this particular family? Are they available for support in times of need? If so, how? By mobile or land phones, e-mail, Webcam, texting, Skype, iChat, FaceTime, and Internet chat groups? Are they in physical proximity?

Questions to Ask the Family. Where do your parents live, Michiko? How often do you have contact with them? What about your brothers, sisters, step-relatives? Which family members do you never see? Which of your relatives are you closest to? Who phones who? With what frequency? Who do you ask for help when problems arise in your family, Zabin? What kind of help do you ask for? Would your family in Shanghai be available if you needed their help? Would you feel more comfortable contacting them by e-mail or in a chat room?

Larger Systems
The subcategory "larger systems" refers to the larger social agencies and personnel with whom the family has meaningful contact. Larger systems generally include work systems, and for some families, they include public welfare, child welfare, foster care, courts, and outpatient clinics. There are also larger systems designed for special populations, such as agencies mandated to provide services to the mentally or physically handicapped or the frail elderly. For many families, engagement with such larger systems is not problematic and can be life-affirming. We believe that larger professional systems can be an appreciative audience that supports families' narratives of hope and preferred new lives.

We encourage nurses to watch their language in discussing clients with larger system helpers so as to support family stories of courage, growth, and persistence instead of perpetuating stories of hopelessness and problems. Having family group conferences such as those begun as a legal process in New Zealand can be another way of fostering a participatory model of decision making with families in child protection (Connolly, 2006). Such a practice strengthens families. We are particularly drawn to clinicians who engage families as experts and create community-based programs for families using a collaborative family program development model. We advocate that professionals adopt the stance of being respectful learners and form collaborative professional relationships with families. The work of Looman (2011) reminds us of the importance of understanding the family-community interface—that is, some individualistic societies focus on loose ties between individuals, groups, and families, whereas collectivist societies are associated with a sense of duty toward one's group and social harmony.

Some families and larger systems may develop difficult relationships that exert a toll on normative development for family members. Some health-care professionals in larger systems contribute to families being labeled *multiproblem, resistant, noncompliant,* or *uncooperative.* These health-care professionals limit their perspective by using these labels. In their study evaluating the quality of care coordination provided for children with developmental disabilities, Nolan, Orlando, and Liptak (2007) found that 50% of the 83 families said that medical personnel never or rarely communicated with schools, and 27% never or rarely involved families in decision making. Communication about care across systems was key to satisfaction with service.

Another larger system relationship that nurses should consider is the computer network. Social media, electronic bulletin boards, chat rooms, blogs, texting, and discussion groups abound. Internet infidelity, pornography, and cybersex as a prelude to affairs and often sexual addiction are hot topics of conversation for many couples and nurses. We believe that infidelity consists of taking energy of any sort (thoughts, feelings, and behavior) outside of the committed relationship in such a way that it damages the relationship. Internet romance may begin outside any real-life context, but it quickly can escalate to a context all its own.

But the Internet can offer families valuable assistance in terms of information, validation, empathy, advice, and encouragement. Some have used e-mail, blogs, and online resources to augment, extend, deepen, inform, enrich, and prepare for in-person psychotherapy. However, we have found that online dialogues can sometimes be more sustaining than transformative—in other words, these dialogues tend to support the status quo rather than stimulate change.

Vigorous attention should be given to ways that professional expertise and electronic connectivity can be combined. Telenursing is one such example. Questions for consideration in providing family-centered telehealth care include how do health professionals ensure that the voices of *all* family members are part of the discussion between the nurse and the family? Using videoconferencing or Skype to gather all the larger system helpers in one space with the family to discuss, plan, and evaluate care can be a solution. We believe that increasingly health care will be provided in people's homes. Equipment necessary for such care continues to decline in price and simultaneously is easier to use. In working with technology and larger systems, nurses need to continue to find ways to address such challenges as telehealth infrastructure changes, reimbursement for services, liability, and licensing issues.

In our clinical supervision with nurses, we encourage them to discover whether the *meaningful system* is the family alone or the family *and* its larger system helpers. Nurses can ask themselves questions such as: Who are the health-care professionals involved? What is the relationship between the family and the larger system? How regularly do they interact? Is their relationship symmetrical or complementary? Are the larger systems overconcerned? Overinvolved? Underconcerned? Underinvolved? Does the larger system blame the family for its problems? What do the helpers desire for the family? Is the nurse being asked to take responsibility for another system's task? How do the family and helpers define the problem? When one young woman suffering from metastases from breast cancer was asked, "Who do you think of as family?" she answered, "I have three families: my own family, my church family, and my 'family' at the cancer center."

Questions to Ask the Family. What agency professionals are involved with your family, Mr. Rajwani? How many agencies regularly interact with you? Has your family moved from one health-care system to another? Who most thinks that your family needs to be involved with these systems? Who most thinks the opposite? Would there be agreement between your definition of the problem and the system's definition of the problem? How about between the definitions of the solution? What has been the best or worst advice you have been given by professionals for this issue, Atul? How is our working relationship going so far, Laura? If it were not going well, would you tell me?

Context

Context is explained as the whole situation or background relevant to some event or personality. Each family system is itself nested within broader systems, such as neighborhood, class, region, and country, and is influenced by these systems. The connectivity experienced by persons using the Internet is another context to be considered. Because the context permeates and circumscribes both the individual and the family, its consequences are pervasive. Context includes but is not limited to these five subcategories:

1. Ethnicity
2. Race
3. Social class
4. Spirituality and/or religion
5. Environment

Ethnicity

Ethnicity refers to the concept of a family's "peoplehood" and is derived from a combination of its history, race, social class, and religion. It describes a commonality of overt and subtle processes transmitted by the family over generations and usually reinforced by the surrounding community. Ethnicity is an important factor that influences family interaction. We believe that nurses must be aware of the great variety within and between ethnic groups. Some people are second-, third-, or fourth-generation immigrants, with ancestors who were born in a foreign country. Others may be from "recently arrived" (either legally or undocumented) immigrant families, of whom some are refugees. Another category is "immigrant American" families, in which the parents were born in a foreign country but their children were born in the United States.

The U.S. Census Bureau reports that 12% of the nation's population were foreign-born and another 11% were native-born with at least one foreign-born parent in 2009, making one in five people either first- or second-generation U.S. residents (United States Census Bureau, 2010b). Many were separated from one or both parents for extended periods. Suarez-Orozco, Todorova, and Louie (2002) report that results from their study of 385 early adolescents originating from China, Central America, the Dominican Republic, Haiti, and Mexico indicate that "children who were separated from their parents were more likely to report depressive symptoms than children who had not been separated" (p. 625). The immigration experience is central, not incidental, to health care.

For some immigrant families, the impact of cultural adjustment can be seen as a transitional difficulty, with issues such as economic survival, racism, and changes in extended family and support systems needing to be addressed. Specific life experiences, such as a trade school or college education, financial success in business, or family intermarriage, can encourage assimilation into a dominant culture, whereas isolation in a rural area or an urban ghetto tends to foster continuity of ethnic patterns. It is important, though, to recognize that these views of assimilation and isolation are from our "observer perspective." What matters is the family's cultural narrative, how it is deconstructed and co-constructed.

Ethnic differences in family structure and their implications for intervention have often been highlighted in a stereotypical manner. For example, Italians in North America usually have strong extended family connections and loyalties. African American families tend to have flexible family boundaries, and some may include the grandmother in child-rearing. Members of some Latin American cultures encourage emotionality between relatives and between generations, whereas the Irish in North America tend to have more strictly defined boundaries between generations.

In our clinical work, we have found it essential to recognize the infinite variety and lack of stereotypes among families from various ethnic groups. This is particularly important as Internet dating sites and more frequent opportunities for intermingling in the workplace and socially are introducing more diverse singles than ever before. Immigration and intermarriage (e.g., interracial) are shifting demographics in the United States. Cultural diversity is a matter of balance between validating the differences among us and appreciating the forces of our common humanity. We believe our own cultural narratives help us to organize our thinking and anchor our lives, but they can also blind us to the unfamiliar and unrecognizable and can foster injustice. For example, the importance of listening to history and context in caring for refugee immigrant women cannot be overestimated.

Nurses should sensitize themselves to differences in family beliefs and values and be willing to alter their "ethnic filters." We believe it is important for nurses to recognize their own ethnic blind spots and adjust their interventions accordingly. We are never "expert," "right," or in full possession of the "truth" about a family's ethnicity. Also, if we engage a translator to assist us with family work, we should not assume that the translator is an expert on this particular family's ethnicity. Rather, we and the translator should strive to be informed and curious about ourselves and others' diversity as we collaborate in health care.

The importance of participatory models of knowledge transfer and exchange cannot be underestimated whether in working with aboriginal communities or with other ethnic groups. For example, the findings from the study by Hiott and colleagues (2006) of gender differences in anxiety and depression among immigrant Latinos suggest that clinicians should ask questions about social isolation and separation from family. Answers to such questions may provide insights into stress and its contribution to significant anxiety and depression; these should also be considered when devising a treatment plan.

Some questions that we have found useful to ask ourselves include, What is the family's ethnicity? Have the children and parents had periods of separation in their immigration experience? If so, with what impact? Is their social network from the same ethnic group? Do they find that helpful or not? If the available economic, educational, health, legal, and recreational services were similar to the family's ethnic values, how would our conversation be different? Are the assessment and testing instruments we use in our clinic relevant for this ethnic group? Do they match the values and beliefs of this particular family?

Questions to Ask the Family. Could you tell me about your Japanese cultural practices or traditions regarding illness? How does being an immigrant from Iran influence your beliefs about when to consult with health professionals? What does health mean to you? How would you know that you are healthy? How would I know that you are healthy? As a second-generation Chinese family, how are your health-care practices similar to or different from those of your grandparents? Which practices seem most useful to you at this point in your family's life?

Race

The subcategory of race is a basic construct and not an intermediate variable. Race influences core individual and group identification; it both constrains and empowers identities. Contributors to an empowering identity include the participants having multiple reference group orientations, being strong, and refusing to take sides with, for example, blacks or whites. Race intersects with mediating variables such as class, religion, and ethnicity. Racial attitudes, stereotyping, and discrimination are powerful influences on family interaction and, if left unaddressed, can be negative constraints on the relationship between the family and the nurse.

The "myth of sameness" (Hardy, 1990) has been challenged and the uniqueness of various family forms emphasized more so in the last decade, especially with increased use of the Internet and other social media. Many college-age and younger Americans are rejecting the color lines that once defined racial identity in favor of a much more fluid identity. The crop of students moving through college right now includes the largest group of mixed-race people ever to come of age in the United States, and they are only the vanguard (Saulny, 2011). Saulny states that "nearly 9% of all marriages in the U.S. in 2009 were interracial or interethnic, more than double the percentage 30 years ago. Gender, race, and ethnicity are important influential variables. For example, black men marry someone from a different group twice as often as black women do while among Asians, the gender pattern is reversed" (2011, p. 21).

Family clinicians appreciate that the variations in family structure and development of African Americans, Asians, Hispanics, whites, and others are potential strengths in helping these families to function under various economic and social conditions. There is a dearth of literature on potential relationship strengths in intercultural and interracial relationships. We encourage nurses to elicit strengths rather than challenges in working with these couples.

The rapid change in racial patterns in the United States is important to note. Hispanics or Latinos constitute 16% of the total U.S. population, forming the second largest ethnic group after non-Hispanic white Americans (a group composed of dozens of subgroups, as are Hispanic and Latino American groups; Humes, Jones, & Ramirez, 2011). Mexican Americans, Cuban Americans, Columbian Americans, Dominican Americans, Puerto Rican Americans, Spanish Americans, and Salvadoran Americans are some of the larger national origin groups. The black or African American group represented 13% of the total U.S. population in the 2010 census, while 5% of all respondents identified as Asian alone (Humes, Jones, & Ramirez, 2011).

Racial differences, whether intracultural or intercultural, are not problems per se. Rather, prejudice, discrimination, and other types of intercultural aggression based on these differences are problems. With the number of interracial families continuing to rise in the United States, we believe race will become less divisive than it was. About 8% of U.S. marriages are mixed race, a rise of 20% since 2000, although a marked drop-off from the 65% increase between 1990 and 2000. Interracial families are quietly eroding many assumptions that have guided America's politics, customs, and habits for many decades.

For some persons, whether of the majority or minority race, the word *race* is very distasteful, as we are all members of the human race. They feel that the word itself implies harsh borders between groups of people in the human race and is therefore not very constructive in binding us together.

It is important for nurses to understand family health beliefs and behaviors influenced by racial identity, privilege, or oppression. In our clinical work with families, we have found it very useful to critically reflect on our own ideas about our race, marginalization, invisible and visible minorities, and "the myth of sameness" and to vigorously pursue the differences between and within various racial groups. For example, we ask ourselves how a Jamaican American family might differ from an African American family in their beliefs about hospitalization or how a Vietnamese couple might differ from a Japanese couple in their beliefs about whether to institutionalize an aging grandmother.

We believe health professionals should be racially and culturally competent. For example, non–African Americans working with African American families should not assume familiarity but should address issues of racism, intervene multisystemically, use a problem-solving and solution focus, and acknowledge strengths. These guidelines apply equally well for all races working with each other.

Questions to Ask the Family. What differences do you notice between, for example, your Hong Kong relatives' child-rearing practices and your own? If you and I were the same race, would our conversation be different? How? Would our different type of conversation be more or less likely to assist you in regaining your health? Could you help me to understand what I need to know to be most helpful to you?

Social Class

Social class shapes educational attainment, income, and occupation. It is frequently confused with socioeconomic status (SES). Kliman (2011) points out that SES is typically a decontextualized and hierarchical formula of education, occupation levels, and income dividing people into upper-upper, lower-upper, upper-middle, lower-middle, upper-lower, or lower-lower segments. Without taking into account the family's context, SES can obscure more than shed light on how a family has access to resources, information, privilege, and power. For example, an undocumented young man earning $20,000 in a full-time job has access to different resources than a graduate student working part-time, earning the same amount of money, and enjoying the privileges of his parents' accumulated wealth. Each class position has its own clustering of values, lifestyles, and behavior that influences family interaction and health-care practices. Social class affects how family members define themselves and are defined; what they cherish; how they organize their day-to-day living; and how they meet challenges, struggles, and crises. Class position can intensify or soften the impact of crises at each family life cycle stage. For example, middle-class seniors are likely to help their adult children, whereas working-class older adults are more likely to receive help.

Social class has been referred to as one of the prime molders of the family value and belief system. Much of the sociological and psychological research has been confounded by social class differences among ethnic groups. We believe that, in a racist and classist society, class and race are not inseparable. Because poverty is disproportionately concentrated among racial minorities, many professionals have considered the African American statistical subgroup to represent the lower-income class and the white statistical subgroup to represent the middle- or upper-income class. Furthermore, although Hispanics, including Mexicans, Puerto Ricans, Cubans, and people from South and Central America, have increased substantially in number to become a sizable group within the United States, until recently, data about marriage and family have excluded them. Such data have generally been limited to blacks and whites, without taking into account Hispanics or Asians. Much of the literature confounds the effects of race and class, not to mention the "myth of sameness" about families within each race or class.

Just as nursing has often been presented as intercultural, it has also been presented as interclass and nonpolitical. We believe that many nurses have pursued sickness in families to the exclusion of obtaining the *meaning* people give to events; their day-to-day living standards; and their access to employment, income, and housing. Social class issues have often been considered to be of little consequence to the "serious talk" about illness. This viewpoint has enabled nurses to sidestep many class issues associated with inequality and injustice. However, treatment must take into account the cultural, social, and economic context of the people seeking help. From factory workers to farmers to business executives, families are trying to cope with higher health-care costs and threats of losing insurance coverage. They continually make decisions based on which health care they can afford.

With higher prescription drug costs and a growth in the aging population, many families are anxious about their long-term care and ability to provide for their loved ones. Economic uncertainty, tsunamis, wars, fears of terrorism, and the aftereffects of 9/11 have created increased difficulties for the working poor. We have found in our clinical work that particularly in low-income situations, parents have to embed family time in other activities such as meal preparation, shopping, or driving, and not in leisure activities or time "off the clock" from mundane daily caretaking of children or elders.

Assessment of social class helps the nurse understand in a new way the family's stressors and resources. Generally speaking, women move down in social class following a divorce, whereas men do not. Recognizing differences in social class beliefs between themselves and families may encourage nurses to utilize new health promotion and intervention strategies. It is important for health-care delivery that nurses be aware of such influences as the "glass ceiling", the "glass escalator", and part-time temporary work versus full-time permanent work with benefits. The upward mobility risks of harassment faced by women entering some male-dominated work environments, such as the military, should also be known to health-care professionals.

In our clinical work, we have often asked ourselves how a family's social class might influence their health-care beliefs, values, utilization of services, and interaction with us. Serious illness can intensify financial problems, diminish the capacity to deal with them, and call for solutions at odds with conventional financial wisdom. We have wondered about the intrafamilial differences with respect to class and how these might help or hinder a family coping with, for example, chronic illness.

Questions to Ask the Family. How many times have you moved within the past 5 years? Have these moves had a positive or negative influence on your ability to deal with your son's AIDS? How many schools has your daughter, Frishta, attended? How does your money situation influence your use of health-care resources? What impact does Nuar's shift work have on your family's stress level?

Spirituality and/or Religion

Family members' spiritual and religious beliefs, rituals, and practices can have a positive or negative influence on their ability to cope with or manage an illness or health concern. Therefore, nurses must explore this previously neglected area. Emotions such as fear, guilt, anger, peace, and hope can be nurtured or tempered by one's spiritual or religious beliefs. Wright (2005) encourages distinguishing between spirituality and religion for the purposes of assessment and believes that doing so has the potential to invite more openness by family members regarding this potentially sensitive domain of inquiry. *Spirituality* is defined as whatever or whoever gives ultimate meaning and purpose in one's life and invites particular ways of being in the world toward others, oneself, and the universe (Wright, 2005). Religion is defined as an affiliation or a membership in a particular faith community that shares a set of beliefs, rituals, morals, and sometimes a health code centered on a defined higher or transcendent power most frequently referred to as *God* (Wright, 2005).

We recommend that assessment of religion's influence is most critical at the time a chronic or life-threatening illness has been diagnosed and/or when illness, disability, or loss has changed a family's life and relationships *forever.* Assessment is especially important and relevant when crises have occurred that may cause extreme suffering, such as a traumatic death caused by a motor vehicle accident; sudden death due to illness, violence, or abuse; or a life-threatening diagnosis. In these situations, it is critical that the nurse ascertain what meaning the family gives to their suffering due to these tragic events and ultimately how family members make sense of their suffering (Wright, 2005). This type of exploration about meaning and purpose in one's life following profound changes in family life opens the domain into spirituality. We prefer this more indirect method of inquiry about suffering than directly asking about spiritual and religious beliefs. We think that beliefs, spirituality, and transcendence are keys to family resilience.

Spirituality and religion also influence family values, size, health care, and socialization practices. For example, individualism is intricately related to the Protestant work ethic. Community and family support, on the other hand, is evident in the Mormon and Jewish religions, which foster intergenerational and intragenerational support. Folk-healing traditions that combine health and religious practices are quite common in some ethnic groups. In some spiritualistic practices, a medium, or counselor, helps to exorcise the spirits causing illness. For example, *espiritistas,* or healers, can be found in many Cuban and other Latino communities. Such healers, religious leaders, shamans, and clergy can be invaluable resources for families dealing with crises and with long-term needs such as caregiver support.

We encourage nurses visiting families' homes to note signs of religious influence in the home—for example, statues; candles; flags; and religious texts, such as the Bible, Torah, or Koran. We have been curious about dietary restrictions and habits and about traditional or alternative health practices influenced by religious beliefs. However, we have been cautious not to assume that strong spiritual or religious beliefs enhance marital happiness or interaction, although they may diminish the possibility of divorce. It is interesting to note, though, that the work of Parker and colleagues (2011) found that parents raising typically developing children scored higher on private and public religiosity and marital satisfaction than parents raising a child with a disability. Our clinical work with families has taught us that the experience of suffering frequently becomes transposed to one of spirituality as family members try to find meaning in their suffering (Wright, 2005).

If nurses are to be helpful, they must acknowledge that suffering, and in many cases the senselessness of it, is ultimately a spiritual issue. Therefore, in our clinical work, we have asked ourselves about the influence of religion and spirituality on the family's health-care practices. For a more in-depth discussion of clinical ideas and examples addressing the connection between spirituality and suffering, as well as how to assess and intervene, we encourage readers to peruse the 2005 text *Spirituality, Suffering, and Illness: Ideas for Healing* by Lorraine M. Wright.

Questions to Ask the Family. What meaning does spirituality or religion have for you in your everyday life? Are you involved with a mosque, temple, or synagogue? Can you tell me if there are ceremonies or spiritual practices that help keep your family strong and healthy or that you believe inhibit your family? Would it help if we arranged for a visit from a tribal elder or medicine man? Are your spiritual beliefs a source of support for you in coping with your illness? A source of stress for you? For other family members? Who among your family members would most encourage your use of spiritual beliefs to cope with Perminder's cancer? What are your sources of hope? Have you found that prayer or other religious practices help you cope with your son Surinder's schizophrenia? If so, may I ask what you pray for? Have your prayers been answered? What does your religion say about gender roles? Ethnicity? Sexual orientation? How have these beliefs affected you, Davinderpal?

Environment

The subcategory environment encompasses aspects of the larger community, the neighborhood, and the home. Environmental factors such as adequacy of space and privacy and accessibility of schools, day care, recreation, and public transportation influence family functioning. These are especially relevant for older adults, who are more likely to remain in a poor environment even if it has become dangerous to live there. Epstein (2003) raises a disturbing issue about the environment: "In America's rundown urban neighborhoods, the diseases associated with old age are afflicting the young. Could it be that simply living there is enough to make you sick?" Some of these neighborhoods have the highest mortality rates in the country owing to the prevalence of chronic diseases rather than gunshot wounds or drugs. Epstein comments that "the grinding everyday stress of living in poverty in America is 'weathering,' a condition not unlike the effect of exposure to wind and rain on houses" (p. 76). We have adjusted our perceptions of homelessness and come to grips with the idea that families with children are the fastest-growing homeless group. Homelessness is neither an urban nor a regional problem but rather one that is pervasive throughout North America.

In clinical work with families, nurses can ask themselves whether the home is adequate for the number of people living there. What health and other basic services are available within the home? Within the neighborhood? How accessible in terms of distance, convenience, and so forth are transportation and recreation services? How safe is the area? By asking in an open-ended way what other contextual forces may influence the family, it is possible to obtain a much broader range of responses.

Questions to Ask the Family. What community services does your family use? Are there community services you would like to learn about but do not know how to contact? On a scale of 1 to 10, with 10 being most comfortable, how comfortable are you in your neighborhood? What would make you more comfortable so that you can continue to function independently at home?

Structural Assessment Tools

The genogram and the ecomap are two tools that are particularly helpful in outlining a family's internal and external structures. Each is simple to use and requires only a piece of paper and a pen. The genograph designed by Duhamel and Campagna (2000) can also be used to draw the genogram (to obtain the genograph, visit www.familynursingresources.com). Alternatively, some computer programs (www.genopro.com) have genograms as a feature.

The *genogram* is a diagram of the family constellation. The *ecomap* is a diagram of the family's contact with others outside the immediate family. It pictures the important connections between the family and the world. We are aware of the arbitrariness of the distinction for some cultural groups between a genogram and an ecomap. For example, the standard genogram may be inadequate for African Americans or other racial or ethnic groups because of its underlying assumption that family is strictly a biological entity. We encourage nurses to develop a fit between these tools to depict specific family compositions.

These tools have been developed as family assessment, planning, and intervention devices. They can be used to reframe behaviors, relationships, and time connections within families and to detoxify and normalize families' perceptions of themselves. By pointing to the future and to the past and the present, genograms facilitate alternative interpretations of family experience. They can help the nurse and the family see the larger picture and view problems in both a historical and current context. Genograms can also be used to foster the training of culturally competent clinicians and to help nurses increase their self-awareness.

We agree with McGoldrick (2011a) that although much can be said about expanding genograms to include issues from larger social contexts (i.e., the sexual, cultural, religious, or spiritual genogram), realistically such mapping is extremely difficult to accomplish. Gendergrams have been developed to map gender relationships over the life cycle. At best, we can probably explore only a few dimensions at a time, and we recommend that these dimensions be directly connected to the purpose of the family's encounter with the nurse. For example, a nurse meeting with a couple in a rehabilitation treatment center for sexual addiction might reasonably explore a family's sexual and addiction history on a genogram. This content area would likely not be appropriate for a nurse meeting with a family in an intensive care unit.

Important issues that are difficult to capture on genograms include family members involved in family business; family members' relationships to the health-care system; cultural issues; family secrets; particular family-relationship nuances, including power, patterns of avoidance, and so on; patterns of friendship; relationships with work colleagues; spiritual and community connections; and medical and psychological stressors.

Genograms do not typically show the emotional connections among family members, present or past. The complex relationships of those who have warmed our hearts, mentored and nurtured us, aggravated us, or caused us severe trauma are not generally depicted. This is both a limitation of genograms and an asset; genograms tend to be a quick snapshot of the present.

With the help of computers, we can make three-dimensional maps that enable us to track complex genogram patterns. We caution practicing nurses to use the genogram as a clinically relevant tool, not as a map or data-collection sheet. Computerized genograms enable us to explore specific family patterns, resiliencies, and symptom constellations. Gathering, mapping, and tracking family history is much easier using a computer database. We urge nurses to ask themselves, What is the purpose of collecting vast amounts of information about this family's history, and how will this information be helpful for the purpose of my work with this family? Using computers and genogram information will provide rich data for family research, but it is unknown how useful this will be for immediate family care. Of course, by using computer genogram software, there will be many more possibilities for depicting family issues at different moments in family history. Clinicians and family members will have the opportunity to choose what aspects of a genogram they want to display for a particular purpose and at the same time create a database of a family's whole history.

Genogram

Genograms convey a great deal of information in the form of a visual gestalt. When one considers the number of words it would take to portray the facts thus represented, it becomes clear how simple and useful these tools are. Genograms, when placed on patients' charts, act as constant visual reminders for nurses to "think family." Sigurdardottir and Sveinbjarnardottir (2011) have described their use of genograms in the electronic health record as a way of supporting family nursing implementation and increasing family documentation. As an engagement tool, it is helpful to use during the first meeting with the family. It provides rich data about relationships over time and may also include small amounts of data about health, occupation, religion, ethnicity, and migrations. The genogram can be used to elicit information helpful to both the family and the nurse about development and other areas of family functioning. It is a tool that enables clinicians to develop hypotheses for additional evaluation in a family assessment.

The skeleton of the genogram tends to follow conventional genetic and genealogic charts. It is a family tree depicting the internal family structure. It is usual practice to include at least three generations. Family members are placed on horizontal rows that signify generational lines. For example, a marriage or common-law relationship is denoted by a horizontal line. Children are denoted by vertical lines. Children are rank-ordered from left to right, beginning with the eldest child. Each individual is represented. A blank genogram is shown in Figure 3–2.

Some authors differ slightly in the symbols they use to denote the details of the genogram. The symbols in Figure 3–3, however, are generally agreed upon. With increased use of computer genograms, symbols and color-coding will become standardized.

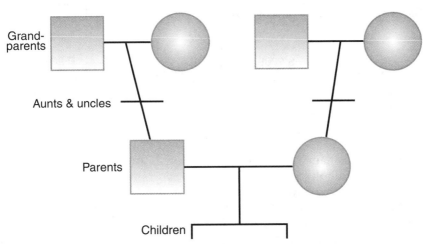

FIGURE 3-2: Blank genogram.

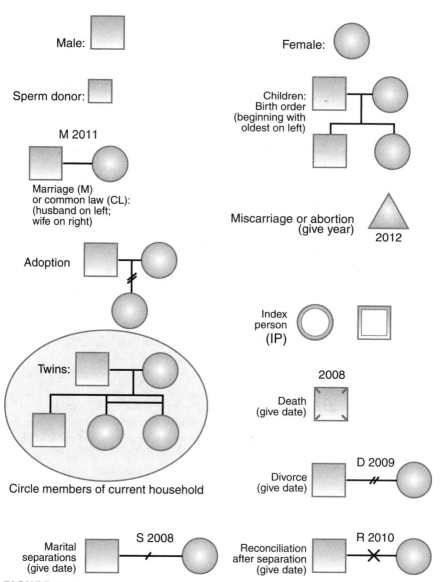

FIGURE 3-3: Symbols used in genograms.

The person's name and age should be noted inside the square or circle. Outside the symbol, significant data gathered from the family (e.g., travels a lot, depressed, overinvolved in work) should be noted. If a family member has died, the year of his or her death is indicated above the square or circle. When the symbol for miscarriage is used, the sex of the child should be identified if it is known. A small square is used to denote a sperm donor (McGoldrick, 2011a). It is helpful to draw a circle around the different households. We find that when children have lived in several contexts (e.g., immediate biological family, foster family, grandparents, adoptive family), separate genograms can help to show the child's multiple families over time. McGoldrick (2011a) offers an expanded description of symbols that could be used in drawing genograms if the clinician so desired. We find it best to keep the genogram symbols fairly simple so as to facilitate their adoption in busy clinical settings.

An example of a nuclear and extended family genogram is given in Figure 3–4 for the Lamensa family. Raffaele, age 47, has been married to Silvana, age 35, since 2000. They lived common-law for 2 years prior to their marriage. They have two children: Gemma, age 14, who is in grade 8, and Antonio, age 7, who is repeating grade 1. Raffaele is employed as a machinist, and Silvana refers to him as an "alcoholic." Silvana is a homemaker and states that she has been "depressed" for several years. Both of Raffaele's parents are deceased. His father died in 2010, and his mother died in 2008 of a stroke. Raffaele's older brother also has a drinking problem. Young

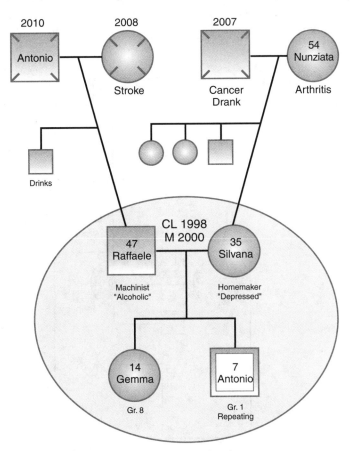

FIGURE 3-4: Sample genogram: The Lamensa family.

Antonio was named for his grandfather. Silvana's mother, Nunziata, age 54, has arthritis, which has been getting progressively worse since her husband died in 2007. Silvana has two older sisters and a brother.

Figure 3–5 illustrates a lesbian couple with a child born to one of them, Jennifer (age 30), and adopted by the other, Amanda (age 28). Jennifer and Amanda have lived as a couple since 2009 and have been married since 2011. Jennifer's biological son, Griffin (age 8), was conceived by artificial insemination. The unknown sperm donor is depicted as a small square. Jennifer's mother, Adrienne, a Jamaican retired nurse (age 65), divorced Jennifer's father in 1986, remarried in 1987, had another daughter, Mitzi, by her second husband and became a widow when he died in 1993. Mitzi is considering transgender surgery. Amanda's parents are separated, and her father is living common-law with Dan, his business partner. Amanda has no siblings. Jennifer has a younger brother, Spencer (age 28), and her half sister, Mitzi (age 25).

How to Use a Genogram

At the beginning of the interview, the nurse engages the family by informing them that they will be having a conversation so that the nurse can gain an overview of who is in the family and their situation. The nurse can then use

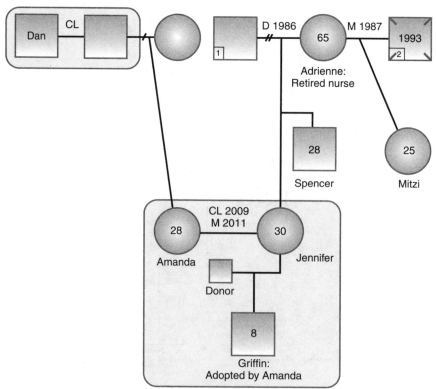

FIGURE 3-5: Sample genogram: Artificial insemination and lesbian couple.

the structure of the genogram to discern the family's internal and external structures as well as its context. Thus, the nurse gains an understanding of the family's composition and boundaries.

Initially, the nurse starts out with a blank sheet of paper and draws a line or circle for the first person in the family to whom a question is directed. Following is a sample interview with the Manuyag family.

Nurse: Elena, you said you were 23, and, Matias, how old are you?

Matias: Thirty-four.

Nurse: How long have you been married?

Matias: This time or the first time?

Nurse: This time. And then the first time.

Matias: Just 2 years for Elena and me.

Nurse: And the first time?

Matias: Ten years for the first one.

Nurse: And, Elena, have you been married before?

Elena: *(Laughs nervously.)* I'm only 23.

Nurse: Sure, it's just that many people have lived together in common-law marriages or were married when they were very young.

Elena: No. I lived with my parents till I met Matias.

Nurse: Do either of you have children from prior relationships? *(Turns to both Matias and Elena.)*

Matias: Yes, I have two sons.

Elena: No.

Nurse: In addition to Teresita here *(looks at infant on couch),* do the two of you have any other children?

Elena: Yes, there's Manandro.

Matias: Old Stinko, you mean.

Nurse: Old Stinko?

Matias: He isn't toilet trained yet.

Nurse: Oh, I see. And he's how old?

Elena: He's almost 3. I've been trying to train him since I knew I was pregnant with Teresita, but he just doesn't seem to want to be trained.

Nurse: *(Nods.)* Mmm.

Matias: Yeah, Old Stinko!

Nurse: And Teresita is how many weeks now?

Elena: She'll be 21 days tomorrow. *(Smiles at infant.)*

Nurse: Does anyone else live with you?

Matias: No. Her parents live next door.

The nurse now has a rudimentary genogram of the Manuyag family (Fig. 3–6) and has gathered information that may or may not be significant, depending on the way in which the family has responded to various events in the history of their family, such as:

- Manandro was conceived before the marriage.
- Manandro is unaffectionately called "Old Stinko" by his father.
- Elena has been trying to toilet train Manandro since he was 24 months old.
- Elena lived with her family of origin before the marriage. They live next door.
- Matias has been married before and has two other sons.

After inquiring about the nuclear family, the nurse can continue to inquire about the extended family. It is generally not very important to go into great detail about these relatives, but clinical judgment should prevail. If, for example, the grandparents are involved in a child's colostomy care, then a three-generational genogram should be constructed. On the other hand, if a child has a sprained wrist, then a two-generational genogram is sufficient. After asking questions about the husband's parents and siblings, the nurse should then inquire about the wife's family of origin. It is important for the nurse to gain an overview of the family structure without getting sidetracked or inundated by a large volume of information. Box 3–1 contains helpful hints for constructing genograms.

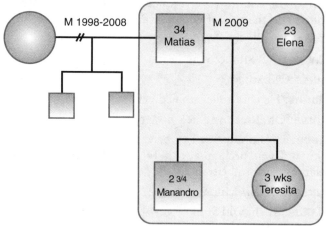

FIGURE 3-6: Genogram of the Manuyag family.

Box 3-1 Helpful Hints for Constructing Genograms

- Determine priorities for genogram construction based on the family situation.
- A three-generational genogram may be useful when the child's health problem (physical or emotional) is influenced by or affects the third generation.
- A brief two-generational genogram is generally most useful initially, especially for a family that has preventive health-care needs (immunizations) or minor health concerns (sports injury). The nurse can always expand to the third generation if needed.
- Invite as many family members to the initial meeting or visit as possible to obtain each family member's view and to observe family interaction.
- Engage the family in an exercise to complete the genogram.
- Use the genogram to "break the ice," provide structure, and introduce purposeful conversation.
- Ask family members how an absent significant family member might answer a question.
- Avoid discussion that is hurtful or blameful, especially of absent family members.
- Take an interest in each family member, and be sensitive to developmental differences.
- Tailor questions to children's developmental stages so that they become active contributors.
- Notice children's nonverbal and verbal comments.
- If some members are shy or seem uninterested in participating directly (such as adolescents), ask other family members about them.
- Begin by asking "easy" questions of individuals followed by exploration of subsystems.
- Ask concrete, easy-to-answer questions of individuals (especially children) about ages, occupations, interests, health status, school grades, and teachers to increase their comfort levels.
- Move the discussion about individuals to subsystems to elicit family relational data. Inquire about parent–child or sibling relationships, depending on parenting concerns.
- With stepfamilies, ask questions about contact with the noncustodial parent, custody, the children's satisfaction with visits, and stepfamily relationships.
- Observe family interactions.
- During genogram construction, note the content (what is said) and the process (how it is said).
- Move from discussion about the present family situation to questions about the extended family if it seems relevant (e.g., "Are Ruhi's parents able to help with the baby's tracheostomy care? What about babysitting?")
- When discussing generations, the nurse may find it useful to ask about psychosocial family health history (e.g., "Is there a history of alcohol abuse [or violence, learning problems, or mental illness] in your family?"). Questions should be tailored to the family's particular area of concern rather than generic exploration.

Levac, A.M., Wright, L.M., & Leahey, M. (2002). Children and families: Models for assessment and intervention. In J. Fox (Ed.): *Primary healthcare of infants, children and adolescents*. St. Louis: Mosby, p. 14. Copyright 2002. Adapted with permission.

The same question format used for nuclear families is used for stepfamilies, with one exception. It is generally easier to ask one spouse about his or her previous relationships before going on to ask the other spouse the same questions. This idea holds true especially in working with complex family situations involving multiple parenting figures and siblings. Again, it is unnecessary to gather specific information on all extended family members. It is useful to draw a circle around the current family members to distinguish among the various households. Usually it is easiest to indicate the year of a divorce rather than the number of years ago that it happened.

Figure 3–7 illustrates a sample genogram of a stepfamily. In this stepfamily, Michael (age 35), has been living in a common-law marriage since 2011 with Melanie (age 33), who is a part-time waitress. Also in the household are Melanie's two children by her first marriage—Kathy (age 11) and Jacob (age 9). Jacob has ADHD and is in a special third-grade class. Michael married his first wife, Laura, in 2001. They were divorced in 2005. Michael and Laura had one son, who is now age 8. Michael is an only child. His father committed suicide in 2008. His mother is still alive. Melanie is the youngest of three daughters, and both of her parents are living. Melanie married David in 2001, separated in 2008, and divorced in 2011. David, age 36, is a mechanic who is presently living in a common-law marriage with Camille and

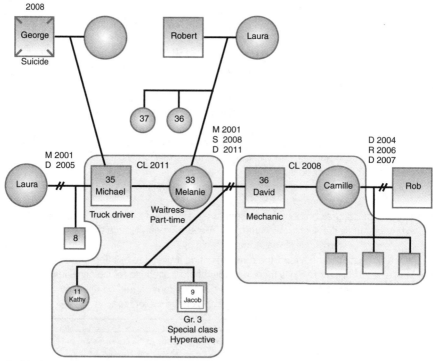

FIGURE 3-7: Sample genogram of a stepfamily.

her three sons. Camille and her first husband, Rob, divorced in 2004, reconciled in 2006, and then divorced in 2007.

There are no specific guidelines for drawing genograms illustrating complex stepfamily situations. Generally, however, it works best if the nurse starts by gathering information about the immediate household. After this, the nurse draws each family's constellation. Whenever possible, it is best to show children from different marriages in their correct birth order, oldest on the left and youngest on the right. We agree with McGoldrick (2011a) that the rule of thumb is, when feasible, that different marriages follow in chronological order from left to right. We have sometimes found it helpful to indicate the number of the relationship or marriage in the lower corner when there have been several relationships. See Figure 3–5, where Adrienne's husbands are indicated as #1 and #2. It can be useful to draw a circle around each separate household. If one member of a couple is involved in an affair, then their relationship is depicted with a dotted rather than a solid line. Additional pertinent information, such as children moving between two households, can be written to the side of the genogram. It is important for the nurse to remember that the purpose of drawing the genogram is to obtain a visual overview of the family. The genogram is not meant to be an exact chart for genetics.

Challenges arise when there are multiple marriages, such as Qatari families who may have one to four wives, intermarriages, and remarriages within the family. For example, when cousins or stepsiblings marry, the clinician should use separate pages to clarify intricacies. With complex family situations, the nurse needs to choose between clarity and level of detail. When computers are used to diagram genograms, complexity can be reduced. We advise nurses to let usefulness be their guide.

Develop a genogram that is useful rather than one that is overly inclusive and too confusing. Sometimes the only feasible way for pediatric nurses to clarify where children were raised is to take chronological notes on each child and draw multiple genograms through time to show the various family constellations the child experienced. With software, specific genograms can be created for specific moments in a person's life. When discrepancies exist in information shared by various family members, we advise nurses to note this on the genogram but not to take on an investigative role. There can be multiple truths and remembrances of information. Cook and Poulsen (2011) have suggested using photographs with genograms as a way of creating a dynamic, information-rich, and experiential environment. We think this might be a useful idea if the nurse is working with patients in a long-term care or rehabilitation facility.

Another, perhaps more typical stepfamily genogram is depicted in Figure 3–8. In this genogram, the Faris family is composed of David (age 42), a software designer who has been living common-law since 2009 with Patti (age 40), a part-time retail associate. They have a daughter, Madison (age 1), who was recently diagnosed with juvenile diabetes. David's twin sons, Jack

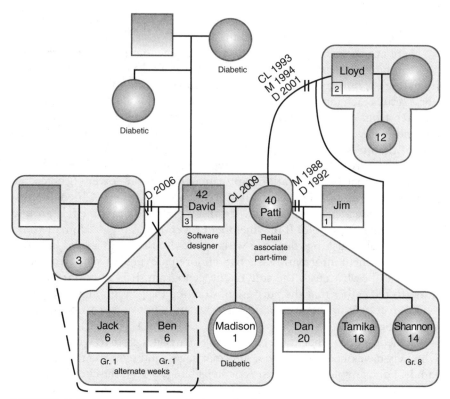

FIGURE 3-8: Sample genogram: Faris stepfamily.

and Ben (age 6), spend alternate weeks at their mom's town house and at their dad's apartment. David was divorced in 2006; his former wife has a daughter, age 3. Patti has a son, Dan (age 20), by her first husband, Jim, who she divorced in 1992. Dan lives alone and works several part-time jobs in bars. Patti also has two other daughters: Tamika (age 16), who recently dropped out of school, and Shannon (age 14), who is in grade 8. They are from her second marriage, to Lloyd, which ended in divorce in 2001. The teenage girls live with their mom and visit Lloyd and his family for 2 weeks most summers. The current health concern is Madison's juvenile diabetes; the current household consists of David, Patti, the three girls, and on alternate weeks the twins. David's mom has diabetes, as does his older sister.

Another sample family situation is the Fitzgerald-Kucewicz family, in which a child lives with the grandmother and her husband. The identified patient, 8-year-old Sophia Kucewicz, lives with her grandmother, 45-year-old Patricia Fitzgerald; Vincent, Patricia's common-law partner of 10 years; and Sophia's 19-year-old aunt, Susan. Patricia was previously married to Steven Fitzgerald for 14 years. Patricia and Steven had three children: 19-year-old Susan, 23-year-old Douglas, and 25-year-old Joan, who is Sophia's mother. Joan became pregnant with Sophia when she was 16. Sophia's father, Michael

Kucewicz, and her mother, Joan, had a brief relationship, through which she was conceived. Although Michael was aware of the pregnancy, he left the city shortly before Sophia was born, never meeting her. When Sophia was 2 years old, Joan had another child, Kayla, who subsequently went to live with her natural father when she was 4. When Sophia was 2.5, her mother moved in with Ben, who Sophia came to know as her father. Joan and Ben had difficulty providing a stable environment for Sophia and Kayla and, from time to time, moved in with Patricia and Vincent. Patricia reports that both Joan and Ben used drugs and alcohol and were often unemployed. Ben was physically and verbally abusive to Joan and, after a particularly frightening episode between Joan and Ben that took place in the basement of Patricia's home, Joan called the police. The child welfare department became involved, leading Patricia and Vincent to take guardianship of Sophia. Joan and Ben moved to a place of their own, agreeing to take Sophia every other weekend. The health concern for this family is Sophia's nightmares, especially after returning from visits to Joan and Ben's trailer. Figure 3–9 shows the Fitzgerald-Kucewicz family genogram.

Most families are extremely receptive to and interested in collaborating with the nurse to complete a genogram. For some, it is the first time that they have ever seen their family life pictured in this manner. Therefore, the nurse needs to be aware that the family may have a reaction to significant events. One family, for example, may express some sensitive material in a

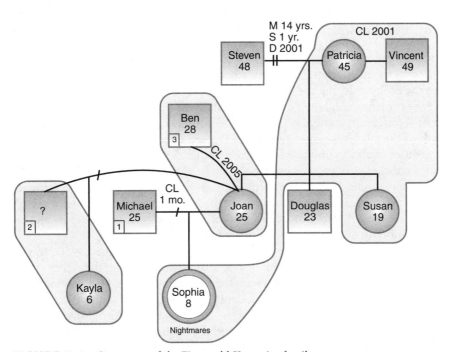

FIGURE 3-9: Genogram of the Fitzgerald-Kucewicz family.

very blasé fashion. If divorce is common in their families of origin, they may not hesitate to discuss their several marriages and those of their siblings. On the other hand, a devout Catholic family may be exquisitely sensitive to seeing the nurse write the word *divorce*.

Ecomap

As with the genogram, the primary value of the ecomap is in its visual impact. The purpose of the ecomap is to depict the family members' contact with larger systems. Hartman (1978) notes:

> The eco-map [sic] portrays an overview of the family in their situation; it pictures the important nurturant or conflict-laden connections between the family and the world. It demonstrates the flow of resources, or the lack of and deprivations. This mapping procedure highlights the nature of the interfaces and points to conflicts to be mediated, bridges to be built, and resources to be sought and mobilized (p. 467).

Ecomaps shift the emphasis away from the historical genogram to the current functioning of the family and its environmental context. This focus on the present is an important message in our outcome-based health-care climate. The ecomap depicts reciprocal relationships between family members and broader community institutions such as schools, courts, health-care facilities, and so forth. Increasingly, the ecomap is being used in a variety of ways to promote family health. For example, Limb and Hodge (2011) have used spiritual ecograms with Native Americans to promote cultural competence.

How to Use an Ecomap

As with the genogram, family members can actively participate in working on the ecomap during the assessment process. The family genogram is placed in the center circle, labeled "Family or household." The outer circles represent significant people, agencies, or institutions in the family's context. The size of the circles is not important. Lines are drawn between the family and the outer circles to indicate the nature of the connections that exist. Straight lines indicate strong connections, dotted lines indicate tenuous connections, and slashed lines indicate stressful relations. The wider the line, the stronger the tie. Arrows can be drawn alongside the lines to indicate the flow of energy and resources. Additional circles may be drawn as necessary, depending on the number of significant contacts the family has.

An ecomap for the Lamensa family is illustrated in Figure 3–10. In this family, Raffaele, Silvana, Gemma, and Antonio are placed in the center circle. Raffaele has strong connections with his workplace, where he is foreman and a union representative. He has moderately strong bonds with his "drinking buddies." However, these relationships are stressful for him. Silvana's connections are mainly with her mother and the health-care system. She sees her family physician every week "for nerves" and sees a community health nurse

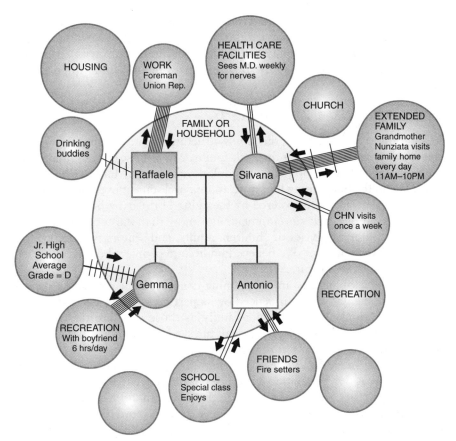

FIGURE 3-10: Lamensa family ecomap.

(CHN) once a week. Silvana's mother, Nunziata, visits Silvana every day from 11:00 AM to 10:00 PM. There is a strong connection between Silvana and her mother, but Silvana says she really "doesn't like Mom coming over so often." Antonio has a few friends, most of whom set fires. He is in a special class for his learning disability and enjoys both the teacher and the school. Gemma is in junior high school, where she maintains an average grade of D. She frequently does not attend school, and when she does attend, she participates little. She spends about 6 hours a day with her boyfriend.

When the CHN completed the ecomap with the Lamensa family, Mrs. Lamensa (Silvana) commented, "I seem to spend all my time with medical or health people." Mr. Lamensa (Raffaele) then said, "You're also so busy with your mother that you don't have time for anybody else." The nurse was able to use this information from the ecomap to discuss further with the family the types of relationships they wanted with those inside their household and with those outside the immediate family.

In summary, the genogram and the ecomap can be used in *all* health-care settings, especially in primary care, to increase the nurse's awareness and "knowing" of the whole family and the family's interactions with larger systems and their extended family. Box 3–2 gives helpful hints for drawing ecomaps.

DEVELOPMENTAL ASSESSMENT

In addition to understanding the family structure, the nurse must understand the developmental life cycle for each family. Most nurses are familiar with the stages of child development and adult development. Many are becoming interested in the burgeoning literature about development in the senior years, an interest that has been fostered by the aging of the baby boomer generation. But what of family development? It is more than the concurrent development at different phases of children, adults, and seniors who happen to call themselves "family." We believe families are people who have a shared history and a shared future.

Family development is an overarching concept, but each family has its own developmental path, influenced by its past and present context and its future aspirations. Some consider family as those who are tied together through their common biological, legal, physical, social, and emotional history and by their implied future together.

There is no single family developmental life cycle or model. This is especially evident as our population ages. The natural sequential phases of generational boundaries are not as clear as in the past with, for example, children maturing at earlier ages but living at home longer, the trend toward later marriages, and seniors continuing to work well into their 70s. This blurring of boundaries can sometimes lead to tension and confusion within families.

In keeping with postmodernist ideas, we believe that there are limits to describing family development in precise, absolute, universal ways. Postmodernists differ from modernists in that exceptions interest them more than rules; specific, contextualized details more than grand generalizations; difference

---

| **Box 3-2** Helpful Hints for Drawing Ecomaps |

Pose questions that explore the family's connections to other individuals or groups outside the family, such as:

- What community agencies are you involved with now? Which are most and least helpful?
- How would you describe your relationship with school staff?
- How did you first become involved with Child Protective Services? What is the nature of your current relationship with them?

Levac, A.M., Wright, L.M., & Leahey, M. (2002). Children and families: Models for assessment and intervention. In J. Fox (Ed.): *Primary Healthcare of Infants, Children and Adolescents*. St. Louis: Mosby, p. 14. Copyright 2002. Adapted with permission.

rather than similarity. We are not concerned with authoritative truth, facts, and rules, but rather with the meaning a family gives to its particular story of development over time.

In our clinical supervision with nurses, we have found it useful to distinguish between "family development" and "family life cycle." *Family development* emphasizes the *unique* path constructed by a family. It is shaped by predictable and unpredictable events, such as illness, catastrophes (e.g., terrorist attacks, fires, earthquakes, hurricanes, floods), and societal trends (e.g., Internet, social media, and smartphone usage; recessions; unemployment; mortgage defaults; stock market fluctuations; company mergers; changes in crime; and birth rates and immigration and migration).

Family life cycle refers to the *typical* path most families go through. The typical life cycle events are connected to the comings and goings of family members. For example, most families experience in their life cycle the events of birth, child-rearing, departure of children from the household, retirement, and death. Such events generate changes requiring formal reorganization of roles and rules within the family. The life cycle course of families evolves through a generally predictable sequence of stages, despite cultural and ethnic variations. Although individual variations, timing, and coping strategies exist, biological time clocks and societal expectations for events such as entrance into elementary school and retirement from work are relatively typical in North America.

Given our keen interest in a particular family's specific development over time, it might be questioned why we include a family developmental section in CFAM at all. We take the position that an informed "not-knowing" stance is useful when working with families—that is, we seek to be informed by the literature, research, and other families' stories of development. Yet, we are "not knowing" but curious about this particular family's developmental story in terms of how they have progressed through time.

A rich history about family development still pervades clinicians' thinking. We believe that it is useful for nurses to have some understanding of this history. The early proponents of the family life cycle (Duvall, 1977) developed a four-stage model that was subsequently expanded into an eight-stage model featuring successive stages in the progression of primary marriages. With the increase in various family forms, more complex designs were created (Carter & McGoldrick, 1988, 1999b; McGoldrick & Carter, 2003; McGoldrick, Carter, & Garcia-Preto, 2011a).

Most early analyses of the family life cycle began with a discussion of the first marriage but also considered activities that preceded the first marriage, such as cohabitation. Lewin (2010) reported that cohabitation is a widely used transitional step to marriage with approximately half of cohabiting couples marrying within 3 years and about two thirds marrying within 5 years, according to the 2010 U.S. Census. Unfortunately, data are now coming forth that indicate cohabiting couples who marry are more likely to divorce than non-cohabiting couples. The median age at first marriage increased to 28.2

for men and 26.1 for women in 2010, an increase from 26.8 and 25.1 in 2000 according to the U.S. Census Bureau (United States Census Bureau, 2010a).

In the field of family therapy, there were "pioneers" in applying the family development framework. Much was written about the interface among family development, functioning, and therapy. Carter and McGoldrick (1988) believed that the family life cycle perspective viewed symptoms in relation to normal functioning over time and that "therapy" helped to reestablish the family's developmental momentum. Family therapists such as Haley (1977), Minuchin (1974), and the Milan Group (Selvini-Palazzoli, et al, 1980) noted the frequency of symptom appearance with the addition or loss of a family member. These therapists worked with families that did not move smoothly or automatically from one stage in the family life cycle to another, and they focused on the stressful transition points between stages. In doing an assessment and in planning interventions, these therapists paid considerable attention to life cycle events as markers of change. Although their approaches differed, these therapists similarly sought to understand the relationship between psychopathology and the family's developmental life cycle stage.

Carter and McGoldrick (1988, 1999b) included the impact of transgenerational stress intersecting with family developmental transitions. They believed that if vertical (transgenerational) stress was too high, a small amount of horizontal (current) stress would lead to great disruption and symptom formation. More recently, McGoldrick, Carter, and Garcia-Preto (2011b) have advocated adding friendship as a component of the family life cycle because it is part of our sense of home and the importance of community. In addition, they recommend clinicians consider the family's sense of what they call *homeplace,* a place of acceptance and belonging essential to developing a solid sense of self as a human being. What is a client's sense of belonging and connection to what is familiar? Clinicians have a significant role to play in encouraging clients to think about the meaning of family and community to them as they go through various life cycle stages.

Over the last decade, there have been a great many changes in the family life cycle. First, there has been an increase in literature discussing families and their developmental phases (e.g., divorce, remarriage, foster families, impact of immigration, chronic illness, terrorism). Second, there has been an increased consciousness of differences in male and female development and a rethinking of the trajectory of various ethnic groups in North American society. Third, there has been a lower birth rate, a longer life expectancy, a change in the roles of women and men, an awareness of microtrends, and increasing divorce and remarriage rates. Fourth, the conception of history as an "objective" ordering of the "facts" of the past has changed. Family development is now seen as an interactive process in which the historian influences which stories of development are told and emphasized. All of these changes have required a critical rethinking of our assumptions about "normality" and the idea of "family" development. The relationship between demographic changes and alterations in the prevalence, timing, and sequencing of some key family transitions must also be noted.

In our clinical work with families presenting in various forms and at all stages of development, we have found it useful to emphasize culture and gender relativity rather than universality, transitions rather than stages, dimensions and processes rather than markers, and a resource rather than a deficit orientation. We believe that a systems approach to family development calls for a dialectical integration of two tendencies: stability and change. The emphasis is therefore on both tendencies rather than on one or the other. Change and stability must be addressed simultaneously. We do not find it clinically useful to think of families as "stuck" and unable to bring about change. Rather, we find it clinically useful to look for patterns of continuity, identity, and stability that can be maintained while new behavioral patterns are changing.

We believe that there is much evidence to support the position that nurses will find heuristic value in the family development category of CFAM. However, they should be aware of some of the problems in its indiscriminate adoption and application. We find it indefensible for some nurses to make sweeping generalizations such as, "The family life cycle is genetically determined," or "The family life cycle is culturally universal." We urge nurses to carefully consider the implication of a family's ethnicity, race, and social class in applying the family development category.

We also caution nurses against *indiscriminately* applying the family development category and overemphasizing *smooth progression.* Contradictions and difficulties inherent in progressing through the life cycle are normal. Families are complex systems that need to deal with many different progressions at once—that is, there are biological, psychological, sociological, and cultural progressions (Nichols, et al, 2000). Tensions and continuing change brought about by contradiction between these progressions are normal. Family life is seldom smooth or bland; rather, it is zestful and active. Therefore, when nurses use the family development category, we encourage them to have families discuss their joys and satisfactions as well as their tensions and stresses.

In addition to delineating stages and tasks implicit in the family life cycle, we have found it useful to notice the attachments between family members. *Attachment* refers to a relatively enduring, unique emotional tie between two specific persons. Each person has the need for emotional connection while also remaining secure in his or her own individuality. There is the need to balance two life forces: (1) togetherness and the capacity for intense intimacy in relationships and individuality, and (2) the capacity for independent thinking and goal-oriented action. Bowlby (1977) notes:

> Affectional bonds and subjective states of a strong emotion tend to go together … Thus many of the most intensive of all emotions arise during the formation, the maintenance, the disruption and renewal of affectional bonds which for that reason are sometimes called emotional

bonds. In terms of subjective experience the formation of a bond is described as falling in love, maintaining a bond as loving someone, and losing a partner as grieving over someone. Similarly the threat of loss arouses anxiety and actual loss causes sorrow, while both situations are likely to arouse anger. Finally the unchallenged maintenance of a bond is experienced as a source of security and renewal of a bond as a source of joy (p. 203).

Although the terms *bonding* and *attachment* are sometimes used to describe different relationships, we have chosen in this book and in our clinical work to make no distinction between these terms. We recognize the complexity of relationships that arise from international connections between family members, the relationship stresses and the hard choices economic and social immigrants face with separations and reunions of parents, young children, and elderly family members. We believe that difficult gender and generational transformations need to be considered when discussing attachments. When working with a family, we tend to pay the most attention to the reciprocal nature of an attachment and the quality of the affectional tie. We illustrate these bonds between family members by drawing attachment diagrams. The symbols used in these diagrams (Fig. 3–11) are similar to those used in the structural assessment diagrams. Again, it is important for us to emphasize that there is no one right level of attachment or best attachment configuration.

We are partial to the idea of the network paradigm as a useful base to integrate attachment and family systems theories. Such a paradigm integrates dyadic and family systems as simultaneously distinct and yet interconnected. The clinician holds multiple perspectives in mind, considers each system level as both a part and a whole, and shifts the focus between levels as required.

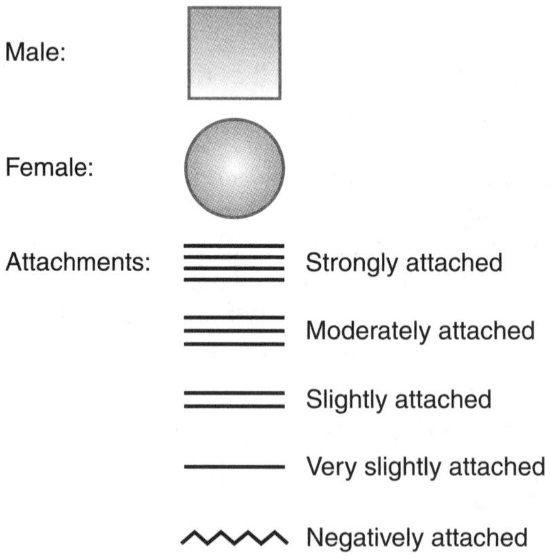

Male:

Female:

Attachments: Strongly attached

Moderately attached

Slightly attached

Very slightly attached

Negatively attached

FIGURE 3-11: Symbols used in attachment diagrams.

We like this concept because it expands attachment to include multiple system levels and networks, which is especially important as the baby boomers increase in age. Attachment theory is relevant to more than just parent-infant bonding; it is important for all ages. We believe that the key elements of attachment processes (i.e., affect regulation, interpersonal understanding, information processing, and the provision of comfort within intimate relationships) are as applicable to family systems as they are to individual development.

In the CFAM developmental category, we discuss family life cycle stages, the emotional process of transition (namely, key principles), and second-order changes—the issues dealt with and tasks often accomplished during each stage. In an effort to emphasize the variability of family development, we discuss six sample types of family life cycles:

1. Middle-class North American

2. Divorce and post-divorce

3. Remarried

4. Professional and low-income

5. Adoptive

6. Lesbian, gay, bisexual, queer, intersexed, transgendered, and twin-spirited

Middle-Class North American Family Life Cycle

We are grateful to Carter and McGoldrick (1988, 1999b) and McGoldrick, Carter, and Garcia-Preto (2011b) for delineating six stages in the North American middle-class family life cycle (Box 3–3). We highlight the expansion, contraction, and realignment of relationships as entries, exits, and development of family members occur. Although the relationship patterns and family themes may sound familiar, we wish to emphasize that the structure and form of the North American family is changing radically. We believe that it is important for nurses to have a positive conceptual framework for what *is*: dual-career families, permanent single-parent households, unmarried couples, homosexual couples, remarried couples, long-distance married couples (commuter marriages), and sole-parent adoptions to list a few.

Transitional crises should not be thought of as permanent traumas. We believe it is imperative that the use of language that links us to stereotypes be dropped. For example, we try to eliminate such phrases as *children of divorce, working mother, out-of-wedlock child, fatherless home,* and so forth, from the language we use about families. Also, we urge nurses to critically reflect on how culture, ethnicity, gender, race, and sexual orientation influence a family's developmental stages and tasks as well as attachments.

Stage One: The Launching of the Single Young Adult

In outlining the stages of the middle-class North American family life cycle, we start with the stage of young adults. The primary task of young adults is to come to terms with their family of origin by remaining connected and yet

Box 3-3 The Stages of the Family Life Cycle		
Family Life Cycle Stage	Emotional Process of Transition: Key Principles	Second-Order Changes in Family Status Required to Proceed Developmentally
Leaving home: emerging young adults	Accepting emotional and financial responsibility for self	a. Differentiation of self in relation to family of origin b. Development of intimate peer relationships c. Establishment of self in respect to work and financial independence d. Establishment of self in community and larger society e. Spirituality
Joining of families through marriage/ union	Commitment to new system	a. Formation of partner systems b. Realignment of relationships with extended family, friends, and larger community and social system to include new partners
Families with young children	Accepting new members into the system	a. Adjustment of couple system to make space for children b. Collaboration in child-rearing, financial, and housekeeping tasks c. Realignment of relationships with extended family to include parenting and grandparenting roles d. Realignment of relationships with community and larger social system to include new family structure and relationships
Families with adolescents	Increasing flexibility of family boundaries to permit children's independence and grandparents' frailties	a. Shift of parent-child relationships to permit adolescent to move into and out of system b. Refocus on midlife couple and career issues c. Begin shift toward caring for older generation d. Realignment with community and larger social system to include shifting family of emerging adolescent and parents in new formation pattern of relating
Launching children and moving on at midlife	Accepting a multitude of exits from and entries into the system	a. Renegotiation of couple system as a dyad b. Development of adult-to-adult relationships between parents and grown children

Box 3-3	The Stages of the Family Life Cycle—cont'd	

Family Life Cycle Stage	Emotional Process of Transition: Key Principles	Second-Order Changes in Family Status Required to Proceed Developmentally
		c. Realignment of relationships to include in-laws and grandchildren
		d. Realignment of relationships with community and larger social system to include new structure and constellation of family relationships
		e. Exploration of new interests/career given the freedom from childcare responsibilities
		f. Dealing with care needs, disabilities, and death of parents (grandparents)
Families in late middle age	Accepting the shifting generational roles	a. Maintenance of own and/or couple functioning and interests in face of psychological decline: exploration of new familial and social role options
		b. Supporting more central role of middle generations
		c. Realignment of the system in relation to community and larger social system to acknowledge changed pattern of family relationships of this stage
		d. Making room in the system for the wisdom and experience of the elders
		e. Supporting older generation without overfunctioning them
Families nearing the end of life	Accepting the realities of limitations and death and the completion of one cycle of life	a. Dealing with loss of spouse, siblings, and other peers
		b. Making preparations for death and legacy
		c. Managing reversed roles in caretaking between middle and older generations
		d. Realignment of relationships with larger community and social system to acknowledge changing life cycle relationships

McGoldrick, Monica; Carter, Betty; Garcia-Preto, Nydia. (Eds.). (2011). Overview: The Life Cycle in Its Changing Context. *The Expanded Family Life Cycle: Individual, Family and Social Perspectives*, 4th edition, copyright 2011, pp16-17. Reprinted by permission of Pearson Education, Inc.. Upper Saddle River, NJ.

separate, without cutting off or fleeing reactively to a substitute emotional source. The family of origin has a profound influence on who, when, how, and whether the young adult will marry.

A 2010 Pew Research found that millennials (today's 18- to 29-year-olds) value parenthood far more than marriage. Of the millennials, 52% stated being a good parent was one of the most important things in life while only 30% said this about having a successful marriage (Wang & Taylor, 2011).

This stage may last for several years in a family's development. It is an opportunity for young adults to sort out emotionally what values and beliefs they will hold onto from the family of origin, what they will leave behind, and what they will establish for themselves as they progress through succeeding stages of the family life cycle. For both men and women, this is a particularly critical phase. During this stage, men sometimes have difficulty committing themselves to relationships and form a pseudoindependent identity centered around work. Women may choose to define themselves in relation to a male and postpone or forgo establishing an independent identity. Young men choosing to cohabit often do not think of the young woman as the desired marital partner, whereas young woman who cohabit believe their partner is their future marital partner.

In our clinical work, we try to understand the client's views and legacies regarding marital status and the flexibility of the young person's expectations about pathways to adulthood. With approximately one in four single Americans looking for a romantic partner using the 1,000 or more dating Web sites, the previous venues for social networking are being replaced by the Internet and chat rooms. Internet marriage is becoming increasingly common, and this will likely lead to more diverse pairings across race, ethnicity, and nationality.

Tasks

1. **Differentiation of self in relation to family of origin.** The young adult's shift toward adult status involves the development of a mutually respectful form of relating with his or her parents, where the parents can be appreciated for who they are. The young adult adjusts the view of the parents by neither making them into what they are not nor blaming them for what they could not be. The complexity of this task is not to be underestimated. Each ethnic and racial group has norms and expectations regarding acceptable ways to be attached and connected to family and about issues of dependence versus independence.

2. **Development of intimate peer relationships.** The emphasis is on the young adult's passing from an individual orientation to an interdependent orientation of self. There is no single model of social experience for young adults to follow as they develop intimate relationships. During this task, young adults strive to bridge the gap between autonomy and attachment as they share themselves with others rather than using others as the source of self. With the increased use of Internet dating sites,

Facebook, Twitter, Pinterest, and chat rooms, the young adult will be exposed to a wide variety of personal styles and personalities.

3. **Establishment of self in relation to work and financial independence.** In a young adult's 20s and 30s, the "trying on" of various identities to test or refine career skills and interests is typical. Young adults who are committed to a career path or occupational choice by their late 20s or early 30s are less vulnerable to self-doubt or decreased self-esteem than young adults who lack direction. Young adults and their family of origin must sort through issues of competitiveness, expectations, and differences regarding work and financial goals.

Attachments

There are no right or wrong attachments for young adults in stage one. Rather, it is important for the nurse to draw forth from family members their beliefs about attachment to one another and how they regard these attachments. These beliefs are influenced by culture, gender, race, sexual orientation, and social class as well as by whether the young adult lives at home. Some sample attachments for stage one are given in Figure 3–12. The first diagram illustrates a young adult who is bonded equally with her father and mother. The second diagram illustrates a young adult who is more closely attached to each parent than the parents are to each other; the parents are negatively bonded. Of significance in the second diagram is that there was a death during the young adult's childhood. It could be hypothesized that his difficulties in establishing his own identity are related to the family's hesitancy to come to grips with his deceased sister and the parents' living alone without children.

Questions to Ask the Family. Which of your parents is most accepting of your career plans? How does he or she show this? What does your sister, Manal, think of your parents' reaction to your career plans? If your father were more accepting of your desire to move into an independent living situation with people not of the Muslim faith, how do you think your mother would react? If you continue to wear hijab because it is integral to your religious beliefs, would this reassure your parents?

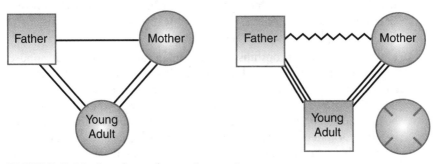

FIGURE 3-12: Sample attachments in stage 1.

Stage Two: Marriage: The Joining of Families

Many couples believe that when they marry, it is just two individuals who are joining together. However, both spouses have grown up in families that have now become interconnected through marriage. Both spouses, although in some ways differentiated from their families of origin in an emotional, financial, and functional way, carry their whole family into the relationship. This is particularly relevant if the marriage is an arranged one. Marriage is a two-generational relationship with a minimum of three families coming together: his family of origin, her family of origin, and the new couple. Given the current prevalence of stepfamilies, the likelihood of several families coming together is increased exponentially. Also, the certainty that the couple will be heterosexual is not evident because, in both the United States and Canada, gay marriages and civil unions have increasingly been formally recognized. In the United States in 2009, the overall national rates of marital events for men were 19.1 marriages, 9.2 divorces, and 3.5 instances of widowhood per 1,000 men. For women there were 17.6 marriages, 9.7 divorces, and 3.5 instances of widowhood per 1,000 women (Elliott & Simmons, 2011).

Tasks

1. **Establishment of couple identity.** The new couple must establish itself as an identifiable unit. This requires negotiation of many issues that were previously defined on an individual level. These issues include routine matters such as eating and sleeping patterns, sexual contact, and use of space and time. The couple must decide about which traditions and rules to retain from each family and which ones they will develop for themselves. They must develop acceptable closeness-distance styles and recognize individual differences in adult attachment styles. Although the majority of studies on the quality and stability of marriage focuses on couple communication, we believe that love is the decisive factor for quality and stability. For some cultures, however, the concept of a "love marriage" as compared with an arranged marriage is quite different.

   The health benefits of a good marriage have been touted and researched over many years, but more nuanced views of the so-called marriage advantage are coming to light (Parker-Pope, 2010). Those individuals in troubled relationships appear far less healthy than if they had never married. Nurses have wonderful opportunities to foster healthy couple identity and relationships.

2. **Realignment of relationships with extended families to include spouse.** A renegotiation of relationships with each spouse's family of origin has to occur to accommodate the new spouse. This places no small stress on both the couple and each family of origin to open itself to new ways of being. Some couples deal with their parents by cutting off the relationship in a bid for independence. Other couples handle this task of realignment by absorbing the new spouse into the family of origin. The third common pattern involves a balance between some contact and some distance.

3. **Decisions about parenthood.** For most couples, happiness is highest at the beginning of the life cycle stage of marriage. Although a small but increasing number of married couples are deciding to be childfree by choice, most still plan on becoming parents. The question of *when* to conceive is becoming increasingly complex, especially with the changed role of women, the widespread use of contraceptives, the availability of a wide range of fertilization strategies, and the trend toward later marriages. Since 2008, there has been a sharp decline in the fertility rate in the United States, and it is linked to the slumping economy (Pew Research Center, 2011). It is interesting for clinicians to note that in the United States, more than a quarter of the unmarried women who gave birth in 2009 were living with a partner (Lewin, 2010). Couples who have evolved more competent marital structures prenatally are more likely to successfully incorporate a child into the family.

Attachments

Figure 3–13 illustrates a sample attachment for a couple in stage two: the development of close emotional ties between the spouses. The first diagram illustrates how they do not have to break ties with their families of origin, but rather maintain and adjust ties with them. A different type of attachment (illustrated in the second diagram) can occur if both members of a couple do not align themselves together. The wife is more heavily bonded to her family of origin than she is to her husband. The husband is more tied to outside interests (such as work and friends) than to his wife. We have found that negative attachment–related events occurring early in the marriage are especially distressing for the couple. These and other attachment injuries can be characterized by a betrayal of trust during a critical moment of need.

Questions to Ask the Family. Which family, Sabeen, was most in favor of your marriage to Hashim? How did you incorporate Pakistani and American traditions in your marriage? How did your siblings show that they supported your marriage? What does your spouse think of your parents' marital relationship? If you two, as a couple, were to use your parents' marriage as

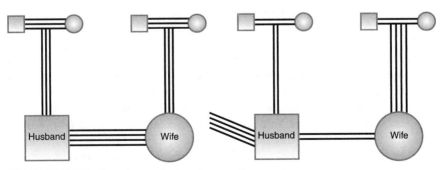

FIGURE 3-13: Sample attachments in stage 2.

a model for your own marriage, what would you incorporate into your marriage? How did the diagnosis of multiple sclerosis influence your bonding as a couple?

Stage Three: Families With Young Children

During this stage, the adults now become caregivers to a younger generation. Family-of-origin experiences can influence the forming of a new family. We have found in our clinical work that individuals who recollect negative qualities in their parents' relationship often report more negative changes in the quality of their own marriages during their first year of transition to parenthood.

The birth and rearing of a baby present varying challenges. Moreover, taking responsibility and dealing with the demands of dependent children are challenging for most families when financial resources are stretched and the parents are heavily involved in career development. Sleep disruption and loss contribute to a decline in marital satisfaction across the transition to parenthood (Medina, Lederhos, & Lillis, 2009). Excessive and inconsolable neonatal crying is one of the most challenging tasks for parents to manage (Patrick, Garcia, & Griffin, 2010). The disposition of childcare responsibilities and household chores in dual-career households is a particular struggle. We have found that men and women often differ in the coping strategies they use to deal with this issue. Women with young children tend to use cognitive restructuring, delegating, limiting avocational activities, and using social support significantly more often than do men.

We believe the work-family issue of juggling childcare and other household accountabilities is a social problem to be dealt with by the couple, not a "woman's problem" for her to struggle with alone. How the increase in "old new dads" in the United States will impact this struggle is unknown. What is evident is that the birth rate between 1980 and 2002 increased 32% among fathers in the United States aged 40 to 44 and increased 21% among fathers aged 45 to 49 (Penn, 2007). It went up almost 10% for dads aged 50 to 54. This trend means that the joys of family life go on well into many dads' 60s. Generational boundaries quickly become blurred with "old new dads" being concerned simultaneously about children's schools and sports and their own retirement finances.

Tasks

1. **Adjusting marital system to make space for a child.** The couple must continue to meet each other's personal needs as well as their parental responsibilities. With the introduction of the first child, challenges for personal space, sexual and emotional intimacy, and socializing exist. Both mothers and fathers are increasingly aware of the need for emotional integration of the child into the family. Children can be brought into three types of environments: (1) there is no space for them, (2) there is space for them, or (3) there is a vacuum that they

are expected to fill. If the child has a handicap, the couple faces more stress as they adjust their expectations and deal with their emotional reactions. We have found that normal family processes in couples becoming parents include shifts in the sense of self, shifts in relationships with families of origin, shifts in relation to the child, changes in stress and social support, and changes in the couple.

2. **Joining in childbearing, financial, and household tasks.** The couple must find a mutually satisfying way to deal with childcare responsibility and household chores that does not overburden one partner. Dealing with finances and juggling family and other responsibilities is a major task. The emotional and financial cost of solutions to deal with childcare responsibilities must be addressed. The influence of illness, such as autoimmune disease, on maternal fatigue and its impact on the caregiving environment, parental discipline style, and daily childrearing practices needs to be considered (White, White, & Fox, 2009).

   Both mothers and fathers contribute to the child's development and can do so in different or similar ways. Physical and playful stimulation of the child complements verbal interaction. Parents can either support or hinder their children's success in developing peer relationships and achieving at school. Some middle-class families, responding to intense pressure from the school system, tend to stress the values of achievement and productivity, whereas some working-class families may respond to this pressure by feelings of alienation. Recent immigration experiences and whether the children are documented or undocumented can also influence peer and school interaction.

3. **Realignment of relationships with extended family to include parenting and grandparenting roles.** The couple must design and develop the new roles of father and mother in addition to the marital role rather than replacing it. Members of each family of origin also take on new roles—for example, grandfather or aunt. In some cases, grandparents who perhaps were opposed to the marriage in the beginning become very interested in the young children. For many older adults, this is an especially gratifying time because it allows them to have intimacy with their grandchildren without the responsibilities of parenting. It also permits them to develop a new type of adult–adult relationship with their children. Opportunities for intergenerational support or conflict abound as expectations about child-rearing and health-care practices are expressed.

Attachments

Parents need to maintain a marital bond and continue personal, adult-centered conversations in addition to child-centered conversations. Space for privacy and time spent together are important needs. Gottman and Notarius (2002) report that for 40% to 70% of couples, marital quality drops following the transition to parenthood, with people commonly reverting to stereotypic gender roles as they become overwhelmed by the complexity of housework, childcare, and work. Marital conversation and sex sharply decrease. However, joy and pleasure with the baby increase.

Children require security and warm attachments to adults, as well as opportunities to develop positive sibling relationships. We believe teaching interdependence is a central goal of parenting, helping children see themselves as part of a community and living cooperatively with others.

Figure 3–14 provides sample attachment diagrams for this stage. A competitive, negative relationship (illustrated by the wavy line) exists between the children and spouses in the second diagram. The mother is overbonded to the daughter, and the father is underinvolved with the daughter. The father is overattached to the son, and the mother is underinvolved with the son. This is an example of same-sex coalitions existing cross-generationally.

Questions to Ask the Family. What percentage of your time do you spend taking care of your children? What percentage do you spend taking care of your marriage? Is this a comfortable balance for the two of you? What effect does this pattern have on your children? If your children thought that you should be closer, how might they tell you this? What impact did the miscarriages have on your marriage?

Stage Four: Families With Adolescents

This period has often been characterized as one of intense upheaval and transition, in which biological, emotional, and sociocultural changes occur with great and ever-increasing rapidity. Peers, texting, social networks such as Twitter and Facebook, pornography, sports, and other activities all compete for the adolescent's attention. This stage is highly influenced by class. Adolescence can begin early within poor, inner-city communities when, at a very young age, children are often faced with pressures related to sexuality, household responsibility, drugs, and alcohol use. In many middle-class families, adolescence can last well into the young adult's 20s and 30s, with the young person being financially dependent on the parents and continuing to live in the family home.

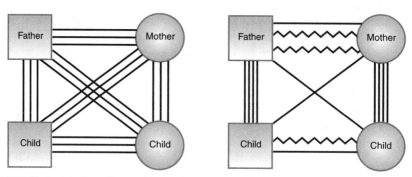

FIGURE 3-14: Sample attachments in stage 3.

Tasks

1. **Shift in parent–child relationships to permit adolescents to move in or out of the system.** The family must move from the dependency relationship previously established with a young child to an increasingly independent relationship with the adolescent. Growing psychological independence is frequently not recognized because of continuing physical dependence. Conflict often surfaces when a teenager's independence threatens the family. For example, teenagers may precipitate marital conflict when they question who makes the family rules about the car: Mom or Dad? Families frequently respond to an adolescent's request for increasing autonomy in two ways: (1) they abruptly define rigid rules and re-create an earlier stage of dependency, or (2) they establish premature independence. In the second scenario, the family supports only independence and ignores dependent needs. This may result in premature separation when the teenager is not really ready to be fully autonomous. The teenager may thus return home defeated. Parents need to shift from the parental role of "protector" to that of "preparer" for the challenges of adulthood.

   The challenge for parents to shift responsibility in a balanced way to their teens is often complicated if there are health problems. For example, Fulkerson and colleagues (2007) found that general family connectedness, priority of family meals, and positive mealtime environment were significantly positively associated with psychosocial well-being in overweight adolescents. These authors also noted that weight-based teasing and parental encouragement to diet were associated with poor psychological health in the 7th to 12th graders they studied. For parents to find a balance between encouraging healthy eating and avoiding encouraging dieting with at-risk-for-overweight or overweight teens is a challenge. Rosenberg and Shields (2009) found intriguing results from their study of parent-adolescent attachment in the glycemic control of adolescents with type 1 diabetes. Mothers' perception of more secure adolescent attachment was associated with better glycemic control. Neither fathers' nor adolescents' reports of attachment were significantly correlated with glycemic control.

2. **Refocus on midlife marital and career issues.** During this stage, parents are often struggling with what Erickson (1963) calls *generativity,* the need to be useful as a human being, partner, and mentor to another generation. The socially and sexually maturing teenager's frequent questioning and conflict about values, lifestyles, career plans, and so forth, can thrust the parents into an examination of their own marital and career issues. Depending on many factors, including cultural and gender expectations, this may be a period of positive growth or painful struggle for men and women.

3. **Beginning shift toward joint caring for older generation.** As parents are aging, so, too, are the grandparents. Parents (especially women)

sometimes feel that they are besieged on both sides: teenagers are asking for more freedom, and grandparents are asking for more support. With the trend of women having children later in life and seniors living longer, this double demand for attention and resources most likely will intensify. Celebrating the wisdom of seniors and intergenerational reciprocity are key tasks.

Attachments

All family members continue to have their relationships within the family, while teenagers become increasingly more involved with their friends than with family members. These transitions through the family life cycle can be stressful because they challenge attachment bonds among family members. We advocate open communication and the addressing of primary emotions. A decrease in parental attachment is normative and developmentally appropriate for adolescents. The young person's widening social network, however, does not preclude strong family relationships, although family relationships are altered. The husband and wife need to reinvest in the marital relationship while this is taking place.

An example of an attachment pattern is illustrated in Figure 3–15. In the second diagram, the mother is overinvolved with the eldest son and has a negative relationship with the husband. The father tends to be minimally involved with all family members. There is conflict between the two sons.

Questions to Ask the Family. What privileges do your teenagers have now that they did not have when they were younger? Ask the adolescents: How do you think your parents will handle it when your younger sister, Nenita, wants to date? Will it be different from when you wanted to date? On a scale of 1 to 10, with 10 being the highest, how much confidence do your parents have in your ability to say no to crystal meth?

Stage Five: Launching Children and Moving On

Many middle-class North Americans whose children are grown up used to assume they would have an empty nest. However, this expectation is in the

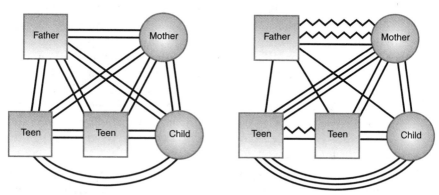

FIGURE 3-15: Sample attachments in stage 4.

process of change. Rising housing costs and beginning pay rates that have not risen as fast as those of more experienced workers have been singled out as some of the causes of this trend. A different explanation is that young North Americans are having difficulty growing up and are unwilling to go out on their own and settle for less affluence than their parents afford them.

Tasks

1. **Renegotiation of marital system as a dyad.** In many cases, a thrust to alter some of the basic tenets of the marital relationship occurs. This is especially true if both partners are working and the children have left home. The couple bond can take on a more prominent position. The balance between dependency, independency, and interdependency must be reexamined.

2. **Development of adult-adult relationships between grown children and their parents.** The family of origin must relinquish the primary roles of parent and child. They must adapt to the new roles of parent and adult child. This involves renegotiation of emotional and financial commitments. The key emotional process during this stage is for family members to deal with a multitude of exits from and entries into the family system.

3. **Realignment of relationships to include in-laws and grown children.** The parents adjust family ties and expectations to include their child's spouse or partner. This can sometimes be particularly challenging if the parents' expectation is for a heterosexual son-in-law or daughter-in-law of the family's race, religion, and ethnicity and the child chooses someone different. The once-prevalent idea that the time after a grown child marries is a lonely, sad time, especially for women, has been replaced. Increases in marital satisfaction have frequently been noted.

4. **Dealing with disabilities and death of grandparents.** Many families regard the disability or death of an elderly parent as a natural occurrence. It can be a time of relishing and finding comfort in the happy memories, wisdom, and contributions of the elder. If, however, the couple and the elderly parents have unfinished business between them, there may be serious repercussions, not only for the children but also for the third generation. The type of disability afflicting the seniors determines the effects on the immediate family. For example, caregivers who do not understand Alzheimer's dementia and its effects on cognitive function and behavior often attempt to deal with inappropriate or disruptive behavior in ineffective and counterproductive ways. Thus, they inadvertently intensify their own stress. We have found that many times female caregivers seek support for depression that often stems from the multiple roles, losses, and guilt they are experiencing.

We recommend that health professionals, in addition to attending to the family's multigenerational legacies of illness, loss, and crisis, also note intergenerational strengths and wisdom. Tracking key events, transitions, and coping strategies helps elicit resiliencies.

Attachments

Each family member continues to have outside interests and establish new roles appropriate to this stage. Sample attachment patterns are illustrated in Figure 3–16. A problem may arise when both husband and wife hold on to their last child. They may avoid conflict by allowing the eldest child to leave home and then focusing on the next child.

Questions to Ask the Family. How did your parents help you to leave home? What is the difference between how you left home and how your son, Zubin, is leaving home? Will your parents get along better, worse, or the same with each other once you leave home? Who, between Mom and Dad, will miss the children the most? As you see your child moving on with a new relationship, what would you like your child to do differently than you did? If your parents are still alive, are there any issues you would like to discuss with them?

Stage Six: Families in Later Life

This stage can begin with retirement and last until the death of both spouses. However, it is hard to say when the stage actually begins for each family, considering that "today there are 5 million people 65 and older in the US labor force, almost twice what there were in the early 1980s and that number is about to explode" (Penn, 2007, p. 29). Potentially, this stage can last 20 to 30 years for many couples. Key emotional processes in this stage are to flexibly adjust to the shift of generational roles and to foster an appreciation of the wisdom of the elders. We agree with Walsh (2011) that as a society we have been gerontophobic, and a larger vision of later life is required to recognize the growth, change, and new learning that can occur at this stage. The idea of dividing up this life cycle stage into extended middle age (to age 75), older seniors (75–85), and old age (85 and older) can be a useful way of "doing hope" for seniors who hold a pessimistic, fearful view of aging.

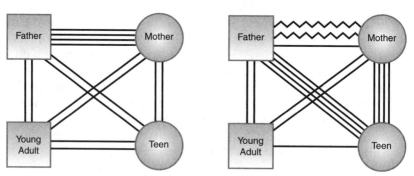

FIGURE 3-16: Sample attachments in stage 5.

Tasks

1. **Maintaining own or couple functioning and interest in the face of physiological decline: exploration of new familial and social role options.** Marital relationships continue to be important, and marital satisfaction contributes to both the morale and ongoing activity of both spouses. We have noted that the husband's morale is often strongly associated with health, socioeconomic status, income, and, to a lesser extent, family functioning. The wife's morale is most strongly associated with family functioning and, to a lesser extent, with health and socioeconomic status.

   As the couple in later life finds themselves in new roles as grandparents and mother-in-law and father-in-law, they must adjust to their children's spouses and open space for the new grandchildren. Difficulty in making the status changes required can be reflected in an older family member refusing to relinquish some of his or her power—for example, refusing to turn over a company or making plans for succession in a family business. The shift in status between the senior family members and the middle-aged family members is a reciprocal one. Difficulties and confusion may occur in several ways. Older adults may give up and become totally dependent on the next generation; the next generation may not accept the seniors' diminishing powers and may continue to treat them as totally competent, or the next generation may see only the seniors' frailties and may treat them as totally incompetent. Another adjustment might be if the older seniors start dating and/or marrying with the middle-aged family members feeling challenged or pressured to be supportive.

2. **Making room in the system for the wisdom and experience of the seniors.** The task of supporting the older generation without overfunctioning for them is particularly salient because, in general, people are living longer. It is not uncommon for a 90-year-old woman to be cared for by her 70-year-old daughter, with both of them living in close proximity to a 50-year-old son and grandson. The phenomena of "seniors caring for seniors" is another emerging area for healthcare providers to address.

   The parents of the baby boomers are the current generation of "young-old." They are highly motivated to participate in self-help groups and are interested in improving their quality of life through counseling, traditional and alternative health activities, and education. Many have found "new" family connections through the use of e-mail, Skype, and smartphones. They do not live by the aging myths of the past. Rather, as consumers, they expect and demand a good quality of life. Many grandparents continue to be involved in childrearing.

3. **Dealing with loss of spouse, siblings, and other peers and preparation for death.** This is a time for life review and taking care of unfinished

business with family as well as with business and social contacts. Many people find it helpful to discuss their life, review and reminisce, and enjoy the opportunity of passing this information along to succeeding generations. Often elders become useful and informative family historians by writing and/or recording their individual or family biographies and collecting and identifying family pictures.

Attachments

The couple reinvests and modifies the marital relationship based on the level of functioning of both partners. Between 1980 and 1990, 17% of those aged 65 and older in the United States lived in a multigenerational family household. Since then, this has increased to 20%. In 2008, a total of 6.6 million older adults lived in a household with one or more children, and in 42% of the situations the child was the head of household (Pew Social Trends Staff, 2010).

This stage is characterized by an appropriate interdependence with the next generation. The concept of interdependence is particularly important for nurses to understand in working with families with adult daughters and their parents. Middle-class older men and women seem equally likely to aid and support their children, especially daughters. Frequency of contact, however, tends to be higher with daughters and daughters-in-law than with sons. Thus, the possibility of strong intergenerational attachments between a daughter and her parents exists. In the attachment pattern illustrated in Figure 3–17, the couple projects their conflicts onto the extended family. This causes difficulty for the succeeding generations.

Questions to Ask the Family. When you look back over your life, what aspects have you enjoyed the most? What has given you the most happiness? About what aspects do you feel the most regret? What would you hope that your children would do differently than you did? Similarly to what you did? As your health is declining, what plans have you and your daughter, Aminah, made for her because of her schizophrenia?

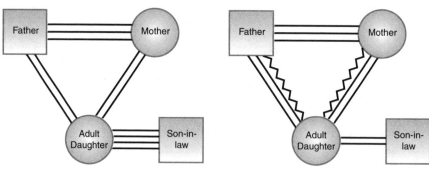

FIGURE 3-17: Sample attachments in stage 6.

Divorce and Post-Divorce Family Life Cycle

Many changes in marital status and living arrangements are prevalent in North America today. Noteworthy is the high level of divorce. In 2005, the divorce rate in the United States was 3.6 per 1,000 population, down from 4.2 in 2000 and 4.4 in 1995 (Daily Almanac, 2007). Whether the divorce rate will level off, climb, or decline is a matter of speculation that can be backed up by various theories. Unstable economic conditions, fear of terrorism, and increased faith-based initiatives may cause divorce rates to decline. Ahrons (2011) believes age is the strongest predictor of divorce, with couples under the age of 20 at the time of marriage having the highest likelihood of divorce. People with less income and less education tend to divorce more frequently with an exception: "well-educated women with 5 or more years of college with good incomes have higher divorce rates than do women who are poorer and less educated" (Ahrons, 2011, p. 293). Single-parent families are on the rise. The number of single-mother families increased from 3 million (12%) in 1970 to 10 million (26%) in 2000 in the United States. Similarly, single-father families grew from 393,000 (1%) to 2 million (5%) in 2000 (Fields & Casper, 2001).

Families experiencing divorce are often under enormous pressure. Single-parent families must accomplish most of the same developmental tasks as two-parent families, but without all the resources. This places extra burden on the remaining family members, who must compensate with increased effort to accomplish family tasks such as physical maintenance, social control, and tension management. However, we caution nurses not to assume that single-parent status alone will influence family functioning. We have found that family composition alone is too broad a variable to predict health outcomes, and we recommend a focus on more specific variables such as parental cooperation in parenting following divorce.

Single-parent households generally experience challenges in managing shortages of time, money, and energy. Some parents voice serious concerns about failure to meet perceived family and societal expectations for living "in a normal family" with two parents. Some women feel they must display behaviors that are contradictory to those they assume they should exhibit if they were to remarry. They perceive ongoing pressure from family, friends, and church to marry again to give their children a "normal" family. These women report being caught in a double bind, trying to demonstrate behaviors such as submissiveness that might attract a new husband while trying to use seemingly opposing behaviors such as assertiveness to successfully manage their lives. We encourage nurses working with single-parent families to explore the parent's feelings about opposing expectations. This is a way of helping these parents plan their responses to various paradoxical situations.

It is also important for nurses engaged in relational family nursing practice to focus on the positive changes experienced by many separated spouses. Separated women often use growth-oriented coping, such as becoming more autonomous and furthering their education, and they experience increased confidence and feelings of control in the post-separation phase.

Resilience in the post-divorce period is another focus for nurses. Resilience commonly depends on the ability of parents and children to build close, constructive, mutually supportive relationships that play a significant role in buffering families from the effects of related adversity. Factors that promote resiliency and positive adjustment to divorce include those associated with children's living arrangements. Kelly's review (2007) of the large empirical research findings indicates "children's contacts with their nonresident parent should not be based on every-other-weekend guidelines but should reflect the diversity of parental interest, capability, and the quality of the parent-child relationship" (p. 47). She recommends that children, depending on their age and developmental capacity, should have input into the living arrangements but not be asked to choose between parents.

It should be noted that approximately 75% of children involved in divorce are resilient and able to move on with their lives; only about 25% experience more lasting problems in adjustment (Greene, et al, 2003). Findings from Baum's (2003) study of former couples in Israel showed that the longer and more conflictual the legal proceedings, the worse the coparental relationship in the view of both parents. Interestingly, Baum also found that the more responsibility the father took for the divorce and the more he viewed himself as the initiator, the more he fulfilled his parental functions.

The findings from Ahrons's longitudinal study (2007) of children 20 years after their parents' divorce showed that children who reported their parents as being cooperative also reported better relationships with their parents, grandparents, stepparents, and siblings. Whether family relationships improve post divorce, remain stable, or get worse is dependent on a complex interweaving of many factors. Many of the problems previously attributed to "the divorce" are now seen to be located in the predivorce family situation; divorce is a long-term process that begins prior to separation and lasts long after the legal event of divorce (Ahrons, 2006, 2011).

In our clinical supervision with nurses, we encourage focusing on the siblings, a subsystem that generally remains undisrupted during the process of family reorganization. Siblings are often the unit of continuity. We also try to notice and support cooperative post-divorce parenting environments such as mutual parental support; teamwork; clear, flexible boundaries; high information exchange; constructive problem solving; and knowledgeable, experienced, involved, and authoritative parenting. Because many fathers are not used to taking care of their children without their wives orchestrating things, fathers often fade out of their children's lives. They want to avoid ex-wives and conflict and may feel uncomfortable if they have an unclear role of authority in their children's lives.

Ahrons found (2007) that when children's relationships with their fathers deteriorated after divorce, their relationships with their paternal grandparents, stepmothers, and stepsiblings were distant, negative, or nonexistent.

Nurses can be extremely helpful in intervening in these situations and fostering mutually agreeable post-divorce arrangements for the benefit of the children. Nurses can help fathers redefine their parental roles and identity in distinction from their spousal role and identity. For families locked in intractable disputes, we encourage them to develop a good-enough climate in which parents maintain distance from each other, thus minimizing conflict and triangulation.

Divorce may occur at any stage of the family life cycle and with any family, regardless of class or race. However, it has a different impact on family functioning depending on its timing and the diversity of individuals involved in the process. The marital breakdown may be sudden, or it may be long and drawn out. In either case, emotional work is required so that the family may deal with the shifts, gains, and losses in family membership.

Some sample phases involved in divorce and post-divorce are depicted in Box 3–4. McGoldrick and Carter (2011) found a clinical usefulness in the distinctions made between the four columns given in the table. Column 1 lists the phase. Column 2 gives the tasks, and Column 3 lists the prerequisite attitudes that will assist family members to make the transition and come

Box 3-4	Additional Stages of Family Life Cycle for Divorcing and Remarrying Families		
Phase	Task	Emotional Process of Transition: Prerequisite Attitude	Developmental Issues
Divorce	The decision to divorce	Acceptance of inability to resolve marital problems sufficiently to continue relationship	Acceptance of one's own part in the failure of the marriage
	Planning breakup of the system	Supporting viable arrangements for all parts of the system	a. Working cooperatively on problems of custody, visitation, and finances b. Dealing with extended family about the divorce
	Separation	a. Willingness to continue cooperative coparental relationship and joint financial support of children b. Working on resolution of attachment to spouse	a. Mourning loss of intact family b. Restructuring marital and parent-child relationships and finances; adaptation to living apart c. Realignment of relationships with extended family; staying connected with spouse's extended family

Continued

Box 3-4		Additional Stages of Family Life Cycle for Divorcing and Remarrying Families—cont'd	
Phase	**Task**	**Emotional Process of Transition: Prerequisite Attitude**	**Developmental Issues**
	The divorce	Working on emotional divorce: overcoming hurt, anger, guilt, etc.	a. Mourning loss of intact family; giving up fantasies of reunion b. Retrieving hopes, dreams, expectations from the marriage c. Staying connected with extended families
Post-divorce family	Single parent (custodial household or primary residence)	Willingness to maintain financial responsibilities, continue parental contact with ex-spouse and his or her family	a. Making flexible visitation arrangements with ex-spouse and family b. Rebuilding own financial resources c. Rebuilding own social network
	Single parent (non-custodial)	Willingness to maintain financial responsibilities and parental contact with ex-spouse and to support custodial parent's relationship with children	a. Finding ways to continue effective parenting b. Maintaining financial responsibilities to ex-spouse and children c. Rebuilding own social network
Remarriage	Entering new relationship	Recovery from loss of 1st marriage (adequate emotional divorce)	Recommitment to marriage and to forming a family with readiness to deal with the complexity and ambiguity
	Conceptualizing and planning new marriage and family	Accepting one's own fears and those of new spouse and children about forming new family Accepting need for time and patience for adjustment to complexity and ambiguity of 1. Multiple new roles 2. Boundaries: space, time, membership, and authority 3. Affective issues: guilt, loyalty conflicts, desire	a. Working on openness in the new relationships to avoid pseudomutuality b. Planning for maintenance of cooperative financial and coparental relationships with ex-spouses c. Planning to help children deal with fears, loyalty conflicts, and membership in two systems d. Realignment of relationships with extended family to include new spouse and children

Box 3-4	Additional Stages of Family Life Cycle for Divorcing and Remarrying Families—cont'd		
Phase	Task	Emotional Process of Transition: Prerequisite Attitude	Developmental Issues
		for mutuality, unresolvable past hurts	e. Planning maintenance of connections for children with extended family of ex-spouses
	Remarriage and reconstruction of family	Resolution of attachment to previous spouse and ideal of "intact" family Acceptance of different model of family with permeable boundaries	a. Restructuring family boundaries to allow for inclusion of new spouse-stepparent b. Realignment of relationships and financial arrangements to permit interweaving of several systems c. Making room for relationships of all children with all parents, grandparents, and other extended family d. Sharing memories and histories to enhance stepfamily integration
	Renegotiation of remarried family at all future life cycle transitions	Accepting evolving relationships of transformed remarried family	a. Changes as each child graduates, marries, dies, or becomes ill b. Changes as each spouse forms new couple relationship, remarries, moves, becomes ill, or dies

through the developmental issues listed in Column 4 en route to the next phase. We believe that clinical work directed at Column 4 will not succeed if the family is having difficulty dealing with the issues in Column 3.

Questions to Ask the Family. How do you explain to yourself the reasons for your divorce? Who initiated the idea of divorce? Who left who? Who was most supportive of developing viable arrangements for *everyone* in the family? How did your ex-husband, Luis, show his willingness to continue a cooperative coparental relationship with you? How did you respond to this? What methods have you found most successful in resolving conflicting issues with Luis? What advice would you give to other divorced parents on how to resolve conflictual issues with their ex-partners? How have your children helped you and your ex-spouse to maintain a supportive environment for them?

Remarried Family Life Cycle

"Stepfamilies are families emerging out of hope" (Visher, Visher, & Pasley, 2003, p. 171). The rise of remarriage and the stepfamily in North America in recent decades has been striking. More than 4 in 10 Americans have at least one steprelative in their families, according to a 2010 Pew Research survey (Parker, 2011). While stepfamilies can be found among all races and socioeconomic and age groups, there are demographic trends. Young people under 30, blacks, and those without a college degree are significantly more likely to report having a steprelative (Parker, 2011).

Although we sometimes use the term *recoupled families* to indicate the centrality of the couple bond and the fact that many couples are not getting married, we have chosen in this edition of our text to continue using the term *remarried families*, as it is more familiar to most people. McGoldrick and Carter (2011) have started using the term *multinuclear families* to depict the fluid boundaries and multiple ties that these families have. It is a term we find appealing because in recoupling there may be three, four, or more households at any one time.

Ahrons's longitudinal study (2007) of children 20 years after parental divorce found that most of the children experienced the remarriage of one or both parents, and one third of her sample remembered the remarriage as being more stressful than the divorce. Two thirds reported their father's remarriage as more stressful than their mother's.

The family emotional process at the transition to remarriage consists of struggling with fears about investment in new relationships: one's own fears, the new spouse's fears, and the fears of the children (of either or both spouses). It also consists of dealing with hostile or upset reactions of the children, extended families, and ex-spouse. Unlike biological families, in which family membership is defined by bloodlines, legal contracts, and spatial arrangements and is characterized by explicit boundaries, the structure of a stepfamily is less clear. Nurses must address the ambiguity of the new family organization, including roles and relationships. Some major issues include dealing with feelings of being outsiders versus insiders, addressing boundary disputes and power issues, handling conflicting loyalties, reducing rigid unproductive triangles, and unifying the couple relationship.

We have found the tips offered by Visher and Visher (stepparents themselves) particularly helpful in our work with stepfamilies (www.smartmarriages.com/stepfamily.tips.html). If a child is diagnosed with a potentially life-shortening disease, such as cancer, then the shifting family boundaries after the diagnosis require particular attention in stepfamilies. The work of Kelly and Ganong (2011) points to the reinforcing that takes place in the biological family boundary and the stress in the stepfamily boundaries as one area for health-care attention and possible intervention.

Attachment theory is a useful framework for conceptualizing the impact of structural change and loss on stepfamily adjustment. We think of the stepfamily as an emerging family system; problem patterns are understood in this context where bids for connection may be missed or misinterpreted. We believe nurses can assist stepfamilies in increasing emotional connectivity and stability. If stepcouples have irresolvable problems, use extreme language, and persist with pervasive chronic problems, then we encourage nurses to consider whether attachment injuries are present and need intervention (Sayre, McCollum, & Spring, 2010). In many cases, parental guilt and concerns about the children are increased, and a positive or negative rearousal of the old attachment to the ex-spouse may occur (McGoldrick & Carter, 2011). Box 3–4 summarizes McGoldrick and Carter's (2011) developmental outline for stepfamily formation.

Having been angered by a predominant emphasis on pathology in the divorce literature, Ahrons (2001) conducted a study over 21 years of what she calls "binuclear families." This term refers to joint-custody families or to families in which the relationship between ex-spouses is friendly, and it also indicates a different familial structure, without inferring anything about the nature or quality of the ex-spouses' relationship. Ahrons and Rodgers (1987), who worked with 98 divorced couples over a 5-year period, produced some interesting relationship types, including "perfect pals," a small group of divorced spouses whose previous marriage had not overshadowed their long-standing friendship. The second group, "cooperative colleagues," was a considerably larger and more typical group found by Ahrons and Rodgers. Although not good friends, they worked well together on issues concerning their children. The third group was the "angry associates," and the fourth group was "fiery foes," who felt nothing but fury for their ex-spouses. Ahrons and Rodgers termed the fifth group "dissolved duos," who after the separation or divorce discontinued any contact with each other. Ahrons (2001) advocates for a normative process model of divorce rather than focusing on evidence of pathology or dysfunction. We agree with this stance, being mindful that approximately 25% of children involved in divorce do seem to have longer-lasting adjustment difficulties (Greene, et al, 2003).

We encourage nurses working with divorced and remarried families to bring to their patients research and clinical knowledge of what works and does not work to foster continuing family relationships. However, nurses should be cautious, because complex problems seldom have simple answers. For example, predictors such as a child's age and gender, the frequency and regularity of father/mother–child visitation, father/mother–child closeness, and the effect of parental legal conflict on the child's self-esteem have different implications for different groups of 6- to 12-year-old children and for children in different situations.

We also encourage nurses working with stepfamilies to increase their knowledge about stepfamily issues and respect the uniqueness of complex stepfamily life. Ganong (2011), for example, has conducted almost 20 studies looking at how marital transitions affect family caregiving responsibilities and whether beliefs about obligation to relatives are based on family structure, family membership, or other contextual factors. He found that adult stepchildren and stepparents agreed that stepchildren have few obligations to assist stepparents. However, the key in deciding whether there was a responsibility to assist was how the relationship was defined. Nurses could assist stepfamilies to discuss topics such as these. We encourage nurses to educate themselves about the beliefs of a particular stepfamily because uninformed clinicians may unwittingly increase rather than decrease family tensions if they communicate to stepfamilies that they should be like biological families.

Questions to Ask the Family. Reeves, what were the differences between you and your wife, Lily, in how you each successfully recovered from your first marriage? What most helped each of you deal with your own fears about remarriage? About forming a stepfamily? How did Lily invite your children to adjust to her? What do your children think was the most useful thing you did in helping them deal with loyalty conflicts? What advice do you have for other stepfamilies on how to create a new family? What are you most proud of in how you have helped your stepfamily successfully make the transition from what they were before to what they are now?

Professional and Low-Income Family Life Cycles

The family life cycle of the poor commonly does not match the middle-class paradigm so often used to conceptualize their situations. Anderson (2003) points out that when poverty is factored out, the differences between the adjustment of children in one- and two-parent families almost disappear. Low-income single parents who are also minorities face special issues. Currently, close to 75% of all single-parent families are minorities (Anderson, 2003). The family life cycle of the poor can be divided into three phases: the unattached young adult (perhaps younger than 12 years old), who is virtually unaccountable to any adults; families with children—a phase occupying most of the life span and including three- and four-generational households; and the final phase of the grandmother who continues to be involved in central childrearing in her senior years. We encourage nurses to consider the effects of ethnicity and religion, socioeconomic status, race, and environment on when and how a family makes transitions in its life cycle. This is especially important in relational family nursing practice in primary care.

Adoptive Family Life Cycle

In adoption, the family boundaries of all those involved are expanded. We think of adoption as providing children with security and meeting their developmental and biopsychosocial-spiritual needs through the legal transfer of ongoing parental responsibilities from the birth parents to the adoptive parents. In doing this, we recognize the creation of a new kinship network that forever links these two families through the child.

As with marriage, the new legal status of the adoptive family does not automatically sever the psychological ties to the earlier family. Rather, family boundaries are expanded and realigned. Multiple statistical systems make it difficult to find concrete data on the number of children adopted each year. About 2% of all U.S. children were adopted according to a National Survey of Adoptive Parents (2007). Of the 1.8 million adopted children in the United States, 37% were adopted from foster care, 38% joined their families through private domestic adoptions, and 25% were adopted internationally. The survey excluded stepparent adoptions.

In their study of 20 families who adopted children from Russian and Romanian institutions, Linville and Lyness (2007) reported that the families described having gone through a metamorphosis particularly in the areas of roles, emotional strain, parenting techniques, resilience, and connection to the children's country of origin. They suggest, and we agree, that the way the story of international or cross-cultural adoption is told and retold in the family can have lasting positive or negative consequences for the child's adjustment and emotional well-being. This is an area in which nurses can have a tremendous positive impact in assisting families.

We believe that nurses should be aware of the trends and special circumstances in forming adoptive families. For example, most agencies offer adoption services along a continuum of openness. Some potential benefits of open adoption for birth parents include increased empathy for adoptive parents, reassurance that the child is safe and loved, and a reduction of shame and guilt. For adoptive parents, benefits include increased empathy for the birth parents, reduced stress imposed by secrecy and the unknown, and an embracing from the start of an affirmative acceptance of the child's cultural heritage. For the child, benefits include increased empathy for the adoptive parents, enriched connections with them, and reduced stress of disconnection. Simultaneously, the child experiences increased empathy for the birth parents, a reduction in fantasies about them, and—with clear, consistent information—increased control in dealing with adoptive issues. We believe that these potential benefits are very significant, especially for families adopting babies from different cultures and races. Adoptive families can include divorced, single-parent, married, or remarried families as well as extended families and families with various forms of open dual parentage.

The adoption process, including the decision, application, and final adoption, can be a stressful and joyful experience for many couples. During the preschool developmental phase, the family must acknowledge the adoption as a fact of family life. The question of the permanency of the relationship sometimes arises from both the child and the parents. Clark, Thigpen, and Yates's study (2006) of 11 families who reported having successfully integrated into their family unit at least one older/special needs adoptive child poignantly shows the process these families underwent. Parental perceptions that facilitated the successful process included finding strengths in the children overlooked by previous caregivers, viewing behavior in context, reframing negative behavior, and attributing improvement in behavior to parenting efforts.

In our clinical work with adoptive families, we have found it useful to consider many aspects of the adoption, including:

1. Genetic, hereditary factors in the child

2. Deficiencies in the child's prenatal and perinatal care

3. Adverse circumstances of adoption, including the child's having had multiple disruptions in early life, such as foster care placements

4. Conditions in the adoptive home, including preexisting and current family resiliencies, problems, and strengths

5. Temperamental similarities and differences between the adoptee and the adoptive parents or family

6. Fantasy system and communication regarding adoption, including parental attitudes about adoption

7. Difficulties establishing a firm sense of identity during adolescence

8. Greater age difference than usual between parents and adoptees

We believe that it is important in relational family nursing practice to recognize adoptive families' strengths and resources as they deal with challenging issues. For example, adopted children in the 2007 U.S. survey of adoptive parents were found to be less likely than children in the general population to excel in reading or math, but family relationship quality between children and parents was more comparable between the groups. The exception is children adopted from foster care, who do show lower relationship quality than other adopted children for some indicators, and also seem to account for much of the difference between adopted children and children generally in school performance (Bramlett, 2011).

During the adolescent stage of family development, a major task is to increase the flexibility of family boundaries. In adoptive families, altercations may give rise to threats of desertion or rejection. During the young adult or launching phase, the young adult may "adopt" the parents in a recontracting phase.

As the adopted child proceeds to develop his or her own family of procreation, the integration of the adoptee's biological progeny can be a developmental challenge for everyone. Adoptive parents may be delighted with the psychological and social continuity. Simultaneously, they may mourn the loss of biological grandchildren and the pain of genealogical discontinuity. For the adoptee, reproduction includes the thrill of a biological relationship and possibly some fears of the unknowns in their own genetic history if there has not been ongoing contact with the biological parents.

We believe that nurses can play an important role in helping families navigate the complexities of the adoption process and life cycle. When complexity is accepted, when the losses are acknowledged and resolved, when parents and their children feel satisfied with adoption as a legitimate route to becoming a family, and when the community of family, friends, and professionals who surround them is affirming, then the outcomes for adoptive families are very positive.

Lesbian, Gay, Bisexual, Queer, Intersexed, Transgendered, Twin-Spirited Family Life Cycles

Until recently, popular culture has ignored LGBQITT people in couple or family relationships or has portrayed them as part of an invisible subculture. Much of what we see, read, and hear in the media and society at large expresses a patriarchal, Anglo-Saxon, white, Christian, male, middle-class, ableist, and heterosexual view of the world. More recently, with open discussion about same-sex marriage or union, more attention is being focused on these relationships, their structures, developmental life cycles, challenges, strengths, and issues. Long and Andrews (2007) point out that for same-sex couples, the family functions of formation and membership, nurturance and socialization, and protection of vulnerable members are particularly important. We believe that the popular family life cycle model does not apply to lesbians and gays because it is based on the notions that child-rearing is fundamental to family and that blood and legal ties constitute criteria for definition as a family.

Furthermore, the transmission of norms, rituals, folk wisdom, and values from generation to generation is not typically associated with lesbian and gay life. In many cases, the family of origin may not know what name to call their daughter's partner. For example, the term *girlfriend* does not connote the significance of the relationship.

However, we believe that more differences exist *within* traditionally defined families than *between* LGBQITT families and those families designated as traditional. There are also many differing beliefs *within* diverse couples. For example, Shernoff (2006) points out—and we agree—that male couples need to negotiate their views on monogamy. For many clinicians, sexual nonexclusivity challenges fundamental beliefs. Our view of family life is socially constructed, as is the view held by each nurse. Managing multiple views of relationships is an important task for nurses working with families.

The stages of the traditional family life cycle can be applied to lesbians and gays, with some unique differences. During adolescence, which can be a tumultuous time for most families, gays and lesbians face similar identity and individuation tasks as heterosexuals but often without the support of such rituals as proms or "going steady." Parents frequently struggle more with parenting to "protect" than to "prepare" the young person to live in a homophobic social environment.

The stages of leaving home, single young adulthood, and coupling present challenges for the young person who needs to learn from the gay/lesbian world about dating and cannot rely on the family of origin for modeling in this area. Couch-surfing and seeking hospitality from friends' parents, LGBQITT-friendly shelters, and transitional living programs are examples of the living arrangement options for what some have called "throwaway" youth (i.e., LGBQITT youth in crisis). These are young people who have come out to their families and were then pushed out of the family home.

In discussing their homosexual relationship with their parents, many lesbian and gay couples have found it useful to focus on the strengths of their relationship. When parents see that the relationship has such strengths and can be beneficial for their son or daughter, they often adjust more easily. Dealing with the core issues of coupling—money, work, and sex—involves addressing gender scripts. Sample issues unique to parenting by lesbian and gay couples include the limited options available for getting pregnant by such means as artificial insemination owing to biases by fertility clinics, difficulties with health insurance, the reaction of the family of origin and relatives to the news about parenting, and the often blurred role of the nonbiological parent (Ashton, 2011).

During middle and later life, the LGBQITT family continues to adapt and renegotiate with their families of origin. These relationships may be influenced by illness within either the aging family or the midlife chosen family. Intergenerational responsibility for caregiving and legacy issues may need to be addressed. We believe nurses engaged in relational practice can be helpful in providing a context for these conversations between family members.

We recommend an oppression-sensitive approach to working with LGBQITT families. This approach invites a stance of respectful curiosity for exploring domains of convergence and difference. For nurses working with these couples, some questions that might be useful to ask include:

- In what area do you feel privileged? Oppressed? How do you as a couple deal with these similarities and differences? How does the more privileged one respond to the other's sense of oppression?

- How does each member of the couple deal with heterosexism? With your families of origin? With the dominant gay culture?

- What are your strengths as a couple? How does spirituality influence your relationship?

We encourage nurses to avoid the alpha bias of exaggerating differences between groups of people and the beta bias of ignoring differences that do exist. In their privileged role working with families who are dealing with health issues, nurses can play a significant part in modeling inclusivity and respect for diversity.

In this CFAM developmental category, we have presented six sample types of family life cycles. Nursing is beginning to recognize the special characteristics of diverse family forms, such as lesbian and gay couples. We encourage nurses to broaden their perspectives when interacting with various family forms. What we do know is that great variety exists: the poor and homeless family, the lesbian or gay couple, the single parent, the adopted child with parent, the stepfamily, the divorced family, the separated family, the foster family, the nuclear family, the extended family, the household of children raising children without a parent present, the couple childfree by choice and so forth.

FUNCTIONAL ASSESSMENT

The family functional assessment deals with how individuals *actually* behave in relation to one another. It is the here-and-now aspect of a family's life that is observed and that the family presents. There are two basic aspects of family functioning: instrumental and expressive. Each will be dealt with separately.

Instrumental Functioning

The instrumental aspect of family functioning refers to routine activities of daily living, such as eating, sleeping, preparing meals, giving injections, changing dressings, and so forth. For families with health problems, this area is particularly important. The instrumental activities of daily life are generally more numerous and more frequent and take on a greater significance because of a family member's illness. A quadriplegic, for example, requires assistance with almost every instrumental task. If a baby is attached to an apnea monitor, the parents almost always alter the manner in which they take care of instrumental tasks. For example, one parent will leave the apartment to do a load of wash only if the other parent is sufficiently awake to attend to the infant. If a senior family member is unable to distinguish what medication to take at a specific time, other family members often alter their daily routines to telephone, e-mail, text, or drop in on the senior.

The interaction between instrumental and psychosocial processes in clients' lives is an important consideration for nurses. For example, nurses can pay attention to a family's routines around eating and bedtime rituals and incorporate new health-care practices into the family's routine rather than "adding on" to the family's already busy schedule. Denham's 2011 work and the Web site www.diabetesfamily.net are some creative examples of influencing the family's situation and their active behavioral response to the illness.

Buchbinder, Longhofer, and McCue (2009) found that families with young children (ages 2–9) adjusting to life when a parent has been diagnosed with cancer initially focused on disruptions in caregiving routines and changes in rituals such as birthdays and holidays. Developing and stabilizing new routines and rituals were important positive coping mechanisms for them to maintain a sense of normalcy. We recommend that health professionals understand that caregiving, whether given to a spouse who has cancer by an elderly spouse or to a parent by his or her partner, constitutes a major challenge in adaptation. Elderly spouses often rate the overall burden of caregiving and personal strain (the subjective component) as heavier than do their children and the cancer patients themselves. The importance of *family* nursing care is thus highlighted.

As the nurse inquires into the ordinary routines that families living alongside illness have developed, the nurse and family will discover resiliencies and areas for possible assistance. Effective assistance consists of a series of events rather than single interactions. The trajectory of cardiac illness suggests that interventions may be most effective when provided during all stages of illness and may best be tailored to meet the specific needs of individuals and families in each stage.

Expressive Functioning

The expressive aspect of functioning refers to nine categories:

1. Emotional communication
2. Verbal communication
3. Nonverbal communication
4. Circular communication
5. Problem solving
6. Roles
7. Influence and power
8. Beliefs
9. Alliances and coalitions

These nine subcategories are derived in part from the Family Categories Schema developed by Epstein, Sigal, and Rakoff (1968) and later published by Epstein, Bishop, and Levin (1978). These categories were expanded by Tomm (1977) and later published by Tomm and Sanders (1983). Early work (Westley & Epstein, 1969) suggested that several of these categories distinguished emotionally healthy families from those that were experiencing more than the usual emotional distress. A more recent study by Aarons and colleagues (2007) noted that the Family Assessment Device is less applicable for Hispanic Americans than for Caucasian Americans. They suggest, for example, that Hispanic American families often operate according to more stable hierarchical roles, more often encourage the avoidance of interpersonal conflict, and more often stress family collectivism compared to Caucasian American families. The importance of cultural variability is highlighted.

We have expanded on these works in our earlier editions of *Nurses and Families* to include nonverbal and circular communication, beliefs, and power. However, we do not use any of these categories as determinants of whether a family is emotionally healthy. Rather, it is the family's judgment of whether they are functioning well that is most salient. With the exception of issues such as violence and abuse, we encourage nurses to find ways to support the family's definition of health versus imposing their own definition on the family.

Before discussing each subcategory, we would like to point out that most families must deal with a combination of instrumental and expressive issues. For example, when an older woman experiences a burn, the instrumental issues revolve around dressing changes and an exercise program while the expressive or affective issues might center on roles or problem solving. The family might be considering the following questions:

- Whose role is it to change Gram's dressing?
- Are women better "nurses" than men?
- Whose turn is it to call the physical therapist?
- How can we get Jasdev to drive Gram to her doctor's visit?

If a family is not coping well with instrumental issues, expressive issues almost always exist. However, a family can deal well with instrumental issues and still have expressive or emotional difficulties. Therefore, it is useful for the nurse and the family together to delineate the instrumental from the expressive issues. Both need to be explored when the nurse and family have a conversation about family functioning. Robinson (1998) points out the importance of nurses attending to what she calls "illness work" and "illness burden." Making arrangements for managing chronic or life-threatening illness does not just happen. The ordinary context of women generally shouldering the larger burden of housework than men do is the one in which additional illness arrangements are made.

Although both past behaviors and future goals are taken into consideration in the functional assessment, the primary focus is on the here and now. It is helpful for the nurse and the family to identify a family's strengths and limitations in each of the aforementioned subcategories. We find it helpful to remember that the very conversation the nurse and family have about the family system shapes that system. People continually and actively reauthor their lives and stories. Our commitment to families is to show curiosity, delight, interest, and appreciation for their strengths, resources, and resiliency. Naturally, this does not mean that we condone family violence or abuse. Rather, it means that we recognize that families are trying to make sense of their lives and stories.

Patterns of interaction are the main thrust of the expressive part of the functional assessment category. Families are obviously composed of individuals, but the focus of a family assessment is less on the individual and more on the interaction *among* all of the individuals within the family. Thus, the family is viewed as a system of interacting members. In conducting this part of the family assessment, the nurse operates under the assumption that individuals are best understood within their immediate social context. The nurse conceives of the individual as defining and being defined by that context. Each individual's relationships with family members and other meaningful members of the larger social environment are thus very important. If we do not attend to ideas and practices at play in the larger social context, we risk focusing too narrowly on small, rather tight, recursive feedback loops. We have found this to be especially important since we have witnessed 9/11, random acts of terrorism, and mass slayings at schools and universities, and we and families have struggled to adapt to a changed social and political context.

By interviewing family members together, the nurse can observe how they spontaneously interact with and influence each other. Furthermore, the nurse can ask questions about the impact family members have on one another and on the health problem. Reciprocally, the nurse can inquire about the impact of the health problem on the family. If the nurse thinks "interactionally" rather than "individually," each family member's behavior will not be considered in isolation but rather will be understood in context.

It is important for nurses to remember that, if they embrace a postmodernist worldview, they will not be able to conduct an objective family evaluation. Rather, the nurse and the family, in talking about the family's patterns of interacting, will bring forth a new story, rich in contextualized details. Particular attention is paid to the ways that even the small and the ordinary—single words, single gestures, minor asides, trivial actions—can provide opportunities for generating new meanings. Unlike modernist nurses who define themselves as separate from the family with whom they are working, nurses with postmodernist views assume that each participant in the family interview—wife, husband, partner, nurse—makes an equal, valid, but often different contribution to the process. It is the nurse's task to help family members engage in conversations to make sense of their lives in the context of illness, loss, or disability rather than to explain their behavior.

Emotional Communication

This subcategory refers to the range and types of emotions or feelings that families express or the practitioner observes. Families generally express a wide spectrum of feelings, from happiness to sadness to anger, whereas families with difficulties commonly have quite rigid patterns within a narrow range of emotional expression. For example, some families experiencing difficulties almost always argue and rarely show affection. In other families, parents may express anger but children may not, or the family may have no difficulty with women expressing tenderness but feel that men are not permitted to express it.

The feelings of subjective well-being are usually unrelated to socioeconomic status, income, levels of education, gender, or race. Rather, they are related to the genetic lottery and fortune's favors, good or bad. The influence of biology on emotional communication is an intriguing developing area, and families will no doubt have many beliefs about this.

Questions to Ask the Family. Who in the family tends to start conversations about feelings? How can you tell when your dad is feeling happy? Angry? Sad? How about your mom? What effect does your anger have on your son Noah? What does your mom do when your dad is angry? If your grandmother were to express sadness about her upcoming chemotherapy to your parents, how do you think your parents would react? When your brother Hiesem was killed in the accident, what most helped your family to cope with the grief?

Verbal Communication

This subcategory focuses on the meaning of an oral (or written) message between those involved in the interaction—that is, the focus is on the meaning of the words in terms of the relationship.

Direct communication implies that the message is sent to the intended recipient. An elderly woman may be upset by what her husband is saying but corrects her grandson's inconsequential fidgeting with the comment, "Stop doing that to me." This could represent a displaced message, whereas the same statement directed at her husband would be considered direct.

Another way of looking at verbal communication is to distinguish between clear versus masked messages. In a clear message, there is a lack of distortion in the message. A father's statement to his child, "Children who cry when they get shots are babies," may be masked criticism if the child is fighting back tears at the time of his injection. The old child-management strategy of "say what you mean and mean what you say" is a good guideline for clear, direct communication.

Questions to Ask the Family. Who among your family members is the most clear and direct when communicating verbally? When you state clearly to your young adult son that he has to pay you rent, what effect does that have on him? When your teenagers talk directly to each other about the use of condoms, what do you notice? If your adolescents were to talk more with you and your husband about safer sex, what do you think your husband's reaction might be? What ways have you found for you and Manuel to have good, direct conversations? In person? On a smartphone? By e-mail? Through texting or Twitter?

Nonverbal Communication

This subcategory focuses on the various nonverbal and paraverbal messages that family members communicate. Nonverbal messages include body posture (slumped, fidgeting, open, closed), eye contact (intense, minimal), touch (soft, rough), gestures, facial movements (grimaces, stares, yawns), and so forth. Personal space, the proximity or distance between family members, is also an important part of nonverbal communication. Paraverbal communication includes tonality, guttural sounds, crying, stammering, and so forth.

Nurses must remember that nonverbal communication is highly influenced by culture. For example, in Taiwanese Chinese couples, indirect, nonverbal means of communicating and relating serve a positive function but can be viewed among Euro-Caucasian groups in the United States as an indicator of intrusiveness or overinvolvement. Gestures such as hand signs, shrugs, and posture shifts can be specific to different cultures, and as many as 200 of these gestures may exist among all cultures.

Nurses should note the sequence of nonverbal messages as well as their timing. For example, when an older man starts to talk about his terminal illness and his adult daughter turns her head and casts her tear-filled eyes toward the floor, the nurse can infer that the daughter is sad about her father's impending death. Her sequence of nonverbal behavior is congruent with sadness and the topic of conversation. Note, however, that this behavior sequence may not necessarily be the most supportive for her father.

Nonverbal communication is closely linked to emotional communication. We encourage nurses to inquire about the meaning of nonverbal communication when it is inconsistent with verbal communication.

Questions to Ask the Family. Who in your family shows the most distress when your foster father is drinking? How does Sheldon show it? What does your foster mother do when your foster father is drinking? When your sister Seema turns her head and stares out the window as your stepfather is talking, what effect does it have on you? If your dad were to stop talking at the same time as your stepmother, do you think she might move closer to him?

Circular Communication

Circular communication refers to reciprocal communication between people (Watzlawick, Beavin, & Jackson, 1967). A particular interactional pattern exists in most relationship issues. For example, a common circular pattern occurs when a wife feels angry and criticizes her husband; in return, the husband feels angry and avoids both the issues and her. The more he avoids, the angrier she becomes. The wife tends to see the problem only as her husband's, whereas the husband identifies the wife's criticism as the only problem. This type of pattern is often called the *demand/withdraw pattern*. The circularity of this pattern is the most important aspect in understanding interaction in dyads. Each person influences the behavior of the other. More information about this topic is available in Chapter 2.

Circular communication patterns can also be adaptive. For example, an older parent feels competent and negotiates well with the landlord; the adult son feels proud and praises his parent. The more reinforcement the adult son gives, the more confident and self-assured the senior feels. This pattern is diagrammed in Figure 3–18.

Circular pattern diagrams (CPDs) concretize and simplify repetitive sequences noted in a relationship. This method of diagramming interaction patterns, first developed by Tomm in 1980, may be applied to relationships between family members or between the nurse and the family. Because the nurse and the family also mutually influence each other, the nurse is encouraged to think interactionally about situations and offer the family an opportunity to think interactionally.

The simplest CPD includes two behaviors and two inferences of meaning. The inferences can be cognitive, affective, or both. Inferences about cognition refer to ideas, concepts, or beliefs, whereas inferences about affect refer to emotional states. Affect and/or cognition propels the behavior. Figure 3–19 illustrates the relationship between these elements. "The inference is entered inside the enclosure and represents some internal process (what is going on

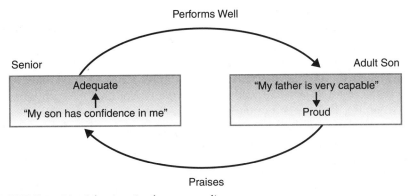

FIGURE 3-18: Adaptive circular pattern diagram.

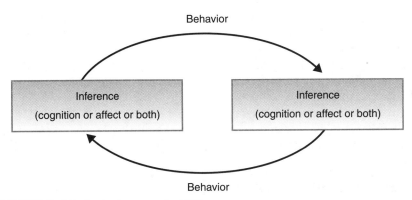

FIGURE 3-19: Basic elements of a CPD.

inside each interactant). The connecting arrows represent information conveyed from each person to the other through behavior. The circular linkage implies an interaction pattern that is repetitive, stable, and self-regulatory" (Tomm, 1980, p. 8). CPDs encourage a position of curiosity rather than a passion for particular values and a stand against others.

Although CPDs can be used to foster circular thinking, one must be mindful of their limitations. CPDs can tempt us to look within families for collaborative causation of problems. This may distract from personal responsibility for unacceptable behavior such as violence. Small, tight feedback loops may be highlighted, and the "big picture" of the negative influence of particular values, institutions, and cultural practices may be forgotten. Another limitation of CPDs is that they may encourage nurses to believe that they are outside the family system. As a participant observer in the larger system, the nurse is shown and hears about circular patterns reflecting family functioning. The interdependence of the nurse interviewer and family must be recognized. Both the nurse and family members cannot be decontextualized from their social and historical surroundings.

In what has come to be called the "feminist critique" of systems, some have taken exception to the simplistic causation ideas advanced by a circular perspective. CPDs, by virtue of their neutral context, ignore power differentials and imply a discourse or relationship between equals. Circularity has been criticized for not being transparent about responsibility and minimizing power differentials in relationships. Of particular concern are such issues as incest, abuse, violence, intimidation, and battering.

Despite these valid criticisms, we believe that it is still useful in clinical work with families to subscribe to the notion of circularity but simultaneously hold to the idea of personal responsibility. Fekete and colleagues (2007) point out the importance of circularity in their study of 243 women experiencing lupus flare-ups and their husbands. They found that more spousal emotional (empathic) support was interpreted as the husband's being more emotionally responsive, which in turn was associated with the wife's greater sense of well-being. In contrast, more problematic (minimizing) spousal support was interpreted as the husband's being less emotionally responsive, which in turn was associated with the wife's poorer sense of well-being. These findings have large implications for helping couples adjust and cope with chronic illness. An example of a circular argument is illustrated in Figure 3–20. Each party blames and threatens the other.

An example of a supportive relationship is illustrated in Figure 3–21. The husband trusts his wife and reveals his needs and fears. She is concerned and so sustains and supports him. This leads him to trust her more, and the relationship progresses.

Sample Conversation With the Family

Nurse: You say your wife "always" criticizes you. (Nurse conceptualizes Fig. 3–22.) What do you do then? (Nurse tries to fill in the husband's behavior in Fig. 3–23.)

Husband: I don't like to discuss things. I avoid conflict. I leave. I go in the other room. What else can I do? She is always telling me what I did wrong. I go to the computer.

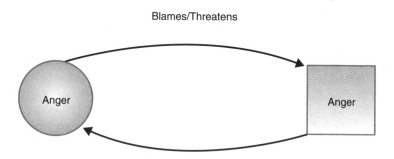

Blames/Threatens

Anger

Anger

Blames/Threatens

FIGURE 3-20: CPD of a circular argument.

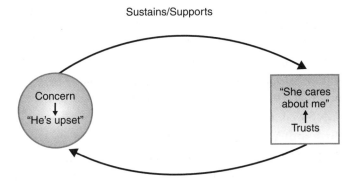

FIGURE 3-21: CPD of a supportive relationship.

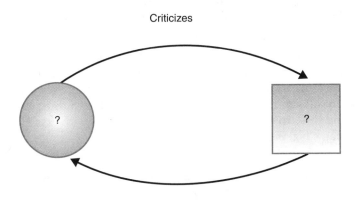

FIGURE 3-22: Beginning conceptualization of CPD.

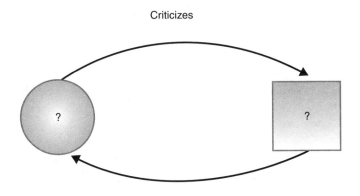

FIGURE 3-23: CPD illustrating husband's and wife's behaviors.

Nurse: So she expresses her needs and you leave. How do you think that makes her feel? (Nurse tries to fill in the inferred emotion in the wife's circle in Fig. 3–24.)

Wife: I'll tell you. I get annoyed. I feel ignored, rejected.

Nurse: So you're annoyed when he leaves and ignores you. And then you become more critical. Is that right?

Wife: Well, I don't really criticize. I just—

Husband: Yeah, you got it, Nurse.

Nurse: So, when you try to express your concerns, how do you think it makes him feel? (Nurse tries to fill in the inference in the square in Fig. 3–24.)

Wife: I don't know.

Nurse: If he thinks you're lecturing and avoids the issues by leaving the room and going to the computer, what effect do you think your talking might be having on him?

Wife: Well, I suppose he could be feeling frustrated. He sulks.

Nurse: So the pattern seems to be that, no matter who starts it, the circle completes itself: Sometimes you're annoyed and you criticize. Your husband feels frustrated and ignores you. He sulks in the other room. Other times he avoids issues, and this arouses your frustration and criticism. (Nurse explains Fig. 3–25.)

Wife: It's a vicious circle.

Husband: I don't want it to go on this way anymore. We both get too upset.

Once the nurse has elicited a CPD, he or she should ask the family members to contextualize their discussion. One context might be that the wife is

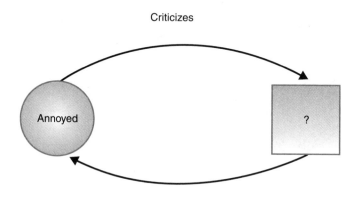

Criticizes

Annoyed

?

Avoids/Ignores

FIGURE 3-24: CPD illustrating wife's emotion.

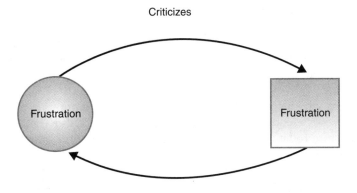

Criticizes

Frustration

Frustration

Avoids/Ignores

FIGURE 3-25: Nurse's conceptualization of this couple's communication pattern.

exhausted by her factory job and all the housework and childcare. The husband does not see why he should change his life because his wife has a stressful job and works long hours. They may engage in this particular negative circular interaction pattern every night while caring for their 3-year-old child with asthma.

Problem Solving

This subcategory refers to the family's ability to solve its own problems effectively. Family problem solving is strongly influenced by the family's beliefs about its abilities and past successes. How much influence the family believes it has on the problem or illness is useful to know. Who identifies the problems is important. Is it characteristically someone from outside the family or from inside the family?

Once the problems are identified, are they mainly instrumental (i.e., routine day-to-day logistics) or emotional problems? Families sometimes encounter difficulties when they identify an emotional problem as an instrumental one. For example, a mother who states that she cannot get her child who has food allergies to maintain the diet is really discussing an emotional issue rather than an instrumental one; she has difficulty influencing her child. As more families cope with issues such as childhood obesity, this is a particularly important distinction for nurses to notice. Is the obesity an instrumental or emotional problem? An individual, family, or societal problem?

What are the family's solution patterns? Are they proactive in planning for issues that might arise? For example, a couple dealing with the wife's myeloma might decide to harvest stem cells as a proactive measure. Many close-knit extended families rely on relatives for assistance in time of need. Others tend to seek help from professionals while others go to the Internet for information and/or support. Knowing a family's usual solution style can give the nurse insight into why this family may seem to be "stuck" at this particular time with this particular issue. For example, older parents move to a retirement community. The wife breaks her hip. The husband is used to being self-reliant or, in a pinch, depending on his middle-aged daughter. The older couple know few people in their new community. The husband is reluctant to accept help from the visiting nurse. He states that he can manage all his wife's care despite the fact that he is losing weight and getting insufficient rest. The husband's solution conflicts with that of the nurse.

Knowing whether a family evaluates the cost of its solutions can be helpful to the nurse. For example, a 68-year-old grandmother tells Kiran, the nurse, "I can't afford to let myself cry about the death of my son's infant. I have to go on for the sake of my other children." Kiran was able to evaluate with the grandmother the cost of her solution pattern. Neither the grandmother nor the son discussed the infant's death with each other. The grandchildren's questions about why the baby did not come home from the hospital were left unanswered. There was considerable tension between the son and the grandmother, and the son was particularly overprotective with his 4-year-old boy (the only surviving male child). By gently exploring the cost of the solution (tension and overprotection), the nurse was able to suggest other solution patterns (e.g., shared grieving).

Holtslander and colleagues (2011) have offered a helpful idea for nurses to use in exploring problem solving solutions. They found that older persons bereaved after caregiving for a spouse with advanced cancer walked a fine line in finding balance between deep grieving and moving forward. We support the notion of asking familiy members about how they find balance in their solutions.

DeJong and Berg (2008) offer many intriguing ideas for interviewing for solutions, such as at the start of a second or third meeting, the clinician can immediately ask clients, "What's better?" This question reflects the notion that clients are competent to have taken steps to progress in the direction they have said they want.

Questions to Ask the Family. Who first noticed the problem? Are you the one who usually notices such things? What most helped you to take the first step toward eliminating the addiction and violence pattern? What effect did it have when Toya also took steps to stop the cycle of violence in your family? How did the relationship between your son Jeremiah and your husband change when the violence stopped? When the addiction stopped? If a violent episode were to occur again, how do you think you and your daughter would deal with it? If his cocaine addiction were to flare up again, what steps would you take to protect your family? Does it usually seem "the punishment fits the crime" in your family? When your brother is punished, does it usually seem he deserves it?

Roles

This subcategory refers to the established patterns of behavior for family members. A role is consistent behavior in a particular situation. However, roles are not static but are developed through an individual's interactions with others. Roles are thus influenced by culture, race, and others' sanctions and norms. In some Hispanic families, for example, *machismo* can be very significant for the hierarchical male role, and *simpatia* or the avoidance of conflict and the ability to get along well, can be often highly valued. That women have a life cycle apart from their roles as wife and mother is a relatively recent one and is still not widely accepted in our culture. The expectation for women has typically been that they would take care of the needs of others, first men, then children, then the older generation.

The psychological cost of providing care for a parent with Alzheimer's disease is often anxiety, depression, guilt, and resentment in the caregiver. The fact that women dominate as adult caregivers reflects a North American pattern. The gender differences clearly profile women's more frequent, intensive, affective involvement with the caregiver role.

Women's roles have changed in recent years and are now less defined by the men in their lives. The birth rate has fallen below replacement levels, and many more women are concentrating on jobs and education. Nevertheless, on average, women still make less than men do for the same job. In many cases, a husband's income is negatively related to role sharing and a wife's education is positively related to role sharing.

Although role change is increasingly prevalent for both men and women in today's society, what is important for nurses to assess is how family members cope with their roles. Does role conflict or cooperation exist? Are roles determined solely by age, rank order, or gender? Do additional criteria, such as social class and culture, influence roles? Are the women in the family more involved with a wider network of people for whom they feel responsible? Do the men hear less than the women in the family about stress in their family network?

Formal roles are those for which the community has broadly agreed on a norm. Examples include the roles of mother, husband, and friend. Informal roles refer to the established patterns of behavior that are idiosyncratic to particular individuals in certain settings. Examples include the roles of "bad kid," "angel," and "class clown." These serve a specific function in a particular family. If Dad is the "softie," most likely Mom is the "heavy." If Giffy is the "good daughter," Kweisi is probably the "black sheep." The roles of "parentified child," "good child," and "symptomatic child" have been identified in many families. Auxiliary roles of "child advocate," "analyst," "peacemaker," and "therapist" have also been described.

It is helpful for the nurse to learn how family roles evolved, their impact on family functioning, and whether the family believes they need to be altered. The findings from a study (Stein, Rotheram-Borus, & Lester, 2007) of adolescents whose parents had HIV/AIDS show that there can be positive effects to what typically might be perceived as a negative role of a "parentified adolescent." Early parentification predicted better adaptive coping skills and less alcohol and tobacco use 6 years later. The authors hypothesized that parentification skills were adaptive in the long run, especially with adolescents who had dying or ill parents, impoverished environments, and family instability.

It is important for nurses to conceptualize the functional assessment category of roles in a family-oriented rather than an individual-oriented way. According to Hoffman (1981):

> The individual-oriented approach badly misrepresents the subject. For instance, to speak of the "role of the scapegoat" is to present the deviant as a person with fixed characteristics rather than a person involved in a process. "Scapegoating" technically applies to only one stage of a shifting scenario—the stage where the person is metaphorically cast out of the village. After all, the term originates from an ancient Hebrew ritual in which a goat was turned loose in the desert after the sins of the people had been symbolically laid on its head. The deviant can begin like a hero and go out like a villain, or vice versa. There is a positive-negative continuum on which he can be rated depending on which stage of the deviation process we are looking at, which sequence the process follows, and the degree to which the social system is stressed.
>
> At the time, the character of the deviant may vary in another direction, depending on the way his particular group does its typecasting. Which symptoms crop up in members of a group is itself a kind of typecasting. Thus the deviant may appear in many guises: the mascot, the clown, the sad sack, the erratic genius, the black sheep, the wise guy, the saint, the idiot, the fool, the imposter, the malingerer, the boaster, the villain, and so on. Literature and folklore abound with such figures (p. 58).

Questions to Ask the Family. To whom do most of you go when you need someone to talk to? What effect does it have on Maxine when Ken helps with the baby's care? When Maxine and Ken collaborate instead of compete, who would be the first to notice? If Ken were to be more responsible for initiating contact with the relatives around Cherie's day-care arrangements and babysitting, how do you think Maxine would feel? Who would your children say is the "favored" child in your family?

Influence and Power

This subcategory refers to behavior used by one person to affect another's behavior. Power is the ability of a person to regulate the criteria by which differing views of "reality"" are judged and resources apportioned. Power addresses hierarchical and egalitarian positions in relationships. In a hierarchical relationship, a person can be in a one-up or a one-down position in the relationship and can be dominant in one context and subordinate in another. In an egalitarian relationship, there is equality in the relationship. In a hierarchical relationship, the needs of the dominant person take precedence while the subordinate person stifles his or her own thoughts and feelings. In a more equal relationship, there is a give-and-take negotiation of individual needs, goals, and desires.

Gender, race, and cultural issues are frequently intermingled with influence and power issues. For example, in many relationships, women tend to raise issues and draw men out in the early phase of a discussion, whereas men tend to control the content and emotional depth of the later discussion phases and largely dominate the outcome. Shifts in power are preceded by changes in "reality," an expansion from a single perspective to a multiverse. We encourage nurses to adopt a postmodernist worldview, because it offers useful ideas about how influence, power, and "truth" are socially constructed, constituted through language, organized, and maintained in families and larger cultural contexts.

A nurse who is unaware of power differences among family members, in terms of roles, gender, economics, or social class, can inadvertently encourage family members in positions of less power to accept goals that decrease their power and constrain their choices. We encourage nurses to discuss with family members areas of power and influence such as decision making about illness management, work, life goals and activities, housework, finances, and sex. How a family member attempts to influence another is important for their relationship and can have consequences for illness management as well. For example, Stephens and colleagues (2010) found that warning and encouragement were two types of negative and positive control strategies used by spouses to urge patients with type 2 diabetes to improve adherence to the diabetic diet. Warning consisted of the spouse emphasizing diabetic complications, demanding dietary adherence, and expressing doubts or concerns. Encouragement, on the other hand, consisted of suggesting alternative healthy foods and complimenting dietary management. Spousal encouragement was significantly and positively associated with patients' reports of dietary adherence.

Miller (2009) noted that even in inherently unequal relationships such as parent-child, there is significant value in collaborative decision making for the management of chronic illness. Asking for other's opinion and sharing information were two factors Miller noted as contributing to beneficial collaboration.

Whether all family members contribute equally to problems and share responsibility for resolution is something that the nurse can pose for consideration. We believe that the most clinically useful stance to take with regard to the idea of power is to say, "Power is...." It can be used positively or negatively, overtly or covertly, to enhance or constrain options. Power relations exist among family members, their health-care providers, and institutions. McGoldrick, Gerson, and Petry (2008, p. 78) have depicted a negative power and control pyramid that includes eight levels and combines racism, heterosexism, and sexism:

1. "Isolation, controlling whom she can see and when and where

2. Sexual abuse, abusive touching, sexual acts against her will, having affairs, exposing her to HIV

3. Using children, being abusive, controlling, guilt-inducing or under-responsible regarding visitation, etc.

4. Physical abuse, hitting, shoving, choking, kicking, grabbing, etc.

5. Economic abuse, controlling her financially, not sharing financial information or resources, challenging her every purchase

6. Threats and intimidation, threatening to hurt her physically, to commit suicide, have an affair, divorce, report her to welfare, take away children or cut off her emotional support system, putting her in fear by looks, actions, destroying property, stalking, driving car too fast

7. Using immigration status, using her undocumented status to threaten deportation, loss of children, job, healthcare, etc.

8. Emotional abuse and use of male privilege, putting her down, name calling, making her think she's crazy, playing mind games, stonewalling, treating her like a servant, assuming right to make all major decisions or to neglect '2nd shift' home responsibilities such as housework and childcare."

Instrumental influence, power, or control refers to the use of objects or privileges (e.g., money; television watching; computer, car, or cell phone use; candy; vacations; etc.) as reinforcers. Psychological influence or power refers to the use of communication and feelings to influence behavior. Examples include directives, praise, criticism, threats, and guilt induction. Corporal control refers to actual body contact, such as hugging, spanking, and so forth. It is important to note the positive and negative influences used in the family, especially with infants and seniors. Abuse of seniors by informal and sometimes formal caregivers is not infrequent.

We have found the most important positive predictors of compliance for children is consistency of enforcement of rules, encouragement of mature action, use of psychological rewards such as praise and approval, and play with the child. The most important negative one is the amount of physical punishment. The use of praise is positively related to success, whereas physical punishment and verbal, psychological punishment are constraining influences.

Questions to Ask the Family. Which of your parents is best at getting Nirmala to take her medication? When Delvecchio dominates the conversation, what effect does that have on Jamilett? What does your mother feel about how your stepfather disciplines your sister? If your stepfather were to be more positive with your sister Tiffany, how might his relationship with your mother change? Whose interests are most reflected in major decisions in the Veliz family? Who is more likely to accommodate the other person, Gustavo or Fines?

Beliefs

This subcategory refers to fundamental attitudes, premises, values, and assumptions held by individuals and families. Beliefs are the blueprint from which people construct their lives and intermingle them with the lives of others.

Families coevolve an ecology of beliefs that arise from interactional, social, and cultural contexts (Wright & Bell, 2009). When illness arises, our beliefs about health are challenged, threatened, or affirmed. During times of illness, nurses may assess patients', family members', or even their own beliefs to be constraining or facilitating. Constraining beliefs can enhance suffering and decrease solution options, whereas facilitating beliefs can soften illness suffering and increase solution options to managing an illness (Wright & Bell, 2009).

It is usually not our actual beliefs that cause suffering but believing that they are true without any self-inquiry. Therefore, when family members express frustration, anxiety, or anger about their illness based on a particular belief, nurses can gently nudge constraining beliefs by simply asking, "Is that true?" followed by "Can you absolutely know that it is true?" (Katie, 2003). Of course, these questions must be asked with a truly genuine, caring, and inquisitive tone so as not to sound insincere or sarcastic.

Which illness beliefs are considered to be constraining or facilitating is determined by the clinical judgment of the nurse in collaboration with the family. However, any healing transaction involves at least three sets of beliefs: those of the ill patient, those of other family members, and those of the nurse (Bell & Wright, 2011; Duhamel & Dupuis, 2003; Hougher Limacher & Wright, 2006; James, Andershed, & Ternestedt, 2007; Marshall, Bell, & Moules, 2010; Moules, 1998; Moules, Thirsk, & Bell, 2006; Watson & Lee, 1993; West, 2011; Wright & Bell, 2009; Wright & Nagy, 1993; Wright & Simpson, 1991; Wright & Watson, 1988). Cousins (1979) offered the poignant idea that what we believe is the most powerful option of all.

Beliefs and behavior are intricately connected. Every action and every choice that families and individuals make evolves from their beliefs. Consequently, beliefs shape the way in which families adapt to chronic and life-threatening illness. For example, if a family believes that the best treatment for colon cancer is a nontraditional approach, it makes good sense for the family to pursue acupuncture. Because North American culture tends to use a paradigm of control about symptoms (e.g., it is good to be in control and bad to be out of control), nurses might find it useful to explore family members' beliefs about control and mastery over their symptoms.

Beliefs are intricately intertwined with familial and socioeconomic contexts. For example, the meaning of pregnancy loss is intricately intertwined with the woman's emotional needs at the time of the loss. If a mother were very happy about being pregnant and felt devastated by her miscarriage, then her emotional needs would differ dramatically from those of another mother who did not want to be pregnant and felt relieved by her miscarriage. Feelings about pregnancy loss can range from feelings of devastation to relief.

In another example, a 51-year-old father of two teenage girls wrote to a nurse about his beliefs about his chronic pain:

> I think each person has a different threshold of pain. Every day I try to disassociate the pain ... I try to "get into" my work and life. I am not always successful ... but I try as hard as I can. The why is because of

my family, friends, and faith (gushy, eh?, but it's true). I think you have to find out what is important in your life and let it motivate you, as terrible as this will be to say, there are always thoughts of "ending it all" … but then you think about the sadness you would leave with the ones you love … it keeps you going. I really think the key is to find one important thing as a start, and let that be the fuel that keeps you motivated to do the things you would like to do. I wish there were more I could say … It's a day to day struggle.

Wright and Bell (2009) have suggested that the most relevant beliefs to explore with patients and their families are beliefs about etiology, diagnosis, prognosis, healing, and treatment; spirituality and religion; mastery and control; role of family members; and role of health-care providers. Box 3–5 provides a list of areas for nurses to explore when assessing family beliefs about the health problem.

Questions to Ask the Family. How do you react when you believe that thought? What do you believe is the cause of your sexual addiction? How much control do you believe your family has over chronic pain? How much control does chronic pain have over your family? What do you believe the

---

Box 3-5 Beliefs About the Health Problem

A. Beliefs about:
 1. Diagnosis
 2. Etiology
 3. Prognosis
 4. Healing and treatment
 5. Mastery, control, and influence
 6. Religion and spirituality
 7. Place of illness in lives and relationships
 8. Role of family members
 9. Role of health-care professionals
B. Influence of the family on the health problem
 1. Resource utilization
  • Internal (to family)
  • External
 2. Medication and treatment
C. Influence of the health problem on the family
 1. Client response to the illness
 2. Family members' responses to illness
 3. Perceived difficulties and changes related to the health problem
D. Strengths related to the health problem at present
E. Concerns related to the health problem at present

Adapted from Family Nursing Unit records, Faculty of Nursing, University of Calgary, Calgary, Alberta.

effect, if any, would be on chronic pain if you and your wife agreed on treatment? Who do you believe is suffering the most in your family because of the changes in your family life due to your war injuries? What do you believe has been the most useful thing health professionals have offered to help you cope with your suffering from PTSD? What has been the least helpful? Have any of your Buddhist beliefs helped you to cope with the tragic loss of your son in Afghanistan?

For a more in-depth reading of the interconnection of the illness beliefs of patients, families, and health-care providers, see *Beliefs and Illness: A Model for Healing,* written by Lorraine M. Wright and Janice M. Bell (2009). Their advanced practice approach, the Illness Beliefs Model, is also offered in their book. Refer to their Web site for more information about the model: www.illnessbeliefsmodel.com.

Alliances and Coalitions

This subcategory focuses on the directionality, balance, and intensity of relationships between family members or between families and nurses. *Complementary* and *symmetrical* are terms used to describe a two-person relationship (see Chapter 2). A term commonly used to distinguish a three-person relationship is *triangle,* a term first coined by Bowen (1978). Bowen, a psychiatrist and family therapist, explains:

> The two-person relationship is unstable in that it has a low tolerance for anxiety and it is easily disturbed by emotional forces within the twosome and by relationship forces from outside the twosome. When anxiety increases, the emotional flow in a twosome intensifies and the relationship becomes uncomfortable. When the intensity reaches a certain level the twosome predictably and automatically involves a vulnerable third person in the emotional issue. The twosome might "reach out" and pull in the other person, the emotions might "overflow" to the third person, or the third person might be emotionally programmed to initiate the involvement. With involvement of the third person, the anxiety level decreases. It is as if the anxiety is diluted as it shifts from one to another of the three relationships in a triangle. The triangle is more stable and flexible than the twosome. It has a much higher tolerance of anxiety and is capable of handling a fair percentage of life stresses (p. 400).

Most family relationships are organized around threesomes or triangles. Triangular alliances can be helpful or unhelpful. We have learned that, in families of combat veterans experiencing post-traumatic stress disorder, the veteran can sometimes become triangulated with a dead buddy without the spouse's knowledge. With soldiers returning from the Iraq or Afghanistan wars, the ongoing impact of their military alliances may be a useful area for the nurse to explore if the family is having difficulty realigning as a unit. Restless days, fractured relationships, and vials of pills that may help with some types of pain have commonly been reported by these families. Relationships are not unidirectional, even if one member of the triangle is an infant, an older person, or a person who has a handicap. The intensity of each relationship and the total amount of interaction is often fairly balanced. If one relationship becomes more intense, another one or two become less intense. Also, if one member of a threesome withdraws, the other two become closer.

We believe that it is important for the nurse to note the degree of flexibility and fluidity within the family as they adjust to new arrivals, death, or illness. Experienced community health nurses have often noticed triangulation in infancy support. For example, if the father acts intrusively while playing with his baby, the infant often averts and turns to the mother. The regulation of this intrusion-avoidance pattern at the family level sheds some light on the couple alliance. When coparenting is supportive, the mother validates the infant's bid for help without interfering with the father. Thus, the problematic pattern is contained within the dyad of father-baby. If coparenting is hostile/competitive, the mother ignores the infant's bid or engages with her in a way that interferes with her play with her father. In this case, triangulation occurs and tension is lessened, but at a cost. The nurse can identify these patterns with the couple and then collaborate with them to design effective interventions.

As nurses address this functional subcategory of alliances and coalitions, they will be aware of its interconnection with structural and developmental categories. The structural subcategory of boundaries is an important part of the alliance or coalition subcategory. The boundary defines who is part of the triangle and who is not. Of course, there are many triangles and many shifting alliances and coalitions within families. What is important for the nurse and family to note, therefore, is whether these are problematic or enriching.

An example of what can inadvertently occur in a family is if a patient's illness is seen as "his problem" versus "our challenge." If the condition becomes defined as the affected patient's problem, a fundamental split occurs between the patient, the well partner, and other family members. By introducing the concept of "our challenge" early on, the nurse can provide an opportunity for all family members to examine cultural and multigenerational beliefs about the rights and privileges of ill and well family members. An alternate example of a positive coalition is when family members join together to help another family member stop smoking or stop drinking alcohol. They collectively voice their concerns to the individual and their intent to provide support and help.

We have observed that cross-generational coalitions sometimes coincide with symptomatic behavior. In addition to noting the connection between the structural subcategory of boundaries and the functional subcategory of alliances and coalitions, nurses should be aware of the interconnection with the developmental subcategory of attachments. Family attachments, or underlying emotional bonds that have an enduring or stable quality, are similar to alliances in that they are both unions. Attachments tend to differ from coalitions, however, in that the latter imply an alignment between two members with a third member being split off or opposed.

Questions to Ask the Family. When Demi and Tyson argue, who is most likely to get in the middle of the fight? If the children are playing very well together, who would most likely come along and *start* them fighting? Who would *stop* them from fighting? What impact has Don's brain tumor had on family members coming together or becoming further distanced?

CONCLUSIONS

The CFAM, although a very comprehensive and inclusive family assessment model, need not be overwhelming if viewed as a "map of the family" from the nurse's and the family's observer perspectives. The model provides a framework that can be drawn on as the nurse and the family discuss and collaborate about the issues. The nurse can use three main categories (structural, developmental, and functional) to obtain a macroassessment of family strengths, resources, problems, and/or suffering. Depending on his or her confidence and competence level, the nurse may also do a microassessment and explore in detail specific areas of family functioning. In either situation, the nurse needs to be able to draw together all relevant information into an integrated assessment. In doing this, the nurse synthesizes information and is not stymied by complexity. It is insufficient to focus on a family's difficulties with problem solving when the specific family structure is unknown. Also, if the nurse focuses too much on previous developmental history, he or she may be ignoring important current functioning issues. Naturally, past history cannot be ignored. It should be integrated, however, only insofar as it helps to explain current functioning and not because of history taking for history's sake.

Once a thorough family assessment has been completed, the nurse and the family may now collaborate to determine whether intervention is needed. However, we wish to emphasize that completing a family assessment utilizing CFAM does not mean that the nurse or the family now has the "truth" about the family's functioning related to a health problem or concern. Rather, the nurse and family members each have their own integrated assessment from their own "observer perspectives" at one point in time.

References

Aarons, G.A., et al. (2007). Assessment of family functioning in Caucasian and Hispanic Americans: Reliability, validity, and factor structure of the Family Assessment Device. *Family Process, 46*(4), 557–569.

Ahrons, C.R. (2001). *Binuclear family study, 1979–2000.* http://dvn.iq.harvard.edu/dvn/dv/cahrons/faces/study/StudyPage.xhtml?globalId=hdl:1902.1/01921&studyListingIndex=0_c01786aa92e03667938b2b0f851f. Accessed October 28, 2011.

Ahrons, C.R. (2006). Long-term effects of divorce on children. *Family Therapy Magazine, 5*(1), 24–27.

Ahrons, C.R. (2007). Family ties after divorce: Long-term implications for children. *Family Process, 46*(1), 53–65.

Ahrons, C. (2011). Divorce: An unscheduled family transition. In M. McGoldrick, B. Carter, & N. Garcia-Preto (Eds.): *The Expanded Family Life Cycle: Individual, Family, and Social Perspectives* (4th ed.). Boston, MA: Allyn & Bacon, pp. 292–306.

Ahrons, C.R., & Rodgers, R.H. (1987). *Divorced Families: A Multidisciplinary Developmental View.* New York: Norton.

American Academy of Pediatrics. (2002). *Technical report: Coparent or second-parent adoption by same-sex parents.* www.aap.org/policy/020008t.html. Accessed October 28, 2011.

Anderson, C.M. (2003). The diversity, strengths, and challenges of single-parent households. In F. Walsh (Ed.): *Normal Family Processes: Growing Diversity and Complexity* (3rd ed.). New York: Guilford Press, pp. 121–152.

Ashton, D. (2011). Lesbian, gay, bisexual, and transgender individuals and the family life cycle. In M. McGoldrick, B. Carter, & N. Garcia-Preto (Eds.): *The Expanded Family Life Cycle: Individual, Family, and Social Perspectives* (4th ed.). Boston, MA: Allyn & Bacon, pp. 115–132.

Baum, N. (2003). Divorce process variables and the co-parental relationship and parental role fulfillment of divorced parents. *Family Process, 42*(1), 117–131.

Beardslee, W.R. (2002). *Out of the Darkened Room: When a Parent Is Depressed.* New York: Hachette Book Group.

Becvar, D.S. (2001). *In the Presence of Grief: Helping Family Members Resolve Death, Dying, and Bereavement Issues.* New York: Guilford Press.

Becvar, D.S. (2003). Introduction to the special section: Death, dying, and bereavement. *Journal of Marital and Family Therapy, 29*(4), 437–438.

Bell, J.M., & Wright, L.M. (2011). Creating practice knowledge for families experiencing illness suffering: The Illness Beliefs Model. In E. Svavarsdottir & H. Jonsdottir (Eds.): *Family nursing in Action.* Reykjavik, Iceland: University of Iceland Press, pp. 15–52.

Bellin, M.H., Bentley, K.J., & Sawin, K.J. (2009). Factors associated with the psychological and behavioural adjustment of siblings of youths with spina bifida. *Families, Systems & Health, 27*(1), 1–15.

Boss, P.G. (2002). Ambiguous loss: Working with families of the missing. *Family Process, 41*(1), 14–17.

Bowen, M. (1978). *Family Therapy in Clinical Practice.* Northvale, NJ: Jason Aronson.

Bowlby, J. (1977). The making and breaking of affectional bonds. *British Journal of Psychiatry, 130,* 201–210.

Bowse, B.P., et al. (2003). Death in the family and HIV risk-taking among intravenous drug users. *Family Process, 42*(2), 291–304.

Bramlett, M.D. (2011). *The national survey of adoptive parents: Benchmark estimates of school performance and family relationship quality for adopted children.* http://aspe. hhs.gov/hsp/09/NSAP/Brief3/rb.shtml#_Toc299603643. Accessed October 28, 2011.

Buchbinder, M., Longhofer, J., & McCue, K. (2009). Family routines and rituals when a parent has cancer. *Families, Systems & Health, 27*(3), 213–227.

Carter, B., & McGoldrick, M. (Eds.). (1988). *The Changing Family Life Cycle: A Framework for Family Therapy* (2nd ed.). New York: Gardner Press.

Carter, B., & McGoldrick, M. (1999a). The divorce cycle: A major variation in the American family life cycle. In B. Carter & M. McGoldrick (Eds.): *The Expanded Family Life Cycle: Individual, Family, and Social Perspectives* (3rd ed.). Boston: Allyn & Bacon, pp. 373–380.

Carter, B., & McGoldrick, M. (Eds.) (1999b). *The Expanded Family Life Cycle: Individual, Family, and Social Perspectives* (3rd ed.). Boston: Allyn & Bacon.

Carter, B., & McGoldrick, M. (1999c). Overview: The expanded family life cycle: Individual, family, and social perspectives. In B. Carter & M. McGoldrick (Eds.): *The Expanded Family Life Cycle: Individual, Family, and Social Perspectives* (3rd ed.). Boston: Allyn & Bacon, pp. 1–26.

Clark, P., Thigpen, S., & Yates, A.M. (2006). Integrating the older/special needs adoptive child into the family. *Journal of Marital and Family Therapy, 32*(2), 181–194.

Connolly, M. (2006). Up front and personal: Confronting dynamics in the family group conference. *Family Process, 45*(3), 345–357.

Cook, J.M., & Poulsen, S.S. (2011). Utilizing photographs with the genogram: A technique for enhancing couple therapy. *Journal of Systemic Therapies, 30*(1), 14–23.

Cousins, N. (1979). *Anatomy of an Illness as Perceived by the Patient: Reflections on Healing and Regeneration.* New York: Bantam Books.

Daily Almanac. (November 22, 2007). *Marriages and divorces, 1900–2005, U.S. statistics.* www.infoplease.com/ipa/A0005044.html. Accessed November 22, 2007.

DeJong, P., & Berg, I.K. (2008). *Interviewing for Solutions.* Belmont: Bantam Books.

Denham, S. (2011). Diabetes: A family matter. In E.K. Svaavarsdottir & H. Jonsdottir (Eds.): *Family Nursing in Action.* Reykjavik, Iceland: University of Iceland Press, pp. 309–332.

Duhamel, F., & Campagna, L. (2000). *Family genograph.* Montreal: Universite de Montreal, Faculty of Nursing. Available from www.familynursingresources.com.

Duhamel, F., & Dupuis, F. (2003). Families in palliative care: Exploring family and health-care professionals. *International Journal of Palliative Nursing, 9*(3), 113–119.

Duvall, E.R. (1977). *Marriage and Family Development* (5th ed.). Philadelphia: Lippincott.

Egan, J. (2002, March 24). The hidden lives of homeless children. *New York Times Magazine*, Section 6, 32–37, 58–59.

Elliott, D.B., & Simmons, T. (2011). *Marital events of Americans*: 2009. www.census.gov/prod/2011pubs/acs-13.pdf. Accessed October 28, 2011.

Epstein, H. (2003, October 12). Enough to make you sick? *New York Times Magazine*, Section 6, 75–81.

Epstein, N., Bishop, D., & Levin, S. (1978). The McMaster model of family functioning. *Journal of Marriage and Family Counseling, 4*, 19–31.

Epstein, N., Sigal, J., & Rakoff, V. (1968). *Family categories schema* [Unpublished manuscript]. Jewish General Hospital, Department of Psychiatry, Montreal.

Erickson, E. (1963). *Childhood and Society* (2nd ed.). New York: Norton.

Fekete, E.M., et al. (2007). Couples' support provision during illness: The role of perceived emotional responsiveness. *Families, Systems & Health, 25*(2), 204–217.

Fields, J., & Casper, L.M. (2001). *America's families and living arrangements: Population characteristics.* U.S. Dept. of Commerce. U.S. Census Bureau, P20–537.

Fulkerson, J.A., et al. (2007). Correlates of psychosocial well-being among overweight adolescents: The role of the family. *Journal of Consulting and Clinical Psychology, 75*(1), 181–186.

Ganong, L.H. (2011). *Who gets custody of Grandma after the divorce? How marital transitions affect family caregiving responsibilities.* Presentation at International Family Nursing Conference, Kyoto, Japan, June 27, 2011.

Gottman, J.M. & Notarius, C.I. (2002). Marital research in the 20th century and a research agenda for the 21st century. *Family Process, 24*(2), 159-197.

Greene, S.M., Anderson, E.R., Hetherington, E.M., Forgatch, M.S., & DeGarmo, D.S. (2003). Risk and resilience after divorce. In F. Walsh (Ed.): *Normal Family Processes. Growing Diversity and Complexity* (3rd ed.). New York: Guilford Press, pp. 96–120.

Haley, J. (1977). Toward a theory of pathological systems. In P. Watzlawick & J.H. Weakland (Eds.): *The Interactional View.* New York: Norton.

Hardy, K.V. (1990). Much more than techniques needed in treating minorities. *Family Therapy News.*

Hartman, A. (1978). Diagrammatic assessment of family relationships. *Social Casework, 59,* 465–476.

Hernandez, B.C., Schwenke, N.J., & Wilson, C.M. (2011). Spouses in mixed-orientation marriage: A 20-year review of empirical studies. *Journal of Marital and Family Therapy, 37*(3), 307–318.

Hiott, A., et al. (2006). Gender differences in anxiety and depression among immigrant Latinos. *Families, Systems & Health, 24*(2), 137–146.

Hoffman, L. (1981). *Foundations of Family Therapy.* New York: Basic Books.

Holtslander, L.F., Bally, J.M.G., & Steeves, M.L. (2011). Walking a fine line: An exploration of the experience of finding balance for older persons bereaved after caregiving for a spouse with advanced cancer. *European Journal of Oncology Nursing,* doi:10.1016/j.ejon.2010.12.004

Hougher Limacher, L., & Wright, L.M. (2006). Exploring the therapeutic family intervention of commendations: Insights from research. *Journal of Family Nursing, 12*(3), 307–331.

Humes, K.R., Jones, N.A., & Ramirez, R.R. (2011). *Overview of race and Hispanic origin: 2010.* 2010 Census Briefs. www.census.gov/prod/cen2010/briefs/c2010br-02.pdf. Accessed October 28, 2011.

James, I., Andershed, B., & Ternestedt, B-M. (2007). A family's beliefs about cancer, dying, and death in the end of life. *Journal of Family Nursing, 13*(2), 226–252.

Katie, B. (2003). *Loving What Is: Four Questions That Can Change Your Life.* New York: Three Rivers Press.

Kelly, J.B. (2007). Children's living arrangements following separation and divorce: Insights from empirical and clinical research. *Family Process, 46*(1), 35–52.

Kelly, K.P., & Ganong, L.H. (2011). "Shifting family boundaries" after the diagnosis of childhood cancer in stepfamilies. *Journal of Family Nursing, 17*(1), 105–132.

Kliman, J. (2011). Social class and the life cycle. In M. McGoldrick, B. Carter, & N. Garcia-Preto (Eds.): *The Expanded Family Life Cycle: Individual, Family, and Social Perspectives* (4th ed.). Boston, MA: Allyn & Bacon, pp. 75–88.

Levac, A.M.C., Wright, L.M., & Leahey, M. (2002). Children and families: Models for assessment and intervention. In J.A. Fox (Ed.): *Primary Health Care of Infants, Children, and Adolescents* (2nd ed.). St. Louis: Mosby, pp. 10–19.

Lewin, T. (2010, November 5). *Census finds single mothers and live-in partners. The New York Times.* www.nytimes.com/2010/11/06/us/06moms.html. Accessed October 28, 2011.

Limb, G.E., & Hodge, D.R. (2011). Utilizing spiritual ecograms with Native American families and children to promote cultural competence in family therapy. *Journal of Marital and Family Therapy, 37*(1), 81–94.

Linville, D., & Lyness, A.P. (2007). Twenty American families' stories of adaptation: Adoption of children from Russian and Romanian institutions. *Journal of Marital and Family Therapy, 33*(1), 77–93.

Livingston, G., & Parker, K. (2010). *Since the start of the great recession, more children raised by grandparents.* http://pewresearch.org/pubs/1724/sharp-increase-children-with-grandparent-caregivers. Accessed October 28, 2011.

Long, J.K., & Andrews, B.V. (2007). Fostering strength and resiliency in same-sex couples: An overview. *Journal of Couple and Relationship Therapy*, 6(1/2), 153–165.

Looman, W.S. (2011). Cross-cultural considerations for measurement in family nursing. In E.K. Svavarsdottir & H. Jonsdottir (Eds.), *Family Nursing in Action*. Reykjavik, Iceland: University of Iceland Press, pp. 85–114.

Marshall, A., Bell, J.M., & Moules, N.J. (2010). Beliefs, suffering, and healing: A clinical practice model for families experiencing mental illness. *Perspectives in Psychiatric Care*, 46(3), 182–196.

McGeorge, C., & Carlson, T.S. (2011). Deconstructing heterosexism: Becoming an LGB affirmative heterosexual couple and family therapist. *Journal of Marital and Family Therapy*, 37(1), 14–26.

McGoldrick, M. (2011a). *The Genogram Journey: Reconnecting With Your Family*. New York: W.W. Norton & Company.

McGoldrick, M. (2011b). Women and the family life cycle. In M. McGoldrick, B. Carter, & N. Garcia-Preto (Eds.): *The Expanded Family Life Cycle: Individual, Family, and Social Perspectives* (4th ed.). Boston, MA: Allyn & Bacon, pp. 42–58.

McGoldrick, M., & Carter, B. (2003). The family life cycle. In F. Walsh (Ed.): *Normal family processes: Growing Diversity and Complexity* (3rd. ed.). New York: Guilford Press, pp. 375–398.

McGoldrick, M. & Carter, B. (2011). Families transformed by the divorce cycle: Reconstituted, multinuclear, recoupled and remarried families. In M. McGoldrick, B. Carter, & N. Garcia-Preto (Eds.): *The Expanded Family Life Cycle: Individual, Family, and Social Perspectives* (4th ed.). Boston, MA: Allyn & Bacon, pp. 317–335.

McGoldrick, M., Carter, B., & Garcia-Preto, N. (Eds.). (2011a). *The Expanded Family Life Cycle: Individual, Family, and Social Perspectives*. Boston, MA: Allyn & Bacon.

McGoldrick, M., Carter, B., & Garcia-Preto, N. (2011b). Overview: The life cycle in its changing context. In M. McGoldrick, B. Carter, & N. Garcia-Preto (Eds.): *The Expanded Family Life Cycle: Individual, Family, and Social Perspectives* (4th ed.). Boston, MA: Allyn & Bacon, pp. 1–19.

McGoldrick, M., Gerson, R., & Petry, S. (2008). *Genograms: Assessment and Intervention* (3rd ed.). New York: WW Norton & Company.

Medina, A.M., Lederhos, C.L., & Lillis, T.A. (2009). Sleep disruption and decline in marital satisfaction across the transition to parenthood. *Families, Systems & Health*, 27(2), 153–160.

Miller, V.A. (2009). Parent-child collaborative decision making for the management of chronic illness: A qualitative analysis. *Families, Systems & Health*, 27(3), 249–266.

Minuchin, S. (1974). *Families and Family Therapy*. Cambridge, MA: Harvard University Press.

Mock, M.R. (2011). Men and the life cycle: Diversity and complexity. In M. McGoldrick, B. Carter, & N. Garcia-Preto (Eds.): *The Expanded Family Life Cycle: Individual, Family, and Social Perspectives* (4th ed.). Boston, MA: Allyn & Bacon, pp. 59–74.

Moules, N.J. (1998). Legitimizing grief: Challenging beliefs that constrain. *Journal of Family Nursing*, 4(2), 138–162.

Moules, N.J., Thirsk, L.M., & Bell, J.M. (2006). A Christmas without memories: Beliefs about grief and mothering—A clinical case analysis. *Journal of Family Nursing*, 12(4), 426–441.

National Survey of Adoptive Parents. (2007). http://aspe.hhs.gov/hsp/09/NSAP/index.shtml. Accessed October 28, 2011.

Neufeld, A., & Kushner, K.E. (2009). Men family caregivers' experience of nonsupportive interactions. *Journal of Family Nursing*, 15(2), 171–197.

Newman, S. (2011). *The Case for the Only Child*. Deerfield Beach, FL: Health Communications.

Nichols, W.C., Pace-Nichols, M., Becvar, D.S., & Napier, A.Y. (Eds.). (2000). *Handbook of Family Development and Intervention* (vol. 1). New York: John Wiley & Sons.

Nolan, K.W., Orlando, M., & Liptak, G.S. (2007). Care coordination services for children with special health care needs: Are we family-centered yet? *Families, Systems & Health, 25*(3), 293–306.

Parker, J.A., Mandleco, B., Roper, S.O., Freeborn, D., & Dyches, T.T. (2011). Religiosity, spirituality, and marital relationships of parents raising typically developing child or a child with a disability. *Journal of Family Nursing, 17*(1), 82–104.

Parker, K. (2011). *A portrait of stepfamilies*. http://www.pewsocialtrends.org/2011/01/13/a-portrait-of-stepfamilies/. Accessed October 28, 2011.

Parker-Pope, T. (2010, April 18). Is marriage good for your health? *New York Times, The Wellness Issue Magazine*, pp. 46–51.

Patrick, S., Garcia, J., & Griffin, L. (2010). The role of family therapy in mediating adverse effects of excessive and inconsolable neonatal crying on the family system. *Families, Systems & Health, 28*(1), 19–29.

Penn, M.J., & Zalesne, E.K. (2007). *Microtrends: The Small Forces Behind Tomorrow's Big Changes*. New York: Hachette Book Group.

Pew Research Center. (2011). *In a down economy, fewer births*. http://pewresearch.org/pubs/2115/births-fertility-rate-economy-recession. Accessed October 28, 2011.

Pew Social Trends Staff. (2010). *The return of the multi-generational family household*. www.pewsocialtrends.org/2010/03/18/the-return-of-the-multi-generational-family-household/. Accessed October 28, 2011.

Robinson, C.A. (1998). Women, families, chronic illness, and nursing interventions: From burden to balance. *Journal of Family Nursing, 4*(3), 271–290.

Rosenberg, T., & Shields, C.G. (2009). The role of parent-adolescent attachment in the glycemic control of adolescents with type 1 diabetes: A pilot study. *Families, Systems & Health, 27*(3), 237–248.

Samir, Y. (2002, October 27). I stand alone. *New York Times Magazine*, Section 6, 98. Frameworks for Practice. Geneva: International Council of Nurses.

Saulny, S. (2011, January 30). Black? White? Asian? More young Americans choose all of the above. *New York Times*, Section 1, 1, 20–21.

Sayre, J.B., McCollum, E.E., & Spring, E.L. (2010). An outsider in my own home: Attachment injury in stepcouple relationships. *Journal of Marital and Family Therapy, 36*(4), 403–415.

Schober, M., & Affara, F. (2001). *The Family Nurse: Frameworks for Practice*. Geneva: International Council of Nurses.

Selvini-Palazzoli, M., et al. (1980). Hypothesizing circularity-neutrality: Three guidelines for the conductor of the session. *Family Process, 19*(3), 3–12.

Shernoff, M. (2006). Negotiated monogamy and male couples. *Family Process, 45*(4), 407–418.

Sigurdardottir, A.O., & Sveinbjarnardottir, E.K. (2011). Family system nursing in Iceland: Follow up strategies to sustain FSN. Presentation at the 10th International Family Nursing Conference, June 25–27, 2011, Kyoto, Japan.

Stein, J.A., Rotheram-Borus, M., & Lester, P. (2007). Impact of parentification on long-term outcomes among children of parents with HIV/AIDS. *Family Process, 46*(3), 317–333.

Stephens, M.P., Rook, K.S., Franks, M.M., Khan, C., & Iida, M. (2010). Spouses use of social control to improve diabetic patients' dietary adherence. *Families, Systems & Health, 28*(3), 199–208.

Suarez-Orozco, C., Todorova, I.L., & Louie, J. (2002). Making up for lost time: The experience of separation and reunification among immigrant families. *Family Process, 41*(4), 625–643.

Toman, W. (1993). *Family Constellation: Its Effects on Personality and Social Behavior* (4th ed.). New York: Springer.

Tomm, K. (1977). *Tripartite family assessment* [Unpublished manuscript]. University of Calgary, Alberta.

Tomm, K. (1980). Towards a cybernetic-systems approach to family therapy at the University of Calgary. In D.S. Freeman (Ed.): *Perspectives on Family Therapy*. Toronto: Butterworths, pp. 3–18.

Tomm, K., & Sanders, G. (1983). Family assessment in a problem oriented record. In J.C. Hansen & B.F. Keeney (Eds.): *Diagnosis and Assessment in Family Therapy*. London: Aspen Systems Corporation, pp. 101–122.

United States Census Bureau. (2010a). Census Bureau News—*America's families and living arrangements*. www.prnewswire.com/news-releases/census-bureau-news-americas-families-and-living-arrangements-2010-107041258.html. Accessed October 28, 2011.

United States Census Bureau. (2010b). *Nation's foreign-born population nears 37 million*. www.census.gov/newsroom/releases/archives/foreignborn_population/cb10-159.html. Accessed October 28, 2011.

USA Today. (2003, August 5). Gay marriage debate clouds real issue of equal treatment. *USA Today*, p. 10A.

Visher, E.B., Visher, J.S., & Pasley, K. (2003). Remarriage families and stepparenting. In F. Walsh (Ed.): *Normal Family Processes: Growing Diversity and Complexity* (3rd ed.). New York: Guilford Press, pp. 153–175.

Walsh, F. (2011). Families in later life: Challenges, opportunities and resilience. In M. McGoldrick, B. Carter, & N. Garcia-Preto (Eds.): *The Expanded Family Life Cycle: Individual, Family, and Social Perspectives* (4th ed.). Boston, MA: Allyn & Bacon, pp. 261–277.

Wang, W., & Taylor, P. (2011). *For millennials, parenthood trumps marriage*. www.pewsocialtrends.org/2011/03/09/for-millennials-parenthood-trumps-marriage/. Accessed October 28, 2011.

Watson, W.L., & Lee, D. (1993). Is there life after suicide? The systemic belief approach for "survivors" of suicide. *Archives of Psychiatric Nursing, 7*(1), 37–43.

Watzlawick, P., Beavin, J.H., & Jackson, D.D. (1967). *Pragmatics of Human Communication: A Study of Interactional Patterns, Pathologies, and Paradoxes*. New York: Norton.

Weber, S. (2010). A stigma identification framework for family nurses working with parents who are lesbian, gay, bisexual, or transgendered and their families. *Journal of Family Nursing, 16*(4), 378–393.

West, C.H. (2011). Addressing illness suffering in childhood cancer: Exploring the beliefs of family members in therapeutic nursing conversations. Unpublished doctoral thesis, University of Calgary, Alberta, Canada.

Westley, W.A., & Epstein, N.B. (1969). *The Silent Majority: Families of Emotionally Healthy College Students*. San Francisco: Jossey-Bass.

White, C.P., White, M.B., & Fox, M.A. (2009). Maternal fatigue and its relationship to the caregiving environment. *Families, Systems & Health, 27*(4), 325–345.

Wright, L.M. (2005). *Spirituality, Suffering, and Illness: Ideas for Healing*. Philadelphia: F.A. Davis.

Wright, L.M., & Bell, J.M. (2009). *Beliefs and Illness: A Model for Healing*. Calgary, AB: 4th Floor Press.

Wright, L.M. & Leahey, M. (2001). Calgary Family Assessment Model: How to Apply in Clinical Practice. DVD available at www.familynursingresources.com

Wright, L.M., & Nagy, J. (1993). Death: The most troublesome family secret of all. In E. Imber-Black (Ed.): *Secrets in Families and Family Therapy*. New York: Norton, pp. 121–137.

Wright, L.M., & Simpson, P. (1991). A systemic belief approach to epileptic seizures: A case of being spellbound. *Contemporary Family Therapy: An International Journal, 13*(2), 165–180.

Chapter **4**

The Calgary Family
Intervention Model

The Calgary Family Intervention Model (CFIM) is a companion to the Calgary Family Assessment Model (CFAM; see Chapter 3). To our knowledge, the CFIM is the first family intervention model to emerge within nursing. The importance and effectiveness of family interventions in health care in the treatment of physical illness is receiving much more recognition in the last few years (Campbell, 2003; Chesla, 2010). In addition, the focus of health-care providers has shifted from deficit- or dysfunction-based family assessments to strengths- and resiliency-based family interventions. For example, the McGill Model of Nursing states that one of its goals is to "help families use the strengths of the individual family members and of the family as a unit, as well as resources external to the family system" (Feeley & Gottlieb, 2000, p. 11). Another example is Rungreangkulkij and Gilliss's (2000) use of the Family Resiliency Model for the study of families that have a member with a severe and persistent mental illness.

The CFIM is a strengths- and resiliency-based model. We believe that this type of shift in emphasis from deficits and dysfunction to strengths and resiliency in family nursing practice greatly influences the types of interventions offered to and chosen by families within our model. It is heartening to note that Gottlieb (2012) has devoted an entire book to the importance of focusing on strengths in nursing care.

Of course, the interventions offered should depend on the nurse's scope of practice, degree of independence, autonomy, and responsibility associated with his or her role in family care (Schober & Affara, 2001). Nursing care may range from "delegated tasks such as wound care in the home, to complex assessment and curative management in health centres and clinics" (Schober & Affara, 2001, p. 23).

This chapter presents our definition and description of the CFIM, examples of interventions in three domains of family functioning, and actual clinical examples using the CFIM. This chapter concludes with intervention ideas for family situations that nurses commonly encounter.

DEFINITION AND DESCRIPTION

If a comprehensive family assessment has been completed and family intervention is indicated, a nurse must then consider how to intervene to facilitate change. The CFIM is an organizing framework for conceptualizing the intersection between a particular domain of family functioning and the specific intervention offered by the nurse (Fig. 4–1). The elements of the CFIM are interventions, domains of family functioning, and "fit" or meshing (i.e., effectiveness). The CFIM visually portrays the fit or meshing between a domain of family functioning and a nursing intervention—that is, it answers the questions, In what domain of family functioning does this intervention intend a change? Is it a fit for this family? The CFIM focuses on promoting, improving, and sustaining effective family functioning in three domains or areas: cognitive, affective, and behavioral.

Interventions can be designed to promote, improve, or sustain family functioning in any or all of the three domains, but a change in one area can affect the other domains. We believe that the most profound and sustaining changes are the ones that occur within the family's beliefs (cognition) (Bell & Wright, 2011; Wright & Bell, 2009). In other words, as a family thinks, so it *is*. In many cases, one intervention can actually simultaneously influence all three domains of family functioning.

We believe that nurses can only offer interventions to the family within a relational stance; they cannot instruct, direct, demand, or insist on a particular kind of change or way of family functioning. Such directive practices by nurses do not result in satisfying family/nurse relationships for either the nurse or the family nor in beneficial outcomes. Families are more open to the ideas offered by a nurse when it is in the context of collaborative interaction (e.g., inviting, asking, encouraging, supporting) rather than instructive interaction (e.g., instructing, directing, lecturing, demanding).

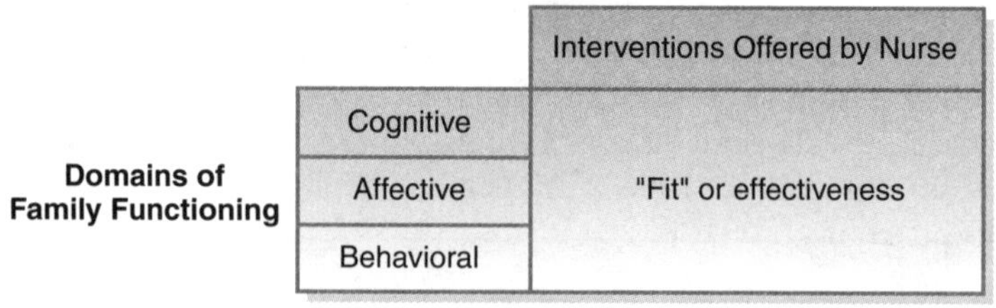

	Interventions Offered by Nurse
Cognitive	
Domains of Family Functioning — Affective	"Fit" or effectiveness
Behavioral	

FIGURE 4-1: CFIM: Intersection of domains of family functioning and interventions.

Whether the family is open to an intervention also depends on its genetic makeup and the family's history of interactions among family members and between family members and health professionals (Maturana & Varela, 1992). Openness to certain interventions is also profoundly influenced by the relationship between the nurse and the family (Bohn, Wright, & Moules, 2003; Duhamel & Talbot, 2004; Houger Limacher & Wright, 2003, 2006; Leahey & Harper-Jaques, 1996; Legrow & Rossen, 2005; McLeod & Wright, 2008; Moules, 2002; Moules, et al, 2004, 2007; Robinson & Wright, 1995; Sveinbjarnardottir, Svavarsdottir, & Saveman, 2011; Tapp, 2001; Thorne & Robinson, 1989) and the nurse's ability to help the family reflect on their health problems (Bell & Wright, 2011; Wright & Bell, 2009; Wright & Levac, 1992). Second-order cybernetics and the biology of cognition (Maturana & Varela, 1992) have influenced our ideas in this area (see Chapter 2).

Intervening in a family system in a manner that promotes or facilitates change and healing is the most challenging and exciting aspect of clinical work with families. The intervention process represents the core of clinical practice with families. It provides an appropriate context in which the family can make necessary changes that enhance the possibilities of healing. Myriad interventions are possible, but nurses need to tailor their interventions to each family and to the chosen domain of family functioning.

An awareness of ethical considerations is necessary. Specific interventions usually vary for each family, although in some instances the same intervention may be used for several families and for different problems. We wish to emphasize, however, that each family is unique and that, although labeling particular interventions is an important part of putting our practice into language, it does not represent a "cookbook" approach. We also wish to emphasize that the interventions we list are examples of interventions that can be used; they are not intended to be all-inclusive. We provide examples of interventions that we have found from our clinical practice and research (Shields, et al, 2012) to be very useful. The interventions that we cite are based on several important theoretical foundations: postmodernism, systems theory, cybernetics, communication theory, change theory, and biology of cognition (see Chapter 2).

In summary, the CFIM is not a list of family functions or a list of nursing interventions. Rather, it provides a means to conceptualize a fit or meshing between domains or areas of family functioning and selected interventions offered by the nurse. The CFIM assists in determining the domain of family functioning that predominantly needs changing, usually where there is the greatest suffering, and the most useful interventions to effect change in that domain. Through therapeutic conversations, the family and nurse collaborate and coevolve to discover the most useful fit (Bell & Wright, 2011; Duhamel & Dupuis, 2004; Holtslander, 2005; McLeod & Wright, 2008; Moules, et al, 2004, 2007, 2009; Wright & Bell, 2009).

We use the qualitative terms *fit* or *meshing* to emphasize whether or not the interventions effect change and/or soften suffering in the presenting problem. *Fit* involves recognizing reciprocity between the nurse's ideas and opinions and the family's illness experience. Therefore, determining fit or meshing may involve some experimentation or trial and error. It also entails a belief by nurses that each family is unique and has particular strengths. In Chapter 7, we outline techniques for enhancing the likelihood that interventions will stimulate change in the desired domain of family functioning.

INTERVENTIVE QUESTIONS

One of the simplest but most powerful nursing interventions for families experiencing health problems is the use of interventive questions. These questions are intended to actively effect change in any or all of the three domains. However, nurses conducting family interviews should remember that knowing when, how, and why to pose questions is more important than simply choosing one type of question over another (Wright & Bell, 2009).

Linear Versus Circular Questions

Interventive questions are usually of two types: linear and circular (Tomm, 1987, 1988). The important difference between these kinds of questions is their intent. Linear questions are meant to inform the nurse, whereas circular questions are meant to effect change (Tomm, 1985, 1987, 1988).

Linear questions are investigative; they explore a family member's descriptions or perceptions of a problem. For example, when exploring parents' perceptions of their daughter Cheyenne's anorexia nervosa, the nurse could begin with linear questions, such as, "When did you notice that your daughter had changed her eating habits?" or "What do you think caused your daughter to stop eating as she normally would?" These linear questions inform the nurse of the history of the young woman's eating patterns and help illuminate family perceptions or beliefs about eating patterns. Linear questions are frequently used to begin gathering information about families' problems, whereas circular questions reveal families' understanding of problems.

Circular questions aim to reveal explanations of problems. For example, with the same family, the nurse could ask, "Who in the family is most worried about Cheyenne's anorexia?" or "How does Mother show that she is the one who worries the most?" Circular questions help the nurse to discover valuable information, because they seek out information about relationships between individuals, events, ideas, or beliefs.

The effect of these different question types on families is quite distinct. Linear questions tend to limit any further understanding, whereas circular questions are generative and open possibilities for new understandings. Circular questions introduce new cognitive connections or a change in the illness beliefs of families, paving the way for new or different family behaviors. Linear questioning implies that the nurse knows what is best for the family and is therefore operating under the "sin of certainty" or objectivity without parentheses (Maturana & Varela, 1992) (see Chapter 2). It also implies that the nurse has become purposive and invested in a particular outcome. Linear questions are intended to correct behavior; circular questions are intended to facilitate behavioral change.

The primary distinction between circular and linear questions lies in the notion that information reveals differences in relationships (Bateson, 1979). With circular questions, a relationship or connection between individuals, events, ideas, or beliefs is always sought and in a context of compassion and curiosity. With linear questions, the focus is on cause and effect. The idea of circular questions evolved from the concept of circularity, and the method of circular interviewing developed by the originators of Milan Systemic Family Therapy (Selvini-Palazzoli, et al, 1980; Tomm, 1984, 1985, 1987) (see Chapters 6, 7, 8, and 10).

Circularity involves the cycle of questions and answers between families and nurses that occurs during the interview process. The nurse's skillful questions are based on thoughtful assessment, conceptualization, and hypotheses that can foster understanding and that can obtain information the family gives in response to the questions the nurse asks, and thus the cycle continues. The family's responses to questions provide information for the nurse and the family. The nurse is not an outside interpreter or narrator in this process but rather a participant in the relationship and interaction (Keeney & Keeney, 2012). Questions in and of themselves can also provide new information and answers for the family, and so they become interventions. Interventive questions may encourage family members to perceive their problems in a new way, which softens their suffering and allows them to see new solutions. Thus, as the family's answers provide information for the nurse, the nurse's questions may provide information for the family.

Circular questions have various applications in family nursing. Loos and Bell (1990) creatively applied the use of circular questions to critical care nursing. Wright and Bell (2009) demonstrated the therapeutic aspect of circular questions with families experiencing chronic illness, life-threatening illness, and psychosocial problems. Utilizing the CFIM, Duhamel and Talbot (2004) found that nurses considered interventive questioning useful because it stimulated discussion on specific topics: "One of the questions was formulated as 'What were the most significant changes that occurred in the family since the onset of the illness?' This question led to the identification of efforts made by the couples to comply with medical recommendations, and of their progress in the rehabilitation process" (p. 23).

Tomm (1987) embellished the types of circular questions used by the Milan Systemic Family Therapy team and identified, defined, and classified various circular questions. The ones we have found most useful in relational clinical practice with families are difference questions, behavioral-effect questions, and hypothetical or future-oriented questions. We have expanded the use of circular questions by providing examples of questions that can be asked to intervene in the cognitive, affective, and behavioral domains of family functioning (Box 4–1).

Box 4-1 Circular Questions to Invite Change in Cognitive, Affective, and Behavioral Domains of Family Functioning

1. Type: Difference Question
Definition: Explores differences between people, relationships, time, ideas, or beliefs.
Examples of intervening in three domains of family functioning:

Cognitive	Affective	Behavioral
• What is the best advice that you have received about managing your son's AIDS? • What is the worst advice? • What information would be most helpful to you about managing the effects of sexual abuse? • Who in the family would benefit most from the information?	• Who in the family is most worried about how AIDS is transmitted? • Who finds your disclosure of sexual abuse most difficult?	• Who in the family is best at getting your son to take his medication on time? • When you first disclosed your sexual abuse, what actions by professionals were most helpful?

2. Type: Behavioral-Effect Question
Definition: Explores the effect of one family member's behavior on another. Examples of intervening in three domains of family functioning:

Cognitive	*Affective*	*Behavioral*
• How do you make sense of your husband not visiting your son in the hospital? • What do you know about the effect of life-threatening illness on children?	• What do you feel when you see your son crying after his treatments? • How does your mother show that she is afraid of dying?	• What do you do when your husband does not visit your son in the hospital? • What could your father do to indicate to your mother that he understands her fears?

3. Type: Hypothetical/Future-Oriented Question
Definition: Explores family options and alternative actions or meanings in the future.
Examples of intervening in three domains of family functioning:

Cognitive	Affective	Behavioral
• What do you think will happen if these skin grafts continue to be so painful for your son? • If the worst occurs, how do you think your family will cope? • If you decide to have your grandmother institutionalized, with whom would you discuss the decision?	• If your son's skin grafts are not successful, what do you think his mood will be? Sad? Angry? Resigned? • If your grandmother's treatment does not go well, who will be most affected?	• How much longer do you think it will be before your son engages in treatment for his contractures? • How long do you think your grandmother will have to remain in the hospital? • If she stays longer, what new self-care behaviors will she be doing?

We have also produced a DVD to demonstrate the use of questions in actual clinical practice as part of the "How to" Family Nursing Series. It is titled *How to Use Questions in Family Interviewing* (Wright & Leahey, 2006). This educational program demonstrates the use of interventive questions in actual clinical interviews. To learn more about this DVD or to view a sample video vignette, visit Family Nursing Resources at www.familynursingresources.com.

In summary, difference questions, behavioral-effect questions, and hypothetical questions can be used to facilitate change in any or all of the domains of family functioning. Figure 4–2 illustrates the intersection of various types of circular questions and the domains of family functioning. We wish to strongly emphasize that the effectiveness, usefulness, and fit of the question, rather than the specific question itself, are most critical in effecting change.

Other Examples of Interventions

To illustrate the intersection of the three domains or areas of family functioning (cognitive, affective, and behavioral) and various interventions, we have chosen a few examples of interventions that can be used in addition to circular questions. This list is not exhaustive; rather, it is a selection of interventions that we have found useful and effective in our clinical practice and research. Examples include:

- Commending family and individual strengths
- Offering information and opinions
- Validating, acknowledging, or normalizing emotional responses
- Encouraging the telling of illness narratives
- Drawing forth family support
- Encouraging family members to be caregivers and offering caregiver support
- Encouraging respite
- Devising rituals

		Interventions Offered by Nurse: Circular Questions			
		Difference	Behavioral Effect	Hypothetical	Triadic
Domains of Family Functioning	Cognitive				
	Affective				
	Behavioral				

FIGURE 4-2: Intersection of circular questions and domains of family functioning.

These interventions can influence change in any or all of the domains of family functioning. For example, the nurse can offer information to promote change in cognitive, affective, or behavioral family functioning (Fig. 4–3).

The following section describes each intervention and offers a case example illustrating its application. We have chosen to cluster the sample interventions around a particular domain of family functioning. However, we do not wish to imply that one intervention can be used to facilitate change in only one domain of family functioning or that one intervention is a "cognitive intervention" and another an "affective intervention." Rather, these are examples of the fit between a specific problem or illness, a particular intervention, and a domain of family functioning.

INTERVENTIONS TO CHANGE THE COGNITIVE DOMAIN OF FAMILY FUNCTIONING

Interventions directed at the cognitive domain of family functioning usually offer new ideas, opinions, beliefs, information, or education on a particular health problem or risk. The treatment goal or desired outcome is to change the way in which a family perceives its health problems so that members can discover new solutions to these problems. The following interventions are examples of ways to change the cognitive domain of family functioning.

Commending Family and Individual Strengths

We routinely commend family and individual strengths, competencies, and resources observed during interviews. Commendations differ from compliments and are instead an observation of *patterns* of behavior that occur across time (e.g., "Your family members are very loyal to one another"), whereas a compliment is usually an observation of a one-time event (e.g., "You were very praising of your son today"). Families coping with chronic, life-threatening, or psychosocial problems commonly feel defeated, hopeless, or unsuccessful in their efforts to overcome or live with these problems. In many cases, families coping with health problems have not been commended

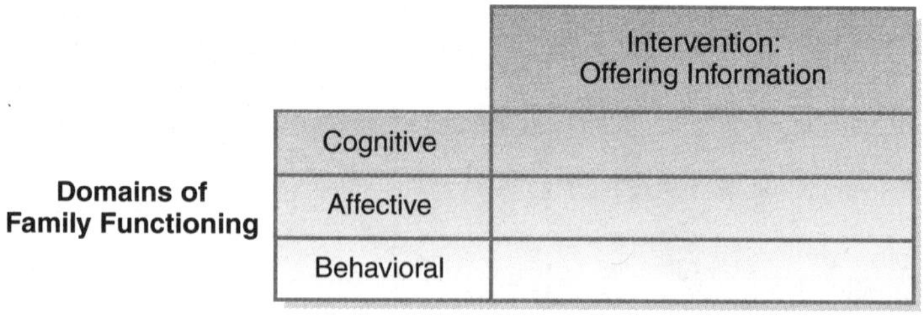

		Intervention: Offering Information
Domains of Family Functioning	Cognitive	
	Affective	
	Behavioral	

FIGURE 4-3: Intersection of intervention (offering information) and domains of family functioning.

for their strengths or made aware of them (McElheran & Harper-Jaques, 1994). We choose to emphasize strengths and resilience rather than deficits, dysfunctions, and deficiencies in family members.

Immediate and long-term positive reactions to commendations indicate that they are effective therapeutic interventions (Bohn, Wright, & Moules, 2003; Houger Limacher, 2008; Houger Limacher & Wright, 2003, 2006; McLeod & Wright, 2008; Moules, 2002, 2009; Moules & Johnstone, 2010; Wright & Bell, 2009). Robinson (1998) offers further credence to this belief with her study that explored the processes and outcomes of nursing interventions with families suffering from chronic illness. The families in this study reported the clinical nursing team's "orientation to strengths, resources, and possibilities to be an extremely important facet of the process" (Robinson, 1998, p. 284). Focusing on strengths was most significant and influential for the women in these families. In addition, families who internalize commendations offered by nurses appear more receptive to other therapeutic interventions that are offered.

Another fluent and moving piece of research focused on the commendation interventions offered in practice at the Family Nursing Unit of the University of Calgary. Both families and nurses reported and reiterated the value and power of commendations that brought forth "goodness" that helped soften suffering (Houger Limacher, 2008; Houger Limacher & Wright, 2003, 2006). This bringing forth of "goodness" becomes a relational phenomenon in the context of the nurse-patient and nurse-family relationship. The routine practice by nurses of commending family and individual strengths is a particular way of being in clinical practice. This notion is best exemplified in the following quote: "We become our conversations and we generate the conversations that we become" (Maturana & Varela, 1992).

In one family, an adopted son's behavioral and emotional problems had kept the family involved with health-care professionals for 10 years. The nurse commended this family by telling them that she believed they were the best family for this boy because many other families would not have been as sensitive to his needs and probably would have given up years ago. Both parents became tearful and said that this was the first positive statement made to them as parents in many years.

By commending a family's competence, resilience, and strengths and offering them a new opinion or view of themselves, a context for change is created that allows families to then discover their own solutions to problems and enhance healing. Offering commendations is a skill that both nonprofessionals and professionals can hone. Hughes, Kay-Raining Bird, and Sommerfeld (2011) found that parents reported peer home visitors were better able to celebrate and enable families after training. Changing the view families have of themselves frequently enables families to view the health problem differently and thus move toward solutions that are more effective. Box 4–2 suggests helpful hints for offering interventions.

Box 4-2 Helpful Hints for Offering Commendations

• Be a "family strengths" detective and look for opportunities to commend families when strengths are discovered and uncovered.
• Ensure that sufficient evidence for the commendation is present; otherwise it may sound insincere and overly ingratiating.
• Use the family's language and integrate important family beliefs to strengthen the validity of the commendation.
• Offer commendations within the first 10 minutes of meeting with a family to enhance the practitioner–family relationship and to increase family receptivity to later ideas.
• Routinely include commendations to families at the end of an interaction or meeting and before offering an opinion.

From Levac, A.M., Wright, L.M., & Leahey, M. (2002). Children and families: Models for assessment and intervention. In J. Fox (Ed.): *Primary Health Care of Infants, Children, and Adolescents* (2nd ed.). St. Louis: Mosby, p. 13. Reprinted by permission.

Offering Information and Opinions

The offering of information and opinions from health-care professionals is one of the most significant needs for families experiencing illness, especially if the illness is complex. The core utility of access to information, skill building, problem solving, and social support cannot be overestimated (Lucksted, McFarlane, Downing, et al, 2012). Families most desire information about developmental issues, health promotion, and illness management (Levac, Wright, & Leahey, 2002; Robinson, 1998). For example, helping parents to understand and help their children is a common but important intervention for families (Levac, Wright, & Leahey, 2002). Nurses can teach families about normal physiological, emotional, and cognitive characteristics and can identify developmental tasks or goals of children and adolescents that can be affected or altered during times of illness (Manassis & Levac, 2004). One family found it useful when the nurse explained that siblings of children experiencing life-shortening illnesses commonly develop symptoms due to feeling lonely because parents are intently focused on their ill child. Box 4–3 suggests helpful hints for offering information and opinions.

Families with a hospitalized member have indicated that obtaining information is a high priority. Many families have expressed to us their frustration at their inability to readily obtain information or opinions from health-care professionals. Nurses can offer information about the impact of chronic or life-shortening illnesses on families. They can also empower families to obtain information about resources. We have learned that this latter approach is even more useful in some circumstances. Offering educational information is an "essential intervention as it reassured family members about certain aspects of the illness and reduced their level of stress" (Duhamel & Talbot, 2004, p. 24).

One complex clinical example concerns a family of two aging parents and their 34-year-old son, who had severe multiple sclerosis. The parents were

---

Box 4-3 Helpful Hints for Offering Information and Opinions

- Use language that is relevant, clear, and specific.
- Provide easy-to-read literature; write out key points on a small card.
- Inform families of community support groups and resources. Determine if these resources have been helpful to families who have used them and how.
- Build on family abilities by encouraging family members to independently seek resources. Inquire about the family's reaction after seeking resources.
- Offer ideas, information, and reflections in a spirit of learning and wondering (e.g., "I wonder what would happen if you tried a slightly different approach to talking with Manisha about sex and birth control. Perhaps you might . . .").
- Do not be invested in the outcome. If the family does not apply the teaching materials, be curious about what did not fit for them rather than becoming judgmental and angry with them.

From Levac, A.M.C., Wright, L.M., & Leahey, M. (2002). Children and families: Models for assessment and intervention. In J. Fox (Ed.): *Primary Health Care of Infants, Children, and Adolescents* (2nd ed.). St. Louis: Mosby, p. 13. Reprinted by permission.

constant, devoted caregivers but had not had any respite for several months. The nurse asked the son if he would be willing to challenge his beliefs about his "helplessness." The nurse asked him to take the leadership role in exploring possible resources for caregivers so that his parents could have a vacation. Because of his search, the son discovered that he was eligible for many financial benefits of which he had previously been unaware, including benefits to hire professional caregivers. Shortly afterward, the son arranged for 24-hour in-home nursing care when his parents took a vacation. His parents reported that they felt much less stressed and that their son was much happier. He began making efforts to walk using parallel bars, which he had not done in several months.

In this case example, the nurse offered an opinion that empowered the son to change his cognitive set. The intervention fit the cognitive domain, and results took place in the affective and behavioral domains of family functioning.

INTERVENTIONS TO CHANGE THE AFFECTIVE DOMAIN OF FAMILY FUNCTIONING

Interventions aimed at the affective domain of family functioning are designed to reduce or increase intense emotions that may be blocking families' problem-solving efforts. The following interventions are examples of ways to change the affective domain of family functioning.

Validating, Acknowledging, or Normalizing Emotional Responses

Validation or acknowledgment of intense affect can reduce or cushion feelings of isolation and loneliness, soften suffering, and help family members to make the connection between a family member's illness and their emotional response (Wright, 2008). For example, after diagnosis of a life-shortening illness, families frequently feel out of control or frightened for a period. It is important for nurses to acknowledge these strong emotions and to reassure and offer hope to families that in time they will adjust and learn new ways to cope. In one clinical example, the nurse normalized changes in sexuality following a couple's experience with a cardiac condition. As a result, the wife reported, "I felt that the question regarding our sexuality was well put, because [the nurse] applied it to couples in general. The fact that others are going through the same experience, well I thought it was good to know. It is a very personal and private question, and you presented it well" (Duhamel & Talbot, 2004, p. 25).

Encouraging the Telling of Illness Narratives

Too often, family members are encouraged to tell only the medical story or narrative of their illness rather than the story of their own unique experience of their illness, or *illness narrative*. However, when nurses encourage family members to tell their illness narratives, not only are stories of sickness and suffering told but also stories of strength and tenacity (Wright & Bell, 2009). Through therapeutic conversations, nurses can create a trusting environment for open expression of family members' fears, anger, and sadness about their illness experience (Tapp, 2001; Wright & Bell, 2009).

These conversations are particularly important for complex family types involving multiple parents and siblings. Having an opportunity to express the illness's impact on the family and the influence of the family on the illness from each family member's perspective validates their experiences. Duhamel and Talbot's (2004) study, which utilized the CFIM and this particular intervention, found that nurses agreed about the importance of encouraging family members to share their experiences of cardiac illness during and after the hospitalization period. Also, family members commented that through these types of clinical sessions, they were able to vent emotions, which provided tremendous relief from suffering, healed psychological wounds, and enabled family members to acknowledge one another's experiences.

Listening to, witnessing, and documenting illness stories can also have a profound impact on the nurse. This approach is very different from limiting or constraining family stories to symptoms, medication use, and physical treatments. By providing a context for family members to share the illness experience, nurses allow intense emotions to be legitimized.

Drawing Forth Family Support

Nurses can enhance family functioning in the affective domain by encouraging and helping family members to listen to each other's concerns and feelings. This technique can be particularly useful if a family member is embracing some constraining beliefs when a loved one is dying or has died (Moules, et al, 2004,

2007; Moules, Thirsk, & Bell, 2006; Wright & Nagy, 1993). By fostering opportunities for family members to express feelings about this painful experience, the nurse can enable them to draw forth their own strengths and resources to support one another. The nurse can be the catalyst that facilitates communication between family members or between the family and other health-care professionals. This type of family support can prevent families from becoming unduly burdened or defeated by an illness. Intervening in this manner is especially important in primary health-care settings.

INTERVENTIONS TO CHANGE THE BEHAVIORAL DOMAIN OF FAMILY FUNCTIONING

Interventions directed at the behavioral domain help family members to interact with and behave differently in relation to one another. This change is most often accomplished by inviting some or all the family members to engage in specific behavioral tasks. Some tasks are given during a family meeting so that the nurse can observe the interaction; other tasks or homework assignments are given for family members to complete between sessions. In some cases, the nurse must review with the family the details of the particular task or experiment in order to verify that the family understands what has been suggested. The following interventions are examples of ways to change the behavioral domain of family functioning.

Encouraging Family Members to Be Caregivers and Offering Caregiver Support

Family members are often timid or afraid to become involved in the care of their ill family member unless a nurse supports them. However, in our experience, we have found that family members greatly appreciate opportunities to help their hospitalized family member. They report that it makes them feel less helpless, anxious, and out of control. Of course, family caregivers are also susceptible to the well-known phenomenon of caregiver burden. Health professionals must be alert to the risks involved in family caregiving and be willing to intervene when necessary by offering caregiver support, which means providing the necessary information, advocacy, and support to facilitate patient care by people other than health-care professionals (Ducharme, 2011). In an informative study about grandparents' experience of childhood cancer, grandparents revealed their often unattended and unacknowledged role of both providing and needing support (Moules, et al, 2012). Therefore, these authors recommended that an inquiry regarding the resources and support needs of grandparents is essential for optimal family care. LeNavenec and Vonhof (1996) offer the notion of "one day at a time" as a useful coping strategy for families with a member experiencing dementia. We encourage nurses to weigh with family members the ethical, emotional, and physical balance between too much caregiving and not enough caregiving.

Encouraging Respite

Family caregivers commonly do not allow themselves adequate respite. Too frequently, family members feel guilty if they need or want to withdraw themselves from the caregiving role, especially female caregivers. Even the ill member must occasionally disengage himself or herself from the usual caregiving and reject another person's assistance. Each family's need for respite varies. Factors affecting respite include the severity of the chronic illness, availability of family members to care for the ill person, and financial resources. All of these issues must be considered before a nurse can recommend a respite schedule. Caregiving, coping, and caring for one's own health need to be balanced. For example, one way to balance needs is to recommend that a family buy a less expensive prosthesis and use the extra money for a family vacation. Another example of encouraging respite is to recommend that a mother and father with a leukemic child have the grandparents babysit for a day while the couple spends time together. Such "time-outs" or "times away" are essential for families facing excessive caregiving demands.

Devising Rituals

Families engage in many types of rituals: daily (e.g., bedtime reading), yearly (e.g., Thanksgiving dinner at Grandma's), and cultural (e.g., ethnic parades). Nurses can suggest therapeutic rituals that are not or have not been observed by the family. Roberts (2003a) defines rituals as:

> co-evolved symbolic acts that include not only the ceremonial aspects of the actual presentation of the ritual, but the process of preparing for it as well. It may or may not include words, but does have both open and closed parts which are "held" together by a guiding metaphor. Repetition can be a part of rituals through the content, the form, or the occasion. There should be enough space in therapeutic rituals for the incorporation of multiple meanings by various family members and clinicians, as well as a variety of levels of participation (p. 9).

Nurses are also contributing to the literature about rituals, as evidenced by a very comprehensive piece about rituals, routines, recreation, and rules by Fomby (2004). She emphasizes the use of family rituals for health promotion and claims the following benefits: cohesiveness among family members, a sense of family pride, continuity, understanding, closeness, and love.

In our clinical practice, we have observed that chronic illness and psychosocial problems frequently interrupt the usual rituals. Roberts (2003b) offers a poignant narrative of her experience with cancer and describes how rituals can "mark the path" of healing when a devastating illness emerges. Rituals are best introduced when there is an excessive level of confusion, and they can provide clarity in a family system. Designing and implementing rituals for new life-cycle transitions can be a helpful intervention offered by the nurse. Imber-Black (2010) suggests "since rituals have the capacity to hold and express differences rather than homogenize them, they are particularly powerful resources for any life cycle transition that differs from the conventional" (p. 439). For example, parents in a new stepfamily who cannot agree on parenting practices commonly give conflicting messages to their families. This can result in chaos and confusion for their children. The introduction of an odd-day/even-day ritual (Selvini-Palazzoli, et al, 1978) can typically assist the family. The mother could experiment with being responsible for the children on Mondays, Wednesdays, and Fridays and the father on Tuesdays, Thursdays, and Saturdays. On Sundays, they could behave spontaneously. On their "days off," parents could be asked to observe, without comment, their partner's parenting.

Another of our educational DVD programs that has been useful to assist nurses in offering interventions is titled *How to Intervene With Families With Health Problems* (Wright & Leahey, 2003). This educational program demonstrates the use of particular interventions in actual clinical interviews. To learn more about this DVD or to view a sample video vignette, go to Family Nursing Resources at www.familynursingresources.com.

CLINICAL EXAMPLES

The following clinical examples illustrate the use of the CFIM. In these real-life examples, interventions were chosen to facilitate change in all three domains (cognitive, affective, and behavioral) of family functioning. Remember, it is not always necessary or efficient to try to "fit" interventions to all three domains of family functioning simultaneously. Whether this can be done successfully depends on how well the family is engaged and on prior assessment of the nature of the illness, problems, or concerns.

Clinical Example 1: Difficulty Putting 3-Year-Old Child to Bed

To illustrate a specific family intervention aimed at all three domains of family functioning, let us consider a parenting problem commonly presented to community health nurses (CHNs): parents having difficulty putting their young children to bed each night. The parents' efforts are generally met with annoyance from the child, then anger, and then tears. In their efforts, the parents also become frustrated and commonly end up angry with each other and with their child. The family intervention offered was in the form of information and opinions. In describing this case example, we will also discuss executive skills the nurse can use to operationalize the intervention. These skills are also outlined in Chapter 5.

Parent-Child System Problem. Parents' chronic inability to get their 3-year-old to go to bed and stay there at required time.

Domains of Family Functioning	Intervention: Offering Information and Opinions
Cognitive	Offer a parenting book that explains what bedtime means to children and suggests how to put children to bed.
Affective	Inform the parents that it is important to admit their frustrations to each other, especially if one spouse made an effort to put the child to bed but was not successful. The other parent may give emotional support (e.g., "You tried real hard, dear; he's a handful").
Behavioral	Teach the parents that, when they put their son to bed, they should not respond to his efforts to gain attention (e.g., asking for a glass of water). Rather, parents should be sure that these needs have been attended to as part of his bedtime rituals. Warn parents that, before they can change their child's behavior of leaving his bed or continually calling them to his bedroom, his behavior will worsen for a few nights while he makes greater efforts to get his parents to respond. If the parents continue in a matter-of-fact way to put him back in his room and respond "no" to any further requests, his behavior should improve dramatically in a few nights.

Clinical Example 2: Elderly Father Complains His Children Do Not Visit Often Enough

Next, let us consider a clinical example that illustrates the intervention of encouraging family members to be caregivers and offering caregiver support. This intervention entails inviting family members to be involved in the emotional and physical care of the patient and offering support. Again, the accompanying executive skills to operationalize the interventions are given.

Parent-Child System Problem. An elderly father wants his adult children to visit more often; the adult children do not enjoy visiting because their father always complains that they do not visit often enough.

We believe very strongly that, in the examples noted in the table, many other interventions and executive skills could have been offered. There is no one "right" intervention, only "useful" or "effective" interventions. How useful or effective an intervention is can be evaluated only after it has been implemented. The element of time must be taken into account. With some interventions, the change or outcome may be noted immediately. However, in many cases, changes (outcomes) are not noticed for a long time. Most

Domains of Family Functioning	Interventions: Encouraging Family Members to Be Caregivers and Offering Caregiver Support
Cognitive	Teach the adult children that their father is having behavioral difficulty remembering their visits (short-term memory deficits), a common phenomenon of aging. Therefore, they need not remind him of when they visited last.
Affective	Empathize with the father, for example, by saying that you understand that it must be lonely at times being a resident in a geriatric care center. The adult children might appreciate knowing that their parent is lonely so that they can respond appropriately. Therefore, advise the father to avoid complaining to the children and instead tell them how lonely he feels sometimes and that he is happy that they come to visit.
Behavioral	Advise the adult children to stop giving excuses for why they cannot visit more often. Instead, obtain a guest book or calendar and write down each visit. Write down who visited, on what day, and perhaps any interesting news so that the aging parent may read this between visits.

problems do not occur overnight; therefore, their resolutions also require reasonable lengths of time. Change can be observed, as Bateson (1972) states, as "difference which occurs across time" (p. 452).

Clinical Example 3: Enuresis and Discipline Problems With Child

To illustrate that change is observed over time, we now offer two more actual case examples of clinical work, from beginning to end, with the emphasis on the interventions that were used. In the first case, a family was referred to one of our graduate nursing students with the complex presenting problems of enuresis and disciplinary problems at school in the eldest child, an 8-year-old boy. The family was composed of the father, age 28, self-employed; the stepmother, age 21, homemaker; and two sons, ages 8 and 6. The couple had been married for approximately 1 year. The family was seen (both as a whole family and in various subsystems) for six sessions over 13 weeks from initial contact to termination. A thorough family assessment (using the CFAM model) revealed problems in the whole family system, in the parent–child subsystem, and at the individual level.

Whole-Family System Problem. Adjustment to being a stepfamily. When the couple married, a new family was formed and all family members had to adjust to a new family structure. After being married for only a short time, the stepmother found herself thrust into a parenting role when she and her husband became responsible for his two children, ages 8 and 6. The birth mother had deserted the children after living with them for 2 years in her home. The children had to adjust to a new set of parents, new surroundings, and no contact with their biological mother.

In the first session, the graduate nursing student acknowledged that the problems the family was experiencing were a usual part of the adjustment process of stepfamilies. The intervention of offering information and opinions was directed at the cognitive area of family functioning. This new information seemed to relieve the parents a great deal. In addition, the student gave advice by encouraging the parents to allow the children to have contact with their biological mother when she again sought them out. Initially, the parents were hesitant about this suggestion, but they later stated that they understood this contact was important for the children. The eldest child's enuresis was conceptualized as a response to the adjustment to a stepfamily and the loss of his mother. This new opinion, also directed at the cognitive domain of family functioning, had a very positive effect on the family. The enuresis improved dramatically over the course of treatment.

Parent-Child Subsystem Problem. Maladaptive interactional pattern between stepmother and eldest son (Fig. 4–4). Because of the initial experience of the loss of their father (as a result of the biological parents' divorce) and then the abandonment by their biological mother, the children, particularly the eldest child, feared being abandoned again. Thus, the eldest child, hoping to be reassured that he would not be abandoned again, frequently reminded his young stepmother that she was not his real mother. Initially, the stepmother made efforts to reassure him, but she eventually withdrew in frustration and felt rejected. This encouraged the child to maintain the maladaptive interactional pattern because he perceived this withdrawal as further evidence that he would again be abandoned. The vicious cycle was evident.

In deciding which interventions to offer the family, the graduate nursing student was at first overwhelmed by the complexity of their situation. Then she considered which area had the most leverage for change. She encouraged the stepmother to stop withdrawing and to offer the child continual and sustained reassurance by stating, "I know I am not your mother, but your father and I love and care for you and want to look after you. We will not leave you." This intervention of parent support and education was aimed at the behavioral, affective, and cognitive domains of family functioning.

The behavioral task proved quite successful. The stepmother reported that when she offered more reassurance to the boy, he stopped rejecting her. With decreased rejection, the stepmother was able to offer even more reassurance. Thus, a virtuous cycle began. The nursing student also offered

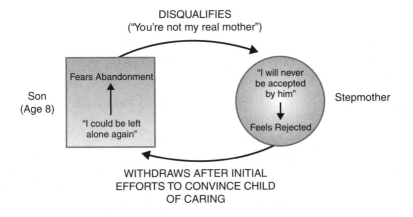

FIGURE 4-4: Circular pattern diagram.

commendations of family strengths (an intervention directed at the cognitive domain of family functioning) to the stepmother for her efforts to fulfill her role, saying that she was an exceptionally warm and caring young mother. The stepmother reported that she felt more relaxed in her parenting after this intervention.

Individual Problem. Eldest child's behavioral problems at school. To further assess this behavioral problem, the graduate nursing student met with the child's teacher at school and discussed the problem twice with the teacher by telephone. The stepmother was also present during the session at school.

The main objective of the interventions was to enhance the eldest child's self-esteem by focusing on his positive behavior. The teacher agreed to implement an intervention focused at the behavioral domain of family functioning: to acknowledge the child's positive behavior in front of his classmates to give him a different status than "class clown." The graduate student also recommended that the stepmother minimize her contact with the school and allow the teacher to assume more responsibility for the boy's behavior in class. Within a few weeks, the teacher reported a positive change in the child's behavior at school. The parents expressed great satisfaction about their child's improvement.

On termination with this family, the graduate student recommended to the parents some readings on stepfamilies and informed them of a self-help group for stepfamilies. These two interventions of offering ideas and opinions in books and providing information on community resources were targeted at all three domains of family functioning: cognitive, affective, and behavioral.

It might seem that the interventions the graduate student chose in this example were "simple." However, we believe that, in many cases, nurses either try to use overly complex interventions to address issues or they have difficulty collaborating with the family to determine areas with leverage for change. In both cases, we have found that nurses commonly become frustrated and immobilized by the complexity of the family situation. A thorough exploration of the presenting issue and then an offering of interventions designed to ameliorate that problem generally works best to foster change.

Clinical Example 4: Social Isolation and Physical Complaints of Elderly Woman

During one of our undergraduate nursing students' field placement in a community-health facility, she encountered a family whose presenting problems were social isolation and frequent physical complaints from the 78-year-old widowed mother. The widow lived in a government-subsidized, one-bedroom apartment. She had 6 adult children (5 sons, ages 51, 48, 41, 37, and 35; and 1 daughter, age 44) and 12 grandchildren. Five of the children were married, and all 6 lived in the same city as their mother. The family was seen as a whole and in various subsystems for eight home visits over a period of 2 months. After a thorough family assessment (using the CFAM model) and individual assessments, the following core problem was identified.

Whole-Family System Problem. The mother's lack of social contact beyond her immediate family. It became apparent that this older woman was overly dependent on her adult children and, therefore, did not make an effort to be involved with her peers or in social activities appropriate to her age group. This resulted in frequent disagreements between the mother and the children over the frequency of visits with the mother. The problem was further exacerbated by the fact that the mother had no friends. After the death of her husband, approximately 10 years earlier, she had lived intermittently with some of her children, but for the past 4 years had been living alone in a one-bedroom apartment. At the time of intervention, the youngest son visited most often and did the mother's grocery shopping.

The nursing student's first significant intervention was to broaden the context in order to expand her view and understanding of this family's concerns. Thus, the student initially interviewed the mother alone and then interviewed her with her youngest son (the adult child who visited most frequently). Then the student took on the ambitious task of arranging an interview with the mother and her six children. This was a significant effort on the student's part to create a context for change by obtaining each family member's view of the problem. In the interview with the mother and her youngest son, the mother agreed to contact the children. However, when the student followed up with the mother, the mother said that she had not called any of her children because she expected her youngest son to do it. This was further evidence of the mother's overdependence on her children. Because the youngest son was anxious to have the meeting take place, he had taken on the task of inviting all of his siblings to an interview with his mother and the student.

At the family interview, all of the siblings were present and two of their spouses attended as well. Interestingly, the daughters-in-law were more vocal than their husbands and stated that they were very involved with their mother-in-law. In this large family interview, the mother's social isolation (apart from her family) was discussed. Through the process of circular questioning, the expectations for family contact of both the mother and children were assessed. Initially, the student encouraged the family to explore solutions to their mother's lack of social activities and peer interactions (an intervention aimed at the behavioral domain of family functioning). To this intervention, the family responded that they had no ideas beyond what they had already tried. Therefore, the student suggested more specific interventions in an attempt to uncover solutions to the mother's social isolation.

This important interview revealed that the woman had always relied on her children for her main social interaction. She had never been a "joiner." In the past few years, she had even discontinued her attendance at church. Throughout her life, she had few close friends. The assessment also revealed that, collectively, the children had generally been supportive of their mother. Each week, she had lunch with one or more of them. They included her in all special family occasions. However, the children always had to initiate contact. They were genuinely concerned about their mother's loneliness and lack of additional social contact but had exhausted their ideas for changing her situation.

One of the first interventions the nursing student attempted was directed at both the cognitive and behavioral domains of family functioning: offering information regarding community resources that are available to older people. Specifically, the student made the family aware of the Community Services Visitor Program. The mother agreed to contact this program, and the children agreed to provide support. The mother also expressed interest in becoming involved in a choir again. The student offered to accompany her to a senior citizens' choir practice and introduce her to other participants.

The final major intervention discussed in that family session was directed at the behavioral domain. The student nurse asked the mother if she would initiate contact with one of her children during the next week. After the contact, the child would ask the mother to come for a visit as soon as possible. This intervention was important because interest of family members in an older parent's activities typically increases the parent's motivation. It is important to emphasize that the mother was involved in and receptive to these interventions.

The effects and outcomes of these interventions were as follows:

- The mother followed through on contacting the Community Services Visitor Program. The coordinator of the program then contacted the mother and arranged for a regular visitor.

- The student nurse accompanied the mother to the senior citizens' choir. The older woman enjoyed the experience and telephoned two of the other women in the choir afterward!

■ The mother took the initiative to contact a couple of her children, and they, in turn, invited her for a family visit, which she accepted. The children reported that they enjoyed having their mother call them, and this new dynamic appeared to increase their own desire to have more frequent contact with her.

In subsequent interviews, the student nurse encouraged the mother to reconnect with her church. The student also solicited the support of the children in this endeavor by requesting that they take an interest in and inquire about their mother's church and choir activities when they called her.

Because this mother was accustomed to a good deal of family support, it was not appropriate to remove that support totally. However, physical instrumental support (i.e., doing things for the mother) was reduced without the mother feeling abandoned. Verbal (emotional) support for the mother's attempts at independence was most appropriate. When the mother began to increase her social contacts and activities, her nonspecific physical complaints decreased.

The student concluded treatment with this woman in a face-to-face interview. To involve the children in the termination process, the student sent a therapeutic letter (Bell, Moules, & Wright, 2009; Hougher Limacher & Wright, 2006; Moules, 2002, 2003; Wright & Bell, 2009) to each of them. This letter, written by the student and her faculty supervisor, is printed below verbatim. It beautifully highlights the major interventions and again solicits further assistance from the children. In addition, the student very nicely included some of the family strengths in the letter. Hopefully, the change process in this particular family will continue to evolve long after this nursing student's termination of the therapeutic relationship with them.

> Dear (real names omitted to preserve confidentiality):
>
> I wish to thank you for your help and cooperation in my family assignment. I enjoyed meeting each of you and appreciated your individual input and assessment of your family. Your willingness to work together is certainly an excellent family strength.
>
> I visited your mother on several occasions during my time with the Outreach Program. She continued to express her desire to be more socially independent. She has been able to make some increased community contact. She attended the choir and several of the choir ladies have called her to encourage her in continued participation. She met with the gentleman from the church and spoke with his wife. The coordinator of the visitor program visited; she is arranging for a friend who will visit with your mother. Hopefully, they will develop some outside interests together. She has also been out to shop on her own on a few occasions.
>
> I did contact Kerby Centre, as well as other seniors from Carter Place who go there, but was unable to find anyone going to the Wednesday lunch or any other suitable transportation. I have discussed this with

your mother and she felt it might be something she could pursue on her own in the future.

Your mother expressed positive feelings about her attempts to be more socially active. However, she still looks to her children for her main support. At times, I found she needed more encouragement not to overly worry about her health to the point that she thinks she is unable to participate in any activities. I believe that each of you may help your mother by encouraging her in this area. I might suggest that if she says that she is unwell that she see her doctor. If there is no serious problem, gentle support for her independent activities might be helpful. This may be somewhat difficult at first, but if you are able to present a united front to your mother and support each other in a mutual approach to her being more socially active, she may be more able to accomplish this.

I am very impressed with the cohesiveness of your family and the continued concern and support you show toward your mother. Thank you very much again for letting me work with you.

Yours truly,
Leslie Henderson
Undergraduate Nursing Student
Faculty of Nursing, University of Calgary

This therapeutic letter sent by the student is an intervention in and of itself (Bell, Moules, & Wright, 2009; Moules, 2002, 2003, 2009; White & Epston, 1990; Wright & Bell, 2009). In addition, several interventions were outlined in the letter. These interventions were aimed at all three areas of family functioning. Specifically, the student offered commendations and opinions directed at the cognitive domain of functioning. She invited the adult children to encourage their mother, which aimed at changes in the behavioral domain. By summarizing the clinical work with the family in the form of a therapeutic letter, the student intended to effect changes in both the affective and cognitive domains of family functioning. This exemplary clinical work is a stellar example of effectively involving families in health care by the use of family assessment and intervention models with clear treatment goals by a student committed to improving family functioning and softening suffering.

CONCLUSIONS

Interventions can be as straightforward and simple or as innovative and dramatic as the nurse deems necessary for the health or illness problems presented. It also depends on the depth and intensity of possible constraining beliefs that are inviting undue suffering. Interventions intended to promote health and manage illness should be based on the assumption that individual health behaviors are strongly influenced by those around us and that family general well-being can promote the physical health of its members. All interventions should be directed toward the healing and treatment goals collaboratively generated by the nurse and the family. The rewarding work of intervening to effect change involves nurses' abilities and skills to actively engage and thoroughly assess families; clearly identify problems, concerns, and suffering; and set healing and treatment goals. The ultimate goal, of course, is to aid family members in discovering new solutions to help soften or alleviate emotional, physical, and/or spiritual suffering.

References

Bateson, G. (1972). *Steps to an Ecology of Mind: Collected Essays in Anthropology, Psychiatry, Evolution, and Epistemology.* New York: Ballantine Books.

Bateson, G. (1979). *Mind and Nature.* New York: E.P. Dutton.

Bell, J.M., Moules, N.J., & Wright, L.M. (2009). Therapeutic letters and the Family Nursing Unit: A legacy of advanced nursing practice. *Journal of Family Nursing, 15*(1), 6–30.

Bell, J.M., & Wright, L.M. (2011). Creating practice knowledge for families experiencing illness suffering: The Illness Beliefs Model. In E. Svavarsdottir & H. Jonsdottir (Eds.) *Family Nursing in Action.* Reykjavik, Iceland: University of Iceland Press, pp 15-51.

Bohn, U., Wright, L.M., & Moules, N.J. (2003). A family systems nursing interview following a myocardial infarction: The power of commendations. *Journal of Family Nursing, 9*(2), 151–165.

Campbell, T.L. (2003). The effectiveness of family interventions for physical disorders. *Journal of Marital and Family Therapy, 29*(2), 545–583.

Chesla, C.A. (2010). Do family interventions improve health? *Journal of Family Nursing, 16(4),* 355-377.

Ducharme, F. (2011). A research program on nursing interventions for family caregivers of seniors: Development and evaluation of psycho-educational interventions. In E. Svavarsdottir & H. Jonsdottir (Eds.): *Family Nursing in Action.* Reykjavik, Iceland: University of Iceland Press, pp. 233–250.

Duhamel, F., & Dupuis, F. (2004). Guaranteed returns: Investing in conversations with families of cancer patients. *Clinical Journal of Oncology Nursing, 8*(1), 68–71.

Duhamel, F., & Talbot, L.R. (2004). A constructivist evaluation of family systems nursing interventions with families experiencing cardiovascular and cerebrovascular illness. *Journal of Family Nursing, 10*(1), 12–32.

Feeley, N., & Gottlieb, L.N. (2000). Nursing approaches for working with family strengths and resources. *Journal of Family Nursing, 6*(1), 9–24.

Fomby, B.W. (2004). Family routines, rituals, recreation, and rules. In P.J. Bomar (Ed.): *Promoting Health in Families: Applying Family Research and Theory to Nursing Practice* (3rd ed.). Philadelphia: Saunders.

Gottlieb, L. (2012). Strengths-based nursing care. New York: Springer Publishing Company.

Holtslander, L. (2005). Clinical application of the 15-minute family interview: Addressing the needs of post-partum fathers. *Journal of Family Nursing, 11*(1), 5–18.

Houger Limacher, L. (2008). Locating relationships at the heart of commending practices. *Journal of Systemic Therapies, 27*(4), 90–105.

Houger Limacher, L., & Wright, L.M. (2003). Commendations: Listening to the silent side of a family intervention. *Journal of Family Nursing, 9*(2), 130–135.

Hougher Limacher, L., & Wright, L.M. (2006). Exploring the therapeutic family intervention of commendations: Insights from research. *Journal of Family Nursing, 12,* 307–331.

Hughes, J., Kay-Raining Bird, E., & and Sommerfeld, D. (2011). The growing together study: NCAST training of non-professionals working with families in two high-risk communities. In E.K. Svavarsdottir & H. Jonsdottir (Eds.): *Family nursing in action.* Reykjavik, Iceland: University of Iceland Press, pp. 333–356.

Imber-Black, E. (2010). Creating meaningful rituals for new life cycle transitions. In M. McGoldrick, B. Carter, & N. Garcia-Preto (Eds.): *The Expanded Family Life Cycle: Individual, Family, and Social Perspectives* (4th ed.). Boston, MA: Allyn & Bacon, pp. 429–439.

Keeney, H. & Keeney, B. (2012). What is systemic about systemic therapy? Therapy models muddle embodied systemic practice. *Journal of Systemic Therapies, 31*(1), 22-37.

Leahey, M., & Harper-Jaques, S. (1996). Family-nurse relationships: Core assumptions and clinical implications. *Journal of Family Nursing, 2*(2), 133–151.

Legrow, K., & Rossen, B.E. (2005). Development of professional practice based on a family systems nursing framework: Nurses and families experiences. *Journal of Family Nursing 11*(1), 38–58.

LeNavenec, C., & Vonhof, T. (1996). *One Day at a Time: How Families Manage the Experience of Dementia.* Westport, CT: Greenwood Publishing Group–Auburn House.

Levac, A.M.C., Wright, L.M., & Leahey, M. (2002). Children and families: Models for assessment and intervention. In J.A. Fox (Ed.): *Primary Health Care of Infants, Children, and Adolescents* (2nd ed.). St. Louis: Mosby, pp. 10–19.

Loos, F., & Bell, J.M. (1990). Circular questions: A family interviewing strategy. *Dimensions of Critical Care Nursing, 9*(1), 46–53.

Lucksted, A., McFarlane, W., Downing, D., Dixon, L., & Adams, C. (2012). Recent developments in family psychoeducation as an evidence-based practice. *Journal of Marital and Family Therapy, 38*(1), 101–121.

Manassis, K., & Levac, A.M. (2004). *Helping Your Teenager Beat Depression: A Problem-Solving Approach for Families.* Bethesda, MD: Woodbine House.

Maturana, H.R., & Varela, F. (1992). *The Tree of Knowledge: The Biological Roots of Human Understanding.* Boston: Shambhala Publications.

McElheran, N.G., & Harper-Jaques, S.R. (1994). Commendations: A resource intervention for clinical practice. *Clinical Nurse Specialist, 8*(1), 7–10.

McLeod, D.L., & Wright, L.M. (2008). Living the as-yet unanswered: Spiritual care practices in family systems nursing. *Journal of Family Nursing. 14*(1), 118–141.

Moules, N.J. (2002). Nursing on paper: Therapeutic letters in nursing practice. *Nursing Inquiry, 9*(2), 104–113.

Moules, N.J. (2003). Therapy on paper: Therapeutic letters and the tone of the relationship. *Journal of Systemic Therapies, 22*(1), 33–49.

Moules, N.J., et al. (2004). Making room for grief: Walking backwards and living forward. *Nursing Inquiry*, 99–107.

Moules, N.J., et al. (2007). The soul of sorrow work: Grief and therapeutic interventions of families. *Journal of Family Nursing, 13*(1), 117–141.

Moules, N.J. (2009). Therapeutic letters in nursing: Examining the character and influence of the written word in clinical work with families experiencing illness. *Journal of Family Nursing, 15*(1), 31–49.

Moules, N.J., & Johnstone, H. (2010). Commendations, conversations, and life-changing realizations: Teaching and practicing family nursing. *Journal of Family Nursing, 16*(2), 146–160.

Moules, N.J., McCaffrey, G., Laing, C.M., Tapp, D.M., & Strother, D. (2012). Grandparents' experiences of childhood cancer, Part 2: The need for support. *The Journal of Pediatric Oncology, 29*(3), 133-140.

Moules, N.J., Thirsk, L.M., & Bell, J.M. (2006). A Christmas without memories: Beliefs about grief and mothering—A clinical case analysis. *Journal of Family Nursing, 12*(4), 426–441.

Roberts, J. (2003a). Setting the frame: Definition, functions, and typology of rituals. In E. Imber-Black, J. Roberts, & R. Whiting (Eds.): *Rituals in Families and Family Therapy*. New York: Norton.

Roberts, J. (2003b). Rituals and serious illness: Marking the path. In E. Imber-Black, J. Roberts, & R. Whiting (Eds.): *Rituals in Families and Family Therapy*. New York: Norton.

Robinson, C.A. (1998). Women, families, chronic illness, and nursing interventions: From burden to balance. *Journal of Family Nursing, 4*(3), 271–290.

Robinson, C.A., & Wright, L.M. (1995). Family nursing interventions: What families say makes a difference. *Journal of Family Nursing, 1*(2), 327–345.

Rungreangkulkij, S., & Gilliss, C.L. (2000). Conceptual approaches to studying family caregiving for persons with severe mental illness. *Journal of Family Nursing, 6*(4), 341–366.

Schober, M., & Affara, F. (2001). *The Family Nurse: Frameworks for Practice*. Geneva: International Council of Nurses.

Selvini-Palazzoli, M., et al. (1978). A ritualized prescription in family therapy: Odd days and even days. *Journal of Marriage and Family Counseling, 4*(3), 3–9.

Selvini-Palazzoli, M., et al. (1980). Hypothesizing circularity-neutrality: Three guidelines for the conductor of the session. *Family Process, 19*(3), 3–12.

Shields, C.G., Finley, M.A., Chawla, N., & Meadors, P. (2012). Couple and family interventions in health problems. *Journal of Marital and Family Therapy, 38*(1), 265–280.

Sveinbjarnardottir, E.K., Svavarsdottir, E.K., & Saveman, B.-I. (2011). Nurses attitudes towards the importance of families in psychiatric care following an educational and training intervention program. *Journal of Psychiatric and Mental Health Nursing, 11*, 1–9.

Tapp, D.M. (2001). Conserving the vitality of suffering: Addressing family constraints to illness conversations. *Nursing Inquiry, 8*(4), 254–263.

Thorne, S., & Robinson, C.A. (1989). Guarded alliance: Health care relationships in chronic illness. *Image: The Journal of Nursing Scholarship, 21*(3), 153–157.

Tomm, K. (1984). One perspective on the Milan systemic approach: Part II. Description of session format, interviewing style and interventions. *Journal of Marital and Family Therapy, 10*(3), 253–271.

Tomm, K. (1985). Circular interviewing: A multifaceted clinical tool. In D. Campbell & R. Draper (Eds.): *Applications of Systemic Family Therapy: The Milan Approach*. London: Grune & Stratton, pp. 33–45.

Tomm, K. (1987). Interventive interviewing: Part II. Reflexive questioning as a means to enable self-healing. *Family Process, 26*(6), 167–183.

Tomm, K. (1988). Interventive interviewing: Part III. Intending to ask linear, circular, strategic, or reflexive questions? *Family Process, 27*(1), 1–15.

White, M., & Epston, D. (1990). *Narrative Means to Therapeutic Ends*. New York: Norton.

Wright, L.M. (2008). Softening suffering through spiritual care practices: One possibility for healing families. *Journal of Family Nursing, 14*(4), 394–411.

Wright, L.M., & Bell, J.M. (2009). *Beliefs and Illness: A Model for Healing*. Calgary, AB: 4th Floor Press.

Wright, L.M., & Leahey, M. (Producers). (2003). *How to Intervene With Families With Health Concerns*. [DVD]. Calgary, Canada. Available at www.familynursingresources.com.

Wright, L.M., & Leahey, M. (Producers). (2006). *How to Use Questions in Family Interviewing*. [DVD]. Calgary, Canada. Available at www.familnursingresources.com.

Wright, L.M., & Levac, A.M. (1992). The non-existence of non-compliant families: The influence of Humberto Maturana. *Journal of Advanced Nursing, 17*, 913–917.

Wright, L.M., & Nagy, J. (1993). Death: The most troublesome family secret of all. In E. Imber-Black (Ed.): *Secrets in Families and Family Therapy*. New York: Norton, pp. 121–137.

Chapter **5**

Family Nursing Interviews: Stages and Skills

Once nurses have a clear, conceptual framework for assessing and intervening with families, they can then begin to consider the various new competencies and skills needed for family interviews. The clinical skills deemed necessary by various authors on family work reflect each author's theoretical orientation and preference regarding how to approach and resolve relational, family, and individual problems. Therefore, the skills delineated in this chapter are based on our postmodernist worldview. This includes, but is not limited to, the theoretical foundations of systems theory, cybernetics, communication theory, biology of cognition, and change theory that inform the Calgary Family Assessment Model (CFAM) and the Calgary Family Intervention Model (CFIM).

We favor an approach that is strengths and resiliency based, problem *and* solution focused, and time effective. We emphasize that families possess the ability to solve their own problems and/or diminish their suffering but often lack the confidence or belief in their strengths due to the oppression felt by families that often follows when illness arises. Our task as nurses is to help families find and facilitate their own solutions to their emotional, physical, or spiritual suffering through compassionate and competent therapeutic conversations. We do not propose that we know what is "best" for families. Rather, we embrace the notion that the world has multiple realities—in other words, that each family member and nurse sees a world that he or she brings forth by interacting with others through language. We encourage openness in ourselves, our students, and our families to the diversity of difference among us. However, to be involved in helping families change requires that nurses possess certain essential competencies and skills.

In the previous chapters, we discussed the theoretical knowledge base that is necessary to begin to competently assess and intervene with families. We also offered two practice models (the CFAM and CFIM) as frameworks to conceptualize family dynamics and offer specific family interventions. This chapter focuses on the specific beginning-level skills necessary for relational family nursing interviews. In Chapter 10 we discuss how to move beyond basic skills and offer ideas for tailoring advanced skills to the unique client and clinical practice setting.

The literature on family work that has appeared in the past 35 years indicates that myriad skills can be used when working with families (Tomm & Wright, 1979; Wright & Bell, 2009). Various professional nursing associations have made efforts to identify the necessary competencies for practice. However, the two most significant documents with regard to the specific development of family nursing skills and competencies are those published by the International Council of Nurses (ICN). The first was titled *The Family Nurse: Frameworks for Practice* developed by Madrean Schober and Fadwa Affara (2001). These ideas were further expanded when on May 12, 2002, the ICN selected the theme for International Nurses Day to be "Nurses Always There for You: Caring for Families" and produced a document with the same title (International Council of Nurses, 2002). In the document is outlined the "nine-star family nurse." We offer it below to demonstrate the vastness of the possibilities of caring for families.

THE NINE-STAR FAMILY NURSE: MULTISKILLED WITH DIVERSE ROLES

Nurses working with families play multiple roles, depending on the family needs and the settings for care, which can include the home, health-care facilities, temporary refugee shelters, or the streets. In an effort to capture the full range of the nurse's work with families, we will refer to the key roles in terms of the nine-star nurse. The roles of the nine-star family nurse include:

- Health educator: Teaching families formally or informally about health and illness and acting as the main provider of health information.

- Care provider and supervisor: Providing direct care and supervising care given by others, including family members and nursing assistants.

- Family advocate: Working to support families and speaking up on issues such as safety and access to services.

- Case finder and epidemiologist: Tracking disease and playing a key role in disease surveillance and control.

- Researcher: Identifying practice problems and seeking answers and solutions through scientific investigation alone or in collaboration.

- Manager and coordinator: Managing, collaborating, and liaising with family members, health and social services, and others to improve access to care.

- Counselor: Playing a therapeutic role in helping to cope with problems and to identify resources.

- Consultant: Serving as consultant to families and agencies to identify and facilitate access to resources.
- Environmental modifier: Working to modify, for example, the home environment so that the disabled can improve mobility and engage in self-care.

The nine-star family nurse uses a number of these roles to identify health risks, a health problem or a need, and to address the situation working singly or in partnership with families, other health professionals, and community groups (p. 10).

Simply stating general skills such as "the student must be able to label interactions accurately" says nothing about how that skill can be achieved. The use of specific learning objectives helps to remove the mystery from what a family nurse interviewer does. Thus, the learning objectives or skills become a tentative "map" for the interview. However, it is essential to highlight that the correlation of skills with client outcomes has not yet been established. The skills described in this chapter emerge from our theoretical orientation and application of the CFAM and CFIM practice models. These skills become the nurse behaviors that are unique to working with families. Of course, each nurse also has a unique genetic and personality makeup and history of interactions, and these personalize the application of these skills.

EVOLVING STAGES OF FAMILY NURSING INTERVIEWS

Within the context of a therapeutic conversation between a nurse and a family, four major stages of family nursing interviews can be identified:

- Engagement
- Assessment
- Intervention
- Termination

These stages evolve throughout the interview. They tend to follow a logical sequence during both the course of a given interview and the overall course of contact. For example, a nurse engages family members and terminates with them at the end of each interview and at the beginning and end of the entire contact. Of course, there are times when a nurse may have to return to a previous stage. For example, interventions may be offered too quickly before a thorough assessment has been completed. Other times, the nurse might want to revisit the engagement stage if a new family member attends a meeting.

In the first stage, *engagement,* the nurse exercises skills that invite him or her and the family to establish and maintain a therapeutic relationship. Our preferred stance or posture with families is to be compassionate, collaborative, and consultative (Leahey & Harper-Jaques, 1996). We also encourage a posture of curiosity and interest in the family. This implies greater equality and respect for the family's resiliency and resourcefulness. As long as there is an atmosphere of curiosity, judgment and blame are kept at bay.

The nurse brings to the relationship expertise about promoting health and managing illness, and family members bring their own expertise about their understanding of health and their illness experiences. It is this synergy of combined expertise that can generate new outcomes to constraining situations. Factors that appear to inhibit engagement by the family interviewer are the lack of creating a context for change, and confrontation or interpretation too early in treatment. (Refer to Chapter 11 for a more in-depth reading about common errors in family interviews and how to avoid or correct them.) Additional ideas and suggestions for the engagement stage are given in Chapters 6 and 7.

Assessment, the second stage, includes the substages of problem identification and exploration plus delineation of a strengths and problems list. During this stage, the nurse enables the family to tell the story about their particular situation. The story is different for each family. It may be an illness story; a story of loss and grief; a story of uncertainty about the health of family members (e.g., a child's developmental delay or undiagnosed symptoms); a story about terror, war, tsunamis, hurricanes, or unwanted migration; or a story of a desire to promote or maintain healthy lifestyles and avoid obesity or alcoholism that has plagued a family. We stress that the conversation between the nurse and the family is in and of itself part of the therapeutic discourse (Wright & Bell, 2009). If the nurse attends only to the signs and symptoms of disease, both the nurse and the family will find themselves in a discourse emphasizing pathology. Alternative discourses that emphasize "right answers" rather than an understanding of the family's frustrations, sufferings, dilemmas, and yearnings would be equally unhelpful.

Beginning nurse interviewers generally lack a clear, stepwise rationale to guide the collecting and processing of data during an interview. Thus, some beginners commonly spend an inordinate amount of time collecting vast amounts of information. Frequently, this information is tangential to the presenting problem and is not usable. Alternatively, beginners sometimes rush into inappropriate treatment because they do not have a clear formulation of the presenting problem. However, it is better for beginners to err on the side of taking longer than usual to complete the initial assessment than to prematurely rush to the intervention stage. Nurses in family work must remember that assessment is an ongoing process. Thus, the strengths and problems list may change over time as the nurse's conceptual understanding of the family becomes more systemic. Ideas for conducting a time-effective 15-minute interview are given in Chapter 9. Information on what areas to assess and how to integrate the data is available in Chapters 3 and 7, respectively.

The third stage, *intervention,* is really the core of clinical work with families. It involves providing a context in which the family may make small or significant changes. There are numerous ways to intervene, and treatment plans should be co-constructed and tailored by the nurse and family to match each family situation. Chapter 4 offers examples of specific interventions that nurses can use, and Chapter 8 gives ideas of the kinds of questions that can be used in family interviewing.

Termination, the last stage, refers to the process of ending the therapeutic relationship between the nurse and the family in a manner that allows the family to maintain and continue constructive changes, new understandings, and facilitating beliefs. Therapeutic termination encourages the family's ability to solve problems in the future. Specific ideas for therapeutic termination are described in Chapter 12.

TYPES OF SKILLS

Each stage of family interviewing requires three types of skills:

- Perceptual
- Conceptual
- Executive

Cleghorn and Levin's (1973) identification and categorization of these three skill types are considered a seminal contribution. Tomm and Wright (1979) used the perceptual, conceptual, and executive skills framework as a guide for their comprehensive outline, which offered examples of therapist functions, competencies, and skills in each category over the evolution of a family interview. In our text, we have kept Wright's previous identification of particular perceptual, conceptual, and executive skills across the four stages of family interviews. However, we have adapted the perceptual, conceptual, and executive skills to be congruent with nurses who are just beginning to practice with families. Although we believe these skills are most descriptive of the work of beginning family nurse interviewers, we do not wish to imply that the skills are used only with "simple" family situations. Rather, we recognize that all nurses, from beginner undergraduates to experienced practicing nurses, deal with complex family situations on a day-to-day basis. These skills provide a framework for relational family nursing practice regardless of the complexity of the family's presenting issue.

The skills that we have identified fit within the context of our particular practice models—namely, the CFAM and CFIM. Perceptual and conceptual skills are paired because what we perceive is so intimately interrelated with what we think; in many cases, separating the perceptual from the conceptual component is difficult. Perceptual and conceptual skills are then matched with executive skills.

Perceptual skills relate to the nurse's ability to make relevant observations. The nurse's age, ethnicity, gender, sexual orientation, race, and class are but a few of the factors that influence his or her perceptions. The perceptual skills required in individual interviewing are much different from those required in family interviewing. This difference can be explained by the fact that, in family interviewing, the nurse is involved in observing multiple interactions and relationships simultaneously; the interaction among family members and the interaction between the nurse and the family are simultaneous.

Conceptual skills involve the ability to give meaning to the nurse's observations. They also involve the ability to formulate one's observations of the family as a whole, as a system. Nurses must always be cognizant that the meanings derived from observations are not "the truth" about the family; instead, they represent efforts to make sense of observations.

We believe that a student entering the nursing profession has intuitive perceptual and conceptual skills that have been learned in other roles in previous life experiences. However, the student is usually unaware of many of these skills. As a nurse, he or she needs to develop an overt awareness of the perceptual process. Perceptual and conceptual skills are the basis of the executive skills.

Executive skills are the observable therapeutic interventions that a nurse carries out in an interview. These skills, or therapeutic interventions, elicit responses from family members and are the basis for the nurse's further observations and conceptualizations. As can be readily seen, the interview process embedded within the therapeutic conversation is a circular phenomenon between the nurse and family. The process is highly influenced by the nurse's and family members' gender, ethnicity, class, and race. Of course, the types of therapeutic interventions the nurse offers are highly dependent on his or her clinical expertise and experience in working with families.

DEVELOPMENT OF FAMILY NURSING INTERVIEWING SKILLS

In the education of nurses developing family nursing skills, emphasis should be placed first on the development of perceptual and conceptual skills. This can be accomplished by several methods. Lectures and readings are helpful. Role-playing, practicing reflective inquiry, and observing and analyzing videos or DVDs of actual family interviews are all useful and effective ways to increase perceptual and conceptual skill accuracy. For this reason, we have developed the "How to" Family Nursing Series, available on DVD at www.familynursingresources.com. This DVD series comprises eight educational programs, which present live clinical scenarios that demonstrate family nursing in actual practice, including interviews with families with young children, middle-aged families, and later-life families. The health problems and health-care settings are varied, as are the ethnic and racial groups. The emphasis is on demonstrating how to practice these skills. The DVD most related to this chapter is *Family Nursing Interviewing Skills: How to Engage, Assess, Intervene, and Terminate* (Wright & Leahey, 2002). See the notice following the Index for a full description of each DVD and for ordering information.

Application of family nursing interview skills is one of the most meaningful skill-development opportunities for both graduate and undergraduate nurses. Moules and Tapp (2003) offer some creative, innovative ideas and exercises for educators conducting family nursing labs for undergraduate students. In their research, they found that experiential and interactive, inquiry-based activities aimed at creating personal, meaningful, relational family nursing practice received positive student feedback. For example, the authors shifted from using role-plays to using a questioning exercise to emphasize reciprocity between the family and the nurse interviewer. After selecting one student in the group, every other student asks questions of that student based on their knowledge and experience of that person as a classmate or friend. The power and timeliness of interventive questions quickly become evident to the students at a very personal level. The exercise continues until each student has had the opportunity to be the questioned member.

Moules and Tapp (2003) also fashioned a commendations exercise aimed at offering students the opportunity to genuinely look for, find, and then offer a sincere acknowledgment to a real student. The exercise was designed in a similar fashion to the questioning exercise, with one student receiving commendations offered by other group members. They reported that the experiential, personal component of these exercises enriched students' valuing of relational family nursing practice. In 2010, Moules and Johnstone reported similar findings of the value of personal reflections, commendations, and life-changing realizations for both students and faculty after a student completed a spontaneous piece of reflective writing.

If a nurse is unable to perform a specific executive skill, it is useful to find out whether he or she has developed a perceptual and conceptual base for that particular skill. This is the value of matching these skills in pairs. We encourage nurses to reflect on their practice to distinguish their areas of strengths and weaknesses in the conceptual, perceptual, or executive areas. Leahey and Harper-Jaques's (2010) work with practicing nurses demonstrates how this can be done in a relational clinical setting. Nurses were asked to create a clinical vignette of a client presenting to their setting and then discuss the conceptual, perceptual, and executive skills involved in that client's care. Nurses shared these vignettes and skill descriptions at their monthly team seminars. This contributed to advancing their personal skill development and increasing team focus on clinical practice.

Family assessment is generally well taught at the baccalaureate level and in masters and doctoral programs specializing in community and/or family nursing in North America. However, family interventions and the accompanying skills at both the undergraduate and graduate levels still need to be greatly enhanced and improved. One of the most exciting new developments in advancing family nursing has been the endowment of $7 million in 2008 to establish the Glen Taylor Nursing Institute for Family and Society (http://ahn.mnsu.edu/nursing/institute/) at the School of Nursing at Minnesota State University, Mankato, Minnesota. Their vision is to create landmark innovations in the scholarship of family and society nursing practice (Eggenberger, 2010). Already they have designed and transformed core curriculum in undergraduate and graduate education emphasizing family nursing practice.

Live supervision of clinical practice with families, particularly at the graduate level, is regularly provided in a very few locations worldwide (Duhamel, 2010; Wright & Bell, 2009). Case discussion and process recording remain the predominant method of supervision in the development of family nursing skills. However, live supervision is essential to developing and achieving therapeutic competence in nursing practice with families (Tapp & Wright, 1996; Wright, 1994; Wright & Bell, 2009). Observing peers as a mirror of one's own development and seeing one's own internal experience as normal were reported as helpful to increasing self-confidence.

A useful study that examined the pedagogical practices in family systems nursing at the Family Nursing Unit, University of Calgary revealed that feeling supported through live and video supervision, having competencies emphasized, and receiving feedback about specific in-session positive behaviors contributed to increased self-confidence and the development of advance practice clinical skills (Moules, Bell, Paton, et al, 2012). However, the study also gleaned that the intensity of the learning process was reported to have both useful and limiting consequences by masters and doctoral students.

Learning from peers is useful in three ways: First, when a novice asks the inexperienced clinician for suggestions, the novice can see that the peer can be a valuable resource. Second, as the inexperienced clinician seeks out consultation from a novice, the novice is able to see himself or herself as competent with the person to whom they are offering consultation. And third, the supervisor gets to hear multiple problem definitions and a variety of solutions. If the treatment team is multidisciplinary, issues of power and hierarchy can become transparent. Different philosophical positions can become overt without attempting to hierarchically position one model over another (Harper-Jaques & Houger Limacher, 2009).

It is especially encouraging to note the increase of nurse educators both in academia and in practice settings enhancing the development of family nursing skills. Specific examples include teaching students to "think family," to offer family nursing workshops within practice settings, and to integrate family nursing into everyday practice in mental health urgent care (Southern, et al, 2007) and in critical care (Nelmes & Eggenberger, 2010). Evidence for the continuing and deepening efforts to enhance and increase nursing students' and practicing nurses' competencies and skills in their care of families is showing up in the literature, conference abstracts, and Listservs. Learning-centered and outcome-based pedagogies in family nursing are part of the trend in multidisciplinary professional education, especially in marriage and family therapy, medicine and psychiatry, psychology, and social work (Gehart, 2011).

Specific skills for interviewing families are listed in logical sequence in Table 5–1. However, during the course of an actual interview, the nurse should not follow this outline rigidly. Rather, this outline serves as a "map

Table 5-1	Family Interviewing Skills for Nurses

STAGE 1: ENGAGEMENT

Perceptual/Conceptual Skills	*Executive Skills*
1. Recognize that an individual family member is best understood in the context of the family.	1. Invite all family members who are concerned or involved with the problem, suffering, or illness to attend the first interview.
That is, no individual exists in isolation.	For example, grandparents or other relatives or friends living inside or outside of the home should also be invited to attend if they are involved with the problem or illness.
2. Appreciate that initial efforts to involve *both* spouses/parents enable (from the onset) a more holistic view of the family and increase engagement,	2. Employ all efforts to initially involve *both* spouses/parents in early sessions.
That is, fathers should definitely be involved for effective family work.	The spouses/parents have the greatest influence on the identification, understanding, and resolution of the problem, softening suffering; and/or managing illness.
3. Recognize that providing a clear structure to the interview reduces anxiety and increases engagement.	3. Explain to family members the purpose, length, and structure of the interview and ask if they have any questions relating to the interview.
That is, people generally feel anxiety related to the uncertainty of being in a new setting and of not knowing how to behave in the situation. Structure is particularly important if the family is experiencing a crisis.	For example, say, "I thought we could spend about 10 minutes together discussing the issues that you are concerned about."
4. Recognize that initially members are most comfortable talking about the structural aspects of the family.	4. Ask each family member to briefly relate information with regard to name, age, work, or school; years married; and so forth.
That is, note nonverbal cues indicating level of comfort, such as taking coat off, adequate versus minimal time spent talking, and participating in versus ignoring conversation.	For example, introduce yourself directly by giving your name and either shaking hands or making some physical contact (such as touching a baby's head). After introductions, ask questions about information that is familiar to all family members, because this type of conversation is least threatening.

STAGE 2: ASSESSMENT

Perceptual/Conceptual Skills	*Executive Skills*
1. Realize the importance of having a conceptual assessment map to understand family dynamics.	1. Explore the components of the structural, developmental, and functional aspects of CFAM to assess strengths and problem areas.
That is, a conceptual assessment map provides the nurse with several possible courses for focused exploration.	Not all components of CFAM need to be explored if they are not relevant to the present issues, problems, or illness.
2. Realize the importance of beginning a family assessment by obtaining a detailed description and history of the presenting problem, concern, or illness.	2. Ask each family member, including the children, to share his or her knowledge and understanding of the presenting concern.

Continued

Table 5-1	Family Interviewing Skills for Nurses—*cont'd*

STAGE 2: ASSESSMENT

Perceptual/Conceptual Skills	*Executive Skills*
That is, the presenting problem usually serves as an entry point for the family to seek help. Focusing on addressing the problem is time-effective.	For example, ask the father, "How do you see the problem?" or ask the whole family, "What is the main problem or issue that each of you would like to see changed?"
3. Realize that the presenting problem is commonly related to other concerns in the family.	3. Explore with the family if there are other problems or concerns connected to the presenting problem.
That is, a child's temper outbursts may be related to family conflict (e.g., the child may be triangulated into a family conflict over caring for the grandmother).	For example, say, "We have been talking for some time about the problem of Theo's refusal to take his meds in the mornings. I am wondering if there are any other problems the family is presently concerned about or that relate to Theo's issue?"
4. Realize that eliciting differences generates more specific information for family assessment.	4. Inquire about differences between individuals, between relationships, and between various points in time.
That is: (a) Clarification of differences between individuals is a significant source of information about family functioning. (b) Clarification of differences between relationships is a significant source of information about family structure and alliances. (c) Clarification of differences in family members or in relationships at various points in time is a significant source of information about family development.	For example: (a) To explore differences between individuals, ask the child, "What is expected of you before you go to bed at night?" and then ask, "Who is the best, mother or father, at getting you to do those things in the evening?" (b) To explore differences between relationships, ask, "Do your father and Ingo argue more or less than your father and Hannah about how to care for your younger sister?" (c) To explore differences before or after important points in time, ask, "Do you worry more, less, or the same about your husband's health since his heart attack?"
5. Use the information obtained from the family assessment to begin formulating hypotheses in the form of a strengths and problems list.	5. Obtain verification of the nurse's understanding of strengths and problems by listing them to the family for their agreement and eventually recording them.
Offering conclusions or a summary of the nurse's assessment ideas enhances engagement and collaboration and allows for self-correction—that is, structural, developmental, and functional strengths and problems may be present at various systems levels. For example, whole family system issues: (a) Structural: Adjusting to new family form of single-parent household. (b) Developmental: Family in life cycle stage of children leaving home. (c) Functional: Family belief that "Father would be displeased with us for still crying about his death."	For example, say, "We have identified that being a new single parent and also having to cope with your child (who has a developmental delay) leaving home are your two major concerns. We have also discussed that your family is very well respected in the Latino community. Have I understood things correctly?"

Table 5-1	Family Interviewing Skills for Nurses—*cont'd*

STAGE 2: ASSESSMENT

Perceptual/Conceptual Skills	*Executive Skills*
6. Assess whether any of the identified problems are beyond the scope of the nurse's competence.	6. Tell the family whether you will continue to work with them on problems. (If a decision is made to refer them to another professional, proceed to Stage 4A: Termination.)
That is, it is appropriate to consider referral when medical symptoms have not been fully assessed or long-standing emotional or behavioral problems exist.	For example, tell the family, "Now that I have a more complete understanding of your concerns, I think it is necessary to have your son's headaches checked out medically. I would like to refer you to a pediatrician."
7. Recognize that a more extensive inquiry into the most pressing problems is necessary before intervention plans can be implemented.	7. Seek the family's opinion of which issue they perceive as most important and/or where there is the greatest suffering, and explore it in depth. If the family cannot agree, then discuss the lack of consensus.
That is, initially families are usually most concerned with the presenting problem or the area of greatest suffering.	For example, ask, "About which of the problems we have discussed today are you most concerned?"
8. Recognize that the assessment is complete when sufficient information has been obtained to formulate a treatment plan.	8. State your integrated understanding of problems to the family and obtain their commitment to work on a specific problem.
That is, nurses sometimes rush into inappropriate treatment because they are without a clear understanding of the presenting problem or other significant related problems.	For example, say, "Because everyone agrees that Soon's bulimia is connected to the other addictions in the family, I would like to suggest that we focus on this problem for three interviews. Would you be willing?"

STAGE 3: INTERVENTION

Perceptual/Conceptual Skills	*Executive Skills*
1. Recognize that families possess problem-solving abilities.	1. Encourage family members to explore possible solutions to problems and to soften suffering.
That is, recognizing that families possess the capability to change and can identify and implement solutions for how to change helps the nurse avoid becoming overcontrolling or over-responsible.	For example, say, "Sanjeshna, you have mentioned that your mother is too blaming of herself. Do you have any ideas of what she could do to blame herself less about experiencing a chronic illness?"
2. Recognize that interventions are focused on the cognitive, affective, and behavioral domains or areas of functioning in families, as described in the CFIM.	2. Plan interventions to influence any one or all three of the domains of functioning described in the CFIM.
That is, it is not always necessary or efficient to design interventions for all three domains of functioning simultaneously.	For example: (a) Cognitive: Invite the family to think differently. (b) Affective: Encourage different affective expression. (c) Behavioral: Ask the family to perform new tasks either within or outside of the interview.

Continued

Table 5-1	Family Interviewing Skills for Nurses—*cont'd*

STAGE 3: INTERVENTION

Perceptual/Conceptual Skills	*Executive Skills*
3. Recognize that lack of information of an educational nature can inhibit the family's problem-solving abilities.	3. Provide information to family members that will enhance their knowledge and facilitate further problem solving.
That is, when given additional information, many families can provide their own creative and unique solutions to problems.	For example, the nurse can ask family members if they would like to hear about some typical reactions of a 3-year-old to a new baby or about the aging process of an older adult with Alzheimer's disease. This type of intervention targets the family's cognitive domain of functioning.
4. Recognize that persistent and intense emotions can often block the family's problem-solving abilities.	4. Validate family members' emotional responses, when appropriate.
That is, families who predominantly experience emotions such as sadness or anger are often unable to deal with problems until the emotional constraint is removed.	For example, family members suppressing grief over the loss of another family member may only need confirmation of the normal grieving process to work through their bereavement. This type of intervention targets the family's affective domain of functioning.
5. Recognize that suggesting specific tasks or assignments can often provide a new way for family members to behave in relation to one another that will improve problem-solving abilities.	5. Assign tasks or assignments aimed at improving family functioning.
That is, some tasks can facilitate changes in the structure of the family or family rules or rituals.	For example, suggest that the father and son spend one evening a week together in a common activity; suggest to the mother and father that one parent put the children to bed on odd days and the other on even days. This type of intervention influences the family's behavioral domain of functioning.

STAGE 4: TERMINATION

A. If Consultation or Referral Is Necessary:

1. Recognize that families appreciate additional professional resources when problems are quite complex.	1. Refer individual family members or the family for consultation or ongoing treatment.
That is, nurses cannot be expected to have expertise in all areas.	For example, say, "I feel that your family needs professional input beyond what I can offer for Tracey's learning disability. Therefore, I would like to refer you to the learning center in the city. They have more expertise in dealing with these types of problems."

B. If Family Interviewing With Nurse Continues:

1. Recognize the importance of evaluating the family interviews or meetings at regular intervals.	1. Obtain feedback from family members about the present status of their problems or level of suffering and initiate termination when the contracted problems have been resolved or sufficient progress has been made.

Table 5-1	Family Interviewing Skills for Nurses—*cont'd*

STAGE 4: TERMINATION

B. If Family Interviewing With Nurse Continues:

That is, evaluating the progress of family interviews leads to more focused and purposeful time spent with the family.	Families normally do not lead problem- or suffering-free lives. Rather, what is important is their feeling of confidence to cope with life's challenges and stresses.
2. Recognize when dependency on the nurse inadvertently may have been encouraged.	2. Mobilize other supports for the family if necessary, and begin to initiate termination by decreasing the frequency of sessions.
That is, many interviews over a prolonged period can foster excessive dependency.	For example, nurses can inadvertently provide "paid friendship," with mothers in particular, unless they mobilize other supports such as husbands, friends, or relatives.
3. Recognize family members' constructive efforts to solve problems or soften suffering.	3. Summarize positive efforts of family members to resolve problems and lessen suffering whether or not significant improvement has occurred.
That is, the family's perception of progress is more significant than the nurse's perception.	For example, comment, "Your family has made tremendous efforts to find ways to care for your elderly father at home while still attending to your children's needs."
4. Recognize that backup support by professional resources is appreciated by individuals and families in times of stress.	4. End the family interviews with a face-to-face discussion when possible. If appropriate, extend an invitation for additional family meetings should problems recur or if the family desires consultation.

of interviewing" that allows considerable flexibility in application. The family's cultural norms for giving and receiving information can provide a guide for the pacing of the meeting. We cannot emphasize enough the importance of the nurse and the family developing a collaborative working relationship during the interview.

CONCLUSIONS

The family interviewing skills (perceptual, conceptual, executive) discussed in this chapter function as a guide or a map for nurses working with families. Thus, through the implementation of these skills, beginning family nurse interviewers can progress through the four stages of the interview by engaging families, assessing strengths and problems, deciding whether to intervene or to refer families, and terminating with the family. These stages of a family interview, with their accompanying skills, are another useful blueprint for nurses working with families. We strongly encourage nurses to tailor the use of these skills to each family's unique context and their relationship with the family. The nurse and family converse and collaborate and bring forth old and new stories of suffering, problems, resiliencies, strengths, competence, and problem resolution. The ethnicity, culture, class, sexual orientation, and race of the nurse and family members will, of course, influence their collaboration.

References

Cleghorn, J.M., & Levin, S. (1973). Training family therapists by setting learning objectives. *American Journal of Orthopsychiatry, 43*(3), 439–446.

Duhamel, F. (2010). Implementing family nursing: How do we translate knowledge into clinical practice? Part II: The evolution of 20 years of teaching, research, and practice to a center of excellence in family nursing. *Journal of Family Nursing, 16*(1), 8–25.

Eggenberger, S. (2010). Glen Taylor nursing institute for family and society: Advancing family nursing. *Journal of Family Nursing, 16*(2), 234–238.

Gehart, D. (2011). The core competencies and mft education: Practical aspects of transitioning to a learning-centered, outcome based pedagogy. *Journal of Marital and Family Therapy, 37*(3), 344–354.

Harper-Jaques, S., & Houger Limacher, L. (2009). Providing marriage and family therapy supervision in a multidisciplinary psychiatric setting: Contextual sensitivity as a cornerstone of supervision. *Journal of Systemic Therapies, 28*(3), 49–58.

International Council of Nurses. (2002). *Nurses Always There for You: Caring for Families*. Geneva, Switzerland: Author.

Leahey, M., & Harper-Jaques, S. (1996). Family-nurse relationships: Core assumptions and clinical implications. *Journal of Family Nursing, 2*(2), 133–151.

Leahey, M., & Harper-Jaques, S. (2010). Integrating family nursing into a mental health urgent care practice framework: Ladders for learning. *Journal of Family Nursing, 16*(2), 196–212.

Moules, N., & Johnstone, H. (2010). Commendations, conversations and life-changing realizations: Teaching and practicing family nursing. *Journal of Family Nursing, 16*(2), 146–160.

Moules, N.J., & Tapp, D.M. (2003). Family nursing labs: Shifts, changes, and innovations. *Journal of Family Nursing, 9*(1), 101–117.

Moules, N.J., Bell, J.M., Paton, B.I., et al. (2012). Examining pedagogical practices in family systems nursing: Intentionality, complexity, and doing well by families. *Journal of Family Nursing, 18*(2), 261–295.

Nelmes, T.P., & Eggenberger, S.K. (2010). The essence of the family critical illness experience and nurse-family meetings. *Journal of Family Nursing, 16*(4), 462–486.

Schober, M., & Affara, F. (2001). The Family Nurse: Frameworks for Practice. Geneva, Switzerland: International Council of Nurses.

Southern, L., et al. (2007). Integrating mental health into urgent care in a community health centre. *Canadian Nurse, 1*, 29–34.

Tapp, D.M., & Wright, L.M. (1996). Live supervision and family systems nursing: Postmodern influences and dilemmas. *Journal of Psychiatric and Mental Health Nursing, 3*, 225–233.

Tomm, K.M., & Wright, L.M. (1979). Training in family therapy: Perceptual, conceptual, and executive skills. *Family Process, 18*(3), 227–250.

Wright, L.M. (1994). Live supervision: Developing therapeutic competence in family systems nursing. *Journal of Nursing Education, 33*(7), 325–327.

Wright, L.M., & Bell, J.M. (2009). Beliefs About Illness: A Model for Healing. Calgary, AB: 4th Floor Press.

Wright, L.M., & Leahey, M. (Producers). (2002). Family Nursing Interviewing Skills: How to Engage, Assess, Intervene, and Terminate With Families. [DVD]. Calgary, AB. Available at www.familynursingresources.com.

6

How to Prepare for Family Interviews

Nurses who work in various types of settings often ask, "How do I prepare for a family interview?" For many nurses, family meetings happen by chance, such as when family members are visiting their loved one in the hospital. For others, family presence in emergency departments or intensive care units is an accepted practice, and nurses are expected to interact with family members as part of their usual practice and supported by institutional and/or administrative policy. However, only 5% of nurses work in units with a written family presence protocol (Duran, et al, 2007). For some nurses, interviews are a planned event and may be initiated by either the family or the nurse. Foucault and colleagues (2008) found that 43% of individual clients would have preferred for a family member to join them for a meeting about mental health issues. Some nurses must overcome the belief that they would be intruding on the family visit if they were present in the patient's room. For many nurses, tension caused by the time required to set up an interview, develop a relationship with the family, and intervene effectively is a major challenge to overcome. Time tension is something that health-care professionals need to learn to manage; otherwise, they can become immobilized by it. We suggest that nurses cannot *not* attend to families!

For both the nurse and the family, the first interview or family meeting is often filled with anxiety often due to lack of experience, skills, or both of how to involve families. We find this to be a natural reaction of nurses who desire and are committed to expand their practice and include families as part of their relational practice. We believe that the less anxious the nurse is, the more he or she invites confidence in family members, thereby reducing their anxiety. The purpose of this chapter is to help reduce the nurse's anxiety by discussing how to plan for the initial and subsequent interviews. First, ideas are offered for the nurse to reflect on the type of relationship that is most desirable to be co-constructed with a family. How to develop hypotheses related to the purpose of the interview is then addressed. Concrete issues are presented, such as deciding on the interview setting, deciding who will be present, and contacting the family by telephone.

IDEAS ABOUT THE NURSE-FAMILY RELATIONSHIP

Since the first edition of this book, there has been a steady increase in the attention paid to the relational aspect of nurse-family encounters. The relationship is actualized through the microcontext of "therapeutic conversations," meaning the nurse clinician acts *with*, rather than on, patients. Madsen (2007) has advocated self-reflection in relation to dominant societal ideas and practices, intimate relationships past and present, the client–health-care professional relationship, gender, sexual thoughts, and strong feelings. We believe that nurses cannot avoid their influence on families, particularly the potential healing power of their words. Nurses and families inevitably influence each other, but not always with predictable results.

Bell (2011) has championed the idea that relationships are the heart of the matter in family nursing: "What would happen if family nurses would continue to focus on families but with a keener interest and heightened sensitivity to relationships?" (p. 3) and "What if, in nursing education, we were to begin instead (of teaching how to do an assessment) to teach about the ways we enter into relationships with the family?" (p. 5). The idea of nurses increasing their attention especially to the first few minutes of an encounter with a client is a powerful one.

We also believe nurses' positive attitudes toward families encourage them to engage more frequently in therapeutic conversations with families. The work of Sveinbjarnardottir, Svavarsdottir, and Saveman (2011) supports this notion that the attitude psychiatric nurses have is fundamental to the quality of interventions offered to families. A revealing study of nurses' attitudes about involving families in nursing care showed that less supportive attitudes existed among the newly graduated, those having no particular approach to the care of families in their workplace, and those who were male nurses (Benzein, Johansson, Arestedt, et al, 2008).

We believe that families and nurses each have their own health-care system. Families provide diagnoses, advice, remedies, and support to their members in both sickness and health. They have constraining and facilitating beliefs about the illness experience (Wright & Bell, 2009). Nurses also have their own constraining and facilitating beliefs, theories, opinions, recommendations, and remedies about managing problems or illness that they share with families. Leahey and Harper-Jaques (1996) have outlined five assumptions relating to the family-nurse relationship and the clinical implications of each assumption. Emphasis is on both the nurse's *and* the family's contribution to establishing and maintaining the relationship. We believe that it is useful for a nurse to reflect on his or her potential contribution to the relationship *before* meeting with a family. It is also helpful for the nurse to reflect with the family about their working relationship at the end of their contract. More ideas on this topic are provided in Chapter 12. The five assumptions related to the family–nurse relationship are detailed in the following sections.

Assumption 1: The Family-Nurse Relationship Is Characterized by Reciprocity. The family and nurse are connected in a pattern that is quite distinct from the positivist-based idea of two separate components, either family or nurse. It is the "fit" between the family and the nurse that is important to foster a collaborative partnership. Sample questions to ask might include:

- What are your thoughts on working together? Is it a good fit so far? What can you imagine will be your preferred way of contributing to our time together?
- What direction do you hope we move in over the next few meetings?
- Is there anything you'd like to know from me to make the conversations easier? (Madsen, 2007)

Trust is a process that evolves over time. Jonsdottir and Ingadottir (2011) offer an example of a nurse clinic in Reykjavik where the focal point is unmet health-care needs of the patients and their families. They stress the importance of recognizing that complementarity of expertise and a holistic approach are essential for success. Collaboration with trust and respect for each other's contribution is essential for action to be taken. If the nurse wishes to foster a reciprocal relationship, he or she can reflect on additional sample questions in Box 6–1.

Box 6-1 Questions About Reciprocity

For the nurse's self-reflection:
To what extent will I:

- Elicit the patient's and family members' expectations, hopes, questions, and ideas?
- Consider the patient's and family members' expectations, knowledge, experience, and desires when planning nursing care?
- Communicate information, ideas, and recommendations to patients and families on a regular basis?
- Involve the patient and family to their satisfaction in making decisions for the overall treatment plan?

To ask the family when evaluating care:
To what extent do you feel that:

- I heard your opinions and ideas?
- I was available and approachable to answer your questions?
- I showed interest in your ideas and experience with illness?

Leahey, M., & Harper-Jaques, S. (1996). Family-nurse relationships: Core assumptions and clinical implications. *Journal of Family Nursing,* 2(2), 133–151. Copyright 1996 by M. Leahey and S. Harper-Jaques. Reprinted by permission of Sage Publications.

Assumption 2: The Family-Nurse Relationship Is Nonhierarchical. Each person's contribution is sought, acknowledged, and valued. A conversation is a co-construction of ideas and mutual discoveries. However, both the nurse and the family remain aware that they are bound by moral, legal, and ethical norms. Tapp's research (2000) identifies useful practices to counterbalance hierarchy and expert professional views: "offering commendations, coevolving a description using the family's language, exploring the illness story and the medical story, asking questions that invite reflection, and initiating conversations about family members' preferences" (p. 69). Madsen (2007) suggests that the clinician examine the stance that clients hold toward problems. Do the clients believe they have some influence over the problem and want to do something about it? Or, perhaps the clients don't see themselves as having a problem? Or, this is a problem, but I have no control over it? Connecting with clients' intentions, hopes, and preferred view of self is a way for the nurse to demonstrate respect and collaboration. (More ideas on this topic are given in Chapter 7.) Box 6–2 contains some sample questions that nurses can ask themselves and the family about hierarchy.

Assumption 3: Nurses and Families Each Have Specialized Expertise in Maintaining Health and Managing Health Problems. Families who live with chronic conditions develop expertise in managing symptoms, adapting their environments, and adjusting their lifestyles. They live "near illness," "alongside of illness," and "with illness" (Wright & Bell, 2009). When they meet with nurses, they bring a wealth of information and personal expertise to the encounter. Nurses, through their education and experience, also bring expertise to the relationship with the family. Out of this mutually respectful encounter, the family members' confidence in self-managing a disease can be enhanced. Diabetes management, for example, depends largely on self-regulation.

| **Box 6-2** | Questions About Hierarchy |

For the nurse's self-reflection:

• To what extent am I imposing my beliefs on the family? Allowing the family to impose their beliefs on me?
• How well do the expectations between the family and I match?
• When there is a mismatch, whose opinion usually predominates?
• How frequently are decisions about the patient's health care made mutually by the patient, family, and me?

To ask the family when evaluating care:

• Overall, what percentage of time were decisions about your health care made in a mutual way between you and me?
• To what extent did I help you feel more in control of your health?

Leahey, M., & Harper-Jaques, S. (1996). Family-nurse relationships: Core assumptions and clinical implications. *Journal of Family Nursing, 2*(2), 133–151. Copyright 1996 by M. Leahey and S. Harper-Jaques. Reprinted by permission of Sage Publications.

We believe that more traditional compliance models relying on pressure to follow recommendations need to be replaced by patient-empowerment models. Nurses risk starting to believe they really know what the best answers are for a family or a particular problem. We agree with Tapp (2000) that "these beliefs can become oppressive when the expert has the expectation that their advice must be obeyed" (p. 81). Nurses can think about their own expertise and the family's expertise as they prepare to meet with a family to discuss managing a particular health problem. Developing and nurturing a kernel of appreciation and respect for the client is foundational to a therapeutic alliance. Box 6–3 provides sample questions that the nurse can consider.

Assumption 4: Nurses and Families Each Bring Strengths and Resources to the Family–Nurse Relationship. Nurses who use a resource-identification lens strive to draw forth the family's cultural, ethnic, spiritual, and other beliefs that have been helpful in dealing with the health problem. Nurses also bring to the relationship their own life experience; clinical intuition; and cultural, ethnic, spiritual/religious, and educational background. Sample questions the nurse could ask the family in evaluating the effectiveness of their relational practice include:

- What have I as a nurse done with you as a family that has made a difference? A positive difference?
- Looking back, what was your preferred way of contributing to our conversations? Is there something in particular that you feel pleased about with the outcome?

Box 6-3   Questions About Expertise

For the nurse's self-reflection:

- What do I know about the family's ideas and plans for care during this course of treatment?
- What can I learn from this family about their experiences in living with this health problem?
- What knowledge and expertise do I have to offer this family?
- How does this family demonstrate its trust in my expertise?
- Who in the family has the most expertise in getting Grandpa to take his medications?

To ask the family:

- What are the things that you or other family members do to help you relieve the pain?
- What ways have you found most useful to invite your father to take care of his own personal needs?

Leahey, M., & Harper-Jaques, S. (1996). Family-nurse relationships: Core assumptions and clinical implications. *Journal of Family Nursing, 2*(2), 133–151. Copyright 1996 by M. Leahey and S. Harper-Jaques. Reprinted by permission of Sage Publications.

Box 6–4 offers sample questions that nurses can ask themselves about how they would like the relationship with the family to be focused on strengths.

Assumption 5: Feedback Processes Can Occur Simultaneously at Several Different Relationship Levels. Nurses have often focused on family dynamics and interactional patterns within family systems. More recently, however, they have begun to address family-nurse relationships and reflect on their own patterns with families (Bergadahl, Benzein, Ternestedt, et al, 2011). Rarely do nurses address the interactive patterns that can simultaneously occur at different relational levels. Box 6–5 offers sample questions that the nurse can consider about the family-nurse relationship.

Box 6-4 Questions About Strengths

For the nurse's self-reflection:

- Will my actions and comments acknowledge the strengths and abilities of this family?
- What interventions can I use to further enhance this family's strengths?
- How am I inviting this family to trust my knowledge and skill in helping them with this health problem?
- What are the strengths that I bring to this relationship?

Leahey, M., & Harper-Jaques, S. (1996). Family-nurse relationships: Core assumptions and clinical implications. *Journal of Family Nursing,* 2(2), 133–151. Copyright 1996 by M. Leahey and S. Harper-Jaques. Reprinted by permission of Sage Publications.

Box 6-5 Questions About the Family–Nurse Relationship

For the nurse's self-reflection:
To what extent did my relationship with the patient and family help to:

- Increase their knowledge? Insight? Coping?
- Increase *my* knowledge? Insight?
- Improve or enhance their emotional well-being? My emotional well-being?
- Improve the patient's physical health?
- Build stronger relationships between the patient and family members?

To ask the family when evaluating care:
To what extent did our meetings together:

- Meet your needs?
- Contribute to your having an increased sense of confidence in living with your illness?

Leahey, M., & Harper-Jaques, S. (1996). Family-nurse relationships: Core assumptions and clinical implications. *Journal of Family Nursing,* 2(2), 133–151. Copyright 1996 by M. Leahey and S. Harper-Jaques. Reprinted by permission of Sage Publications.

HYPOTHESIZING

Before meeting the family for the first time, the nurse should develop an idea of the purpose of the interview and an understanding of the family's context. For example, a nurse in primary care who is conducting an interview to understand how the family is coping with a chronic or life-threatening illness will conduct it differently than a nurse who is trying to assess family violence, abuse, or some other specified problem. In the latter example, either the family or some other agency may have already identified the problem. Also, if a family were in crisis—for example, having just received news of an untimely death of a family member—the context for the interview would be different than if the family were not experiencing a crisis. Another purpose for an interview could be for the nurse to discover parents' desires about whether they want to remain at their child's side during complex invasive procedures and resuscitation. Offering family members a choice is a practice parents often prefer. Inquiring how family members would like to be involved in the patient's home care or hospitalization could be another reason for a family meeting. Depending on the purpose of the interview, the types of questions asked and the flow of the therapeutic conversation may be quite different. See Chapters 4, 7, 8, 9, and 10 for clinical examples of interviews.

We are heartened by the work of Burke and colleagues (2001), who studied the effects of stress-point intervention with families of repeatedly hospitalized children. They hypothesized that each additional hospitalization has unique challenges and could be more stressful than previous ones. A family-focused supportive intervention called Stress-Point Intervention by Nurses (SPIN) was designed to reduce family problems. The findings from a three-site clinical trial with random assignment of nurses and families to experimental (SPIN) and control (usual care) groups indicate that parents who received SPIN were more satisfied with family functioning and had better parental coping after hospitalization than parents who received usual care. The intervention was based partly on CFAM and CFIM and involved " a) identifying the family's own particular stressful issues surrounding the expected or anticipated hospitalization, b) developing a plan with the parents to handle these specific issues and c) following up to praise strengths and successes, modify, and evaluate the success of the intervention" (Burke, et al, 2001, p. 138). It is the follow-through on these types of hypotheses that we find encouraging for the further development of relational family nursing practice.

In our clinical supervision with nurses, we have encouraged them to generate hypotheses related to the purpose of the meeting before the interview. Fleuridas, Nelson, and Rosenthal (1986) define hypotheses as "suppositions, hunches, maps, explanations, or alternative explanations about the family and the 'problem' in its relational context" (p. 115). For them, the purpose of a hypothesis is to connect family behaviors with meaning and guide the interviewer's use of questions. A hypothesis provides order for the interviewing process. It introduces a systemic view of the family and generates new views of relationships, beliefs, and behaviors. Preferably, the hypothesis should be circular rather than linear to maximize the therapeutic potential.

The essence of all these definitions is similar: A hypothesis is a tentative proposition or hunch that provides a basis for further exploration. For example, we know from stress theories and from our own personal and professional experiences that the time of diagnosis of an illness is generally stressful, and in many cases, symptoms temporarily become worse.

Using this as a hypothesis, the nurse can arrange a family interview to discuss the impact of the diagnosis on the family, the family's response to the illness, and the family's expectations of the nurse. In this way, the nurse can explore family patterns of adjusting to the diagnosis and also the family members' ideas of the types of relationships they would like to have with health-care providers. The hypothesis provides general direction for the nurse interviewer in exploring with this particular family their unique adjustment to a diagnosis.

The value of curiosity and naïveté for the nurse working with families, especially in immigrant and marginalized populations, cannot be overestimated. Cultural naïveté and respectful curiosity can be as significant as or more significant than knowledge and skill. It is important for us to point out how our thinking about hypotheses has changed as we work toward operating within a postmodernist paradigm and shift from a modernist point of view. Our attention has shifted from what *we* think about what patients and families are telling us to trying to grasp what *they* think about what they are telling us.

How to Generate Hypotheses

Hypotheses can be formulated from many bases. For example, they can be based on information the family provided or on ideas about the family gathered during hospital admission, during visiting hours, or from the other staff. The information may consist of opinions, observations of behavior or interactive patterns, and other data. In considering this information, we encourage nurses to ask themselves what they think the other staff thinks about what they are saying. We believe the most relevant hypotheses are generally based on information already provided by the family.

Hypotheses can also be based on the nurse's previous experience and knowledge. This experience and knowledge can involve families whom the nurse believes to have similar ethnic, racial, or religious or spiritual backgrounds. The nurse may recall similar problems, symptoms, or situations and similar interactive patterns noticed with previous patients and families. He or she may generate a hypothesis based on knowledge about family development and life-cycle stages, research literature, or another conceptual framework that he or she finds most relevant. We encourage nurses to include in their hypotheses ideas about a family's strong spirit, generosity of heart, devotion to one another, deep caring, and commitment. These are enduring qualities that families can draw upon in times of stress.

In addition to formulating hypotheses based on information from or about the family or from previous experience and knowledge, nurses may develop hypotheses based on whatever is salient or relevant to them about the health problem or risk that is encountered at the time. For example, if a recent tragedy has occurred in the immediate community, the nurse may find such information relevant in generating a hypothesis about what might be most meaningful for this particular family at this point.

We believe that it is important for nurses to state (to themselves) their hypotheses explicitly and consciously before the interview. We do not concur with those who state that hypotheses are unnecessary. Our belief is that a nurse cannot *not* hypothesize or think about a family before the meeting. It is important for nurses to explicate their hunches so that these thoughts may be refined and made transparent as nurse and family engage in the interview process. Hypothesizing before the family meeting is viewed as a way to start focusing on the family, churning up the gray matter, making connections, and generating questions. It should not involve preparing an agenda for the session that is imposed on the family regardless of what the family members desire and despite changes that may have occurred since the last meeting (see Chapter 11 for ideas of how to avoid these kind of mistakes).

The guidelines for designing hypotheses, presented in Box 6–6, have been adapted from the work of Fleuridas, Nelson, and Rosenthal (1986). We encourage nurses to generate hypotheses that are useful. We do not believe that there is one "correct" or "right" hypothesis. Rather, the goal is to generate useful explanations that lead to desired outcomes. We believe that stories

---

Box 6-6 Guidelines for Generating Hypotheses

• Choose hypotheses that are useful.
• Generate the most helpful explanations of the family's behaviors for this particular time.
• Understand that there are no "right" or "true" explanations.
• Include all participants in the "problem-organizing system" to make the hypothesis as systemic as possible.
• Relate the hypothesis to the family's presenting concerns so the interview can proceed along the lines most relevant to the family (versus those relevant to the nurse).
• Make the hypothesis different from the family's hypothesis to introduce new information into the system and avoid being entrapped with the family in solutions that are not working.
• Be as quick to discard unhelpful hypotheses as you are to generate new ones.

are authored through conversations. The story that is co-constructed between the nurse and the family is uniquely personal. We cannot know which hypotheses will fit for a particular family or where people's stories will go. We can only attune ourselves one piece at a time to the story as it unfolds.

We encourage nurses to design hypotheses that are circular rather than linear—that is, a hypothesis that includes all the components of the system (e.g., the family *and* the nurse) is most likely to be more circular than one that includes *either* the nurse *or* the family. (See Chapters 2 and 3 for a more in-depth discussion regarding circularity.) The hypothesis should be related to the family's concerns. This is important because, as previously stated, a hypothesis guides the interview. For example, if the nurse develops a hypothesis that is unrelated to the family's concerns, he or she will ask questions that do not relate to the family's reason for coming to the interview or health-care facility.

The nurse who is attuned to the family's concerns will listen for openings, through questions and reflective discussion, of problem-saturated stories and unique outcomes (see Chapter 7). These outcomes, or "sparkling events," would not have been predicted in light of the problem-saturated story. We remind ourselves that it is the clinician's certainty about her beliefs and opinions that can oppress and constrain opportunities to hear the patient's and family's story as they experience it.

We also encourage nurses to design a hypothesis that is different from the family's explanation or hypothesis. For example, a family may have the explanation that Puichun is a "bad daughter" who is shirking her responsibility by not caring for her elderly mother in her own home. The nurse, on the other hand, may develop an alternate hypothesis that fits the same data. The nurse's hypothesis might be that Puichun is overwhelmed by having to take care of her two preschool children while maintaining a full-time job. Thus, she is stretched to the limit in also trying to take responsibility for her elderly parent. Furthermore, Puichun's elderly mother may be sensitive to her stress and thus may be reluctant to live with her.

Once hypotheses have been designed, the nurse can use them to guide the interview. The nurse can ask questions of each member and note the responses to questions, thus confirming, altering, or rejecting a hypothesis. In conversation with families, the nurse should be sure to pay attention to the small and the ordinary. We agree somewhat with the notion that the starting point for hypotheses is arbitrary and intuitive but that hypotheses are either validated or invalidated by evidence (i.e., they may be confirmed, rejected, or modified). We remain acutely aware that our notion of validation and evidence is just from our "observer perspective."

Hypothesizing and interviewing constitute a reciprocal cycle and are interdependent. The nurse develops a hypothesis, asks questions, converses with the family about the "problem" and its influence on their lives, and gathers evidence that either confirms or refutes the nurse's hypothesis.

Box 6–7 illustrates questions that invite hypothesizing about the system and the problem. As new information is generated, the nurse modifies the previous hypothesis and evolves a more useful one. The goal of the interview is to bring forth the family's resources to deal with the presenting issue. More information about how to conduct family interviews is provided in Chapters 7 to 11.

Box 6-7 | Questions That Invite Hypothesizing About the System and the Problem

Who
Who is in the system? Who are the key players?
Who first noticed the problem?
Who is concerned about the problem?
Who is affected by the problem? (most, least)
Who is interested in keeping things the same? (most, least)
Who referred the system?

What
What is the problem at this time?
What is the meaning that the problem has for the system and for different members of the system?
What solutions have been attempted?
What question(s) do I feel obliged to ask?
What beliefs perpetuate the problem?
What beliefs might be identified as core beliefs?
What beliefs are perpetuated by the problem?
What problems and solutions perpetuate the beliefs?

Why
Why is the system presenting at this time?

Where
Where has the information about this problem come from?
Where does the system see the problem originating?
Where does the system see the problem and the system going if there is no change or if there is change?

When
When did the problem begin?
When did the problem begin in relation to another phenomenon of the system?
When does the problem occur?
When does the problem not occur?

How
How might a change in the problem affect other parts of the system (key players, relationships, beliefs)?
How does a change in one part of the system affect another part of the system or the problem?
How will I know when my work with this system is over?
How might my work with this system constrain the system from finding its solution?

Leahey and Wright (1987) provide an example of how alternative hypotheses can be generated before the first family meeting:

> A nurse working in an extended-care facility noted that the family, especially the 9- and 10-year-old children, avoided visiting their 41-year-old mother who had Huntington's disease, and that the patient's symptoms worsened around visiting days. The children seemed depressed and withdrawn every time they came to the nursing unit on their monthly visits. During case conferences, the staff wondered whether there might be a connection between the family's avoidance and the patient's flailing and head banging. They generated several hypotheses to explain why the family might be avoiding the patient and why the patient's symptoms seem to exacerbate around the time of the family visits.
>
> One hypothesis pertained to the children's belief that head banging and flailing were controllable. Perhaps the children felt that their mother was not trying to control herself so she would not have to return home to care for them. This made them angry and they avoided her. An alternate hypothesis concerned the children's conflicting loyalties toward their mother and the aunt who took care of them. Perhaps they felt that if they visited too often, their aunt might think they did not appreciate her care. Thus they spaced out their visits and seemed depressed and withdrawn. They demonstrated both loyalty to their aunt and affection for their mother.
>
> Yet a third hypothesis involved the children's fears of developing Huntington's disease themselves. They avoided visiting and showed sadness because of their own expectations of contracting the disease (p. 60).

Having generated several hypotheses about the family and the problem in its relational context, the nurse arranged a meeting with the family. The purpose of the interview was to clarify how the family members wanted to be involved with the patient and how the staff could be most helpful to them. The nurse's hypotheses were relevant to the purpose of the interview. She did not know if the frequency of the family visits was a "problem" for either the children or the patient. Rather, the staff had identified the problem. Thus, the nurse chose to frame the purpose of the meeting as one in which the staff wanted to know how they could be most helpful to both the family and the patient during the patient's hospitalization. The patient and family were collaborating with the staff rather than the family being the object of care.

INTERVIEW SETTINGS

A family interview or meeting can take place anywhere: in the home (e.g., kitchen, living room, patient's bedroom), in an institution (e.g., bedside, urgent care center, nurse's clinic or office, used treatment room), or in the community (e.g., interviewing room, school, office, health clinic, on the street where a homeless family "resides"; on Skype for patients/families in remote areas). Depending on the purpose of the clinical interview, some settings are more conducive to beginning a therapeutic conversation than others. Nurses and families, therefore, need to consider the advantages and disadvantages of various settings. They should be flexible in choosing a setting that is appropriate for the specific purpose of the interview. We believe families should be offered a choice of setting whenever possible.

Home Setting

Many nurses interview families in their home setting. There are some concrete advantages to interviewing in the home. Infants, children of all ages, and older family members are able to be present more easily. Chances are increased for meeting significant but perhaps elusive family members, such as boarders, adolescents, or grandparents. Firsthand acquaintance with the physical environment is also possible. For example, the presence of staircases and the display of family photographs can be observed. The nurse can also experience the family's social environment; for example, rituals of eating, challenges with mobility, or who answers the doorbell can be noted.

In addition to the concrete advantages to interviewing in the home, there are also other advantages. These are particularly important if the nurse is from a different social class or ethnic background than the family. Articulate middle-class parents may report only the most exemplary family interactions in the office or school. The nurse may thus have difficulty understanding how the apparent competence of the parents and the banality of the reported parent-child incidents are in such sharp contrast to the degree of behavioral upset manifested by the child.

Lower-class families sometimes have difficulty bridging the gap and explaining their situation to middle-class nurses who are unfamiliar with their home milieu. For example, a nurse suggests that an older woman prepare her husband several small meals a day rather than one very large meal, which he is unable to consume. The nurse did not know (and the family members were too embarrassed to mention) that the family shared cooking facilities with other people in their apartment building. A home interview can thus give the nurse a clearer direction for therapeutic suggestions and can enhance the relationship between the family and nurse.

However, the disadvantages of using the home setting for family interviews are the increased administrative and personal cost involved in the nurse's travel. In addition, the meeting may have far more disruptions and may require the nurse to structure the interview flexibly. Nurses should also be aware that a family's home is their sanctuary. If family members are asked in their own home to share intense and deep emotions, they are often left without a retreat. For example, if abuse is an issue, the nurse should anticipate that the family's affective disclosure would be quite intense. Perhaps they will need more physical and psychological space to deal with the issues than their home permits. On the other hand, if the purpose of the interview is to facilitate shared grieving over the loss of a family member, the home setting might be ideal.

Ideas about therapeutic boundaries and hierarchy, confidentiality, and the timing and pacing of interventions can sometimes be challenged during home interviews. Doubts and confusion about the usefulness of intervention are not uncommon after nurses have experienced firsthand the economic deprivation of their clients. Experiencing families in their homes can teach nurses there are small opportunities even when a client's world seems to go under. It can make them more confident and comfortable to hold clients' hopelessness and helplessness and be with them to develop strategies to get unstuck, rather than trying to rescue them.

The nurse can tell the family that he or she would like to have an interview in the home "to get a better feel for their situation." Explain that, in your experience, there are frequently interruptions to an interview in the home (e.g., telephone calls, texting, neighbors dropping in, children wanting to put on the television or play computer games). Ask, "How should we handle this if it comes up?" In this way, you have already set the stage for work, rather than for visiting, and for a specific purpose to the interview. One way to handle social offerings, such as coffee or a cold drink, is to say, "Thanks, but maybe we could work first and then have coffee afterward." The work and social boundaries are thus clearly identified. Keep in mind that although this boundary might be useful for some nurses working with certain ethnic groups, such a boundary might be offensive to families from other ethnic groups or from rural areas.

Office, Hospital, or Other Work Setting

The greatest advantage of using the work setting for the interview is that the setting is the nurse's base or territory. Therefore, the nurse can capitalize on the opportunity and adapt the setting to the needs of the interview. Fewer telephone calls, mobile phones, and visitor interruptions are also possible. Furthermore, the nurse has a greater opportunity to obtain consultation from colleagues when interviewing the family in the work setting.

Disadvantages of interviewing in the work setting concern issues of context. A family might be intimidated by the professional trappings (e.g., large institution, plush furniture, complicated equipment) of the office and therefore may display anxiety or reluctance to talk. Suggestions for how beginning interviewers can maximize privacy in hospital settings are given later in this chapter.

Another disadvantage of using the institution for interviewing can be the inadvertent fostering of the belief that pathology resides in the individual— for example, "Mom's the sick one. We're only coming to help Mom get over her depression." This attitude is particularly evident if the mother has been hospitalized in a psychiatric unit. This disadvantage can be handled by using the family's willingness to "help Mom." The interviewer can reframe or discuss the mother's hospitalization in a positive light, for example, by saying, "Perhaps your mother's hospitalization has provided the family with an opportunity to all work together in a new way."

How to Use the Work Setting

Some hospitals, clinics, or universities have elaborate interviewing rooms, but most nurses must make do with the usual hospital or clinic facilities. Therefore, they may have to negotiate with coworkers for space and privacy. We recommend that you choose a private place where you will not be interrupted. For example, an unused patient room or an office is often more quiet and private than a four-bed room with curtains, a visitor's lounge, or a waiting area. Remove any important or intimidating equipment (such as machines and monitors). The discussion area should ideally be sparsely furnished with movable chairs and no big desks, couches, or examining tables. This allows family members to control their own space, move closer or farther away from someone, and not worry about children touching hospital equipment. A few quiet toys, such as rubber or cloth hand puppets or paper and crayons, are useful to have readily available in the room. Books and magazines should not be available during the interview because they give a mixed message to the family, especially to adolescents. The participants should expect to discuss issues; they should not expect to read during the interview.

Acquaint yourself with the physical layout of the room before the session. This is likely to increase your feelings of comfort when first meeting the family. At the beginning of the interview, if children are present, you can say to the parents, "I'd like you to handle the children in whatever way you usually do. That will give me a better idea of how things go at home." If the baby starts to cry, observe who comforts the baby. If the noise level gets beyond your tolerance, notice what tolerance level the family has. Unless absolutely necessary, try to avoid giving behavioral directives (e.g., "Watch out for that plant," or "Don't touch Dad's chest tube") during the first interview unless they are required for safety. Valuable information can be lost if you impose your standards of behavior upon family members. At the same time, be sure to structure the interview to avoid chaos and thereby lose your therapeutic leverage.

At the end of the session, assess the influence of the work setting. Ask family members if they behaved differently than they usually do: for example, "Did the children behave better or worse today than they usually do at home?" or "Were family members more or less talkative than usual than they are at home?"

WHO WILL BE PRESENT

Deciding who will be present for the first and subsequent interviews is important. The decision is generally determined together by family members and the nurse. In our early days of working with families, we thought it imperative that *all* family members be present for family interviewing. However, we have significantly changed in our thinking about who should come to the meetings. We now believe that a nurse can develop hypotheses, assess, and intervene with a family regardless of who is in the interviewing room. The number of family members sitting in front of a nurse does not constitute family nursing. Rather, what is more important is how the nurse conceptualizes human suffering, problems, and solutions. See Chapter 10 for a clinical vignette where Dr. Lorraine Wright interviews an individual to gain a family perspective about chronic illness.

We believe that nurses who are beginning to interview families will generally find it easiest to invite everyone living in the household to be present for the first interview. In this way, the nurse can more easily elicit information from members who most likely have a description of the problem, concern, or illness. To begin family work by interviewing just one person reduces the number of perspectives on the concerns, but it is still possible to inquire about family functioning even if seeing only one family member. If the problem concerns a couple, we usually try to have both spouses together for the first meeting. Similarly, if the issue is parenting-related, and it is a heterosexual couple, then the father, mother, and child should all be invited to the meeting.

The more family members present, the more information it is possible to gather. In addition, the more viewpoints and descriptions by family members of the influence of the problem or illness on their lives and relationships can then be considered by the nurse. Family members at the first interview might include the young children, the grandparent "who never has much to say," and the nephew "who just moved in for the weekend." Sometimes the most significant thing that the nurse is able to accomplish in a family interview is just to bring the whole family together in one spot at one time to discuss an important issue. When deciding who to invite to the first meeting, we believe it is very useful to consider the network of professional resources involved with the family as well as the family members themselves. We believe that relational family nursing is best practiced in context.

Nurses frequently question whether they should include in the first interview psychotic family members, those who are mentally or cognitively handicapped, or elderly family members who are experiencing dementia or Alzheimer's disease. Generally, the answer is yes. Including these members provides the nurse with an opportunity to talk with the family about the impact of the psychosis, mental handicap, or dementia on the family. In addition, it shows the nurse how the family and individual interact to deal with the presenting problem. A clinical example may help to illustrate this point. A family requested help for their 6-year-old daughter, who was "regressing, having imaginary friends, and refusing to play with peers or go to school." During the initial interview, the little girl walked over to the door and turned the doorknob. The nurse asked her not to leave the room. In response, the girl's siblings said that she was not leaving but rather "was letting the cat out the door." The nurse looked a bit startled because there was no cat in the room. The nurse then asked the other children how they knew that this was what the little girl was doing and proceeded to inquire if this was how they usually responded to the child's behavior. Had the "psychotic child" not been present, the nurse would have been unaware of the siblings' contribution to perpetuating the presenting problem.

Deciding who should be present for the first meeting is an important indicator of the collaborative nurse–family relationship. It is important for the nurse to be aware of who is in relevant conversation with whom about the problem or illness outside the interview room. Given the ever-increasing use of telecommunication devices such as e-mail, chat rooms, Skype, Facebook, and text messaging, it is useful for nurses to inquire not just about the family contacts in the immediate vicinity but also those online. We must respect family members' ideas about *what* is germane to the conversation and *who* should be involved in it. We recommend that all decisions about who should be involved in meetings, when, and what is talked about are determined collaboratively, one conversation at a time.

FIRST CONTACT WITH THE FAMILY

The way in which the nurse makes the first contact with the family conveys an important message to the parents and the children. We believe that the quality of the nurse's relationship with the family, in addition to manners and etiquette, are important ingredients for accountable and effective therapeutic engagement. Good manners and etiquette may help manage deep currents of tension and ease potentially awkward situations. Manners such as respect, tact, and humility can go a long way in establishing the nurse–family relationship. Madsen (2007) suggests "there is a long history of tension between professionals and poor and working-class people that is often invisible to professionals but painfully apparent to the poor and working classes" (p. 98; see Chapter 9 for more ideas about using manners in relational practice). By inviting each person in the household to the family meeting, the nurse implicitly states that each is a significant family member and each has a role to play in understanding, describing, and dealing with the problem.

The rationale for involving as many family members as possible can be explained in several ways. If a baby is in the intensive care nursery, the nurse might use the following explanation: "When a baby is in the intensive care nursery, we frequently find that family members are concerned and often anxious as well. Bringing family members together results in more information for the whole family on how best to help the baby." Another idea is for the nurse to say, "Years ago, fathers and family members were kept out of the delivery room and out of the hospital units. We've learned, though, how important it is to have family members present for special events such as the birth of a baby. Now we recognize that it is even more important for family members to be present and involved in health care when there is some type of illness. Family members know and care about each other. In many cases, they have a lot to offer each other."

With families experiencing a crisis, such as the diagnosis of a stage 4 glioblastoma in a previously healthy 62-year-old father, nurses may want to focus on providing physical information relating to the patient. Nurses can also see if the family is interested in hearing about services for families coping with the sudden onset of a life-threatening illness. They may state that in times of crisis, families often find comfort in meeting with health professionals so that they can gain accurate, up-to-date patient information. Nurses are aware from their knowledge of crisis theory that the time frame for intervention is limited because crises are self-limiting. Assertiveness and a calm demeanor are generally useful postures for nurses to take when a family is overwhelmed by a crisis.

Spouses sometimes agree to come for an interview but object to either having the children present or taking the children out of school. One way to handle the latter problem is to have meetings before school, during the lunch hour, after school, or in the evening. If this is not possible because of the nurse's work schedule, the nurse may say, "I understand your concern about the children missing school. In my experience, however, children have a tremendous amount to contribute to a family interview. They generally feel quite relieved when they see that the family is dealing with an issue about which they may have been worrying. Schools also are usually quite agreeable to children missing an hour."

How to Set Up an Appointment

On an outpatient basis, the purpose of the initial telephone contact with the family is to set up an appointment for an interview, explain the rationale for involving family members, and determine with the family who will be present at the interview. Naturally, both nurse and family gather much useful information about each other over the telephone. Telephone contact is therefore part of the development of a collaborative working relationship, and the nurse should treat it as such.

Generally, the first telephone contact sets the stage for subsequent interviews. Our advice is to pay careful attention to this contact, whether you call the family to set up an appointment or a family member calls you. The following is a sample first telephone contact:

> **Mother:** Hello.
>
> **Nurse:** Mrs. Garcia, this is Amrita Virk. I'm the community health nurse in your neighborhood.
>
> **Mother:** Yes.
>
> **Nurse:** I understand that you have a new baby. It's our practice to come out and visit all families with new babies.

Mother: Oh, I didn't know that.

Nurse: Yes, we usually do a physical examination of the baby and discuss feeding or other concerns.

Mother: Oh, that seems like a good idea. The doctor didn't tell me much about feeding.

Nurse: Sure, we can get into that during our visit. I was just calling to set up a time that would be convenient for your family and for me. I would like to see the whole family because usually, when a new baby arrives, the child has a great impact, not just on the mother but on the father and other children as well.

Mother: You can say that again! My 2-year-old usually seems to like his baby sister, but last night I saw him pinch her.

Nurse: Yes, these are the kinds of things that we can discuss when the whole family and I get together. The meeting will probably take about an hour. I have some time available on Tuesday at 10:00 or on Thursday at 3:00. Which would be best for you, the baby's father, and the children?

Mother: Tuesday isn't good because my son is going to the doctor that day. Thursday would be better since my husband works shifts and gets off at 2:30. But I should tell you that my husband didn't like the last nurse because she made some negative comments about his tattoos and piercings.

Nurse: Let me reassure you, I'm fine with people expressing themselves in body art. Would a 3:00 appointment give him enough time to get home, or should we make the appointment at 3:15?

Mother: Yes, 3:15 would be better.

Nurse: I look forward to seeing you and the whole family then.

Mother: Yes, me too.

Nurse: Good-bye.

Mother: 'Bye.

In the previous selection, the nurse was clear, confident, focused, and accommodating. She set forth the purpose of the interview and who she thought should be involved. She invited the family to a "meeting" by stating that this is the clinic's usual practice. She responded directly to Mrs. Garcia's concern about tattoos and piercings. Whether the nurse refers to her collaborative time with a family as a "meeting" or an "interview" is arbitrary; it is most important that the nurse use the most palatable language with families based on the context in which she encounters them. The nurse took charge by identifying and introducing herself without apologies and offered specific appointment times. Furthermore, the nurse received much information that can be useful in the family meeting:

"The doctor didn't tell me much about feeding."

"I saw [the 2-year-old] pinch her."

"My son is going to the doctor . . ."

"My husband works shifts . . ."

It is not possible to provide written guidelines to cover all the various situations that nurses will encounter in trying to set up a family interview. Some suggestions for involving fathers include:

- Emphasize the value and importance of fathers' perceptions and observations.

- Demonstrate respect for the father's time by asking if the telephone call was made at a convenient time.

- Use positive verbal cues (e.g., common courtesies, personal titles, a cheerful and interested tone of voice, positive phrases, and affirming remarks) in order to maintain rapport.

Each family presents different challenges for the nurse, and vice versa. Therefore, each interview must be approached with flexibility. A unique approach is always the rule in clinical practice. Each telephone contact demands a slightly different plan of action to invite family members to an interview or to elicit the family's permission for a home visit. We strongly encourage nurses, especially community health nurses, to plan their telephone calls and appointments to maximize efficiency and the possibility of developing a collaborative partnership with the family. We generally do not recommend that appointments be set up by e-mail or text, as there can be issues of confidentiality and ambiguity about how promptly the e-mail or text will be responded to and by whom. However, we do recognize that, in some rural or very remote areas, setting up and even offering family meetings may be done online via Skype, e-mail, or instant messaging. Online family meetings may prove to be very useful if a face-to-face meeting is not possible.

RESISTANCE AND NONCOMPLIANCE

Often in our clinical supervision with nurses, we have been asked how to deal with resistant, difficult, or noncompliant families. When nurses ask this, they are generally referring to families whom they perceive to be "in denial," oppositional, or noncompliant with ideas and advice that they have offered or could offer to promote, maintain, or restore health. The family is designated as noncompliant when they do not respond to particular nursing interventions; nurses often interpret this behavior as unwillingness or a lack of readiness to change (Wright & Levac, 1992).

We do not use the terms *resistance* and *noncompliance,* because we have not found them clinically useful in relational family nursing practice. *Resistance* was initially used to describe a client's reluctance to uncover or recover from some anxiety-filled experience. Resistance is still generally viewed as "located" in the client and is often described as something the client "does." This is a linear view that implies that problems with adherence to treatment regimens reside within individuals and families, not in the interactions or relationships between individuals. However, we see the idea of resistance as a *product* of client–interviewer interaction. We believe that *resistance* and *noncompliance* are not terms describing a unilateral phenomenon but rather an interactional phenomenon.

Rather than using these terms, we have found the multidirectional terms *cooperation* and *collaboration* to be very useful clinically. When nurses think of how they work collaboratively with families, they are less likely to impose their will on them. They tend to open space for the family and to be more tentative and receptive to the family's point of view. For example, they welcome the opportunity to offer their time (Miller, et al, 2011), respond to what they might perceive as challenging questions, sit with the client, not minimize the situation, apologize if indicated, seek solutions (e.g., "What can we do to move forward on this?"), speak in positive terms (e.g., "I will have your lab results by . . ." vs. "I can't get them until . . ."), and so forth.

The theory behind the "death of resistance" has emerged since our first edition of *Nurses and Families.* The result has been a dramatic increase in a solution-focused, strengths-based, and resiliency orientation to family interviewing (Bell & Wright, 2011; Hougher Limacher & Wright, 2006; Madsen, 2007; Walsh, 2011). With emphasis on a solution comes an increasing emphasis on change, cooperation, and collaboration. They open us to reflect on conversation, language, and possibilities rather than pathologizing labels.

We are especially partial to the work of Miller and Duncan (2000), who advocate client-directed, outcome-informed clinical work as compared to a model-driven focus. The "common factors" (Hubble, Duncan, & Miller, 1999) associated with positive outcomes include:

- Extra-therapeutic factors, including clients' beliefs about change, strengths, resiliencies, and chance-occurring positive events in clients' lives (40%)
- The client–therapist relationship experienced as empathic, collaborative, and affirmative in focusing on goals, methods, and pace of treatment (30%)
- Hope and expectancy about the possibility of change (15%)
- Structure and focus of a model or approach in organizing the treatment (15%)

How to Deal With a Hesitant Family Member

A spouse may be hesitant to attend the family session for several possible reasons. Each requires a different approach on the part of the nurse. The following are a few common situations that interviewers encounter:

1. "My husband would never come to a family interview. He thinks that my mother's stroke and how to handle it are my responsibility."

   Ask what the wife thinks about her husband attending the interview. If she believes her mother's chronic illness is *her* responsibility and has very little to do with her husband, she will not be interested in inviting her husband to a family interview. You would need to engage in conversation with the wife to see if she wants to alter *her* cognitive set *before* you start talking to her about her husband.

2. "My husband wouldn't want to come to a family interview. Besides, I wouldn't know how to get him there."

   If the wife would like her husband to attend but does not know how to invite him, you can explore with her why she feels her husband might be hesitant. There could be several reasons:

   - He may view the problem as his wife's, not his own.

   - The timing of the interview might be inconvenient.

   - The thought of going to a hospital might be repugnant ("seeing all those sick people").

   - He may be afraid of being blamed for not taking a more active role in his mother-in-law's care.

You can ask the wife if she thinks any of these feelings or thoughts might be stopping her husband from becoming involved. After she has speculated on the reasons for her husband's hesitance and her own desire for him to be present, you can discuss with her some alternate ways to engage him:

- She can discuss with her husband how *she needs his help* to deal with her mother's illness.

- She can find out convenient times for her husband to come to a half-hour meeting.

- She can tell him exactly where the interview will be held (e.g., not in the patient's room but in an office).

- She can tell him that the nurse is most hesitant to see only parts of the family for a meeting. That is, if you saw only the wife with her mother, there could be a danger that the husband would feel left out and perhaps blamed. If he were present, however, this could not happen. He could help you to understand more fully the relationship between his wife and her mother. The wife can let him know that he has a unique view of the family—a view that only he can provide. Most husbands do not like to be left out of the original planning and decision making.

Once they have a fuller understanding of the purpose of a family interview, they are often quite agreeable to attending.

Although it may involve a little persuasion, when nurse interviewers ask that the husband attend and state that they need him to be there, they are likely to have few problems with absent husbands. Conversely, nurses are likely to have difficulties in this area if they are timid or inconsistent in requesting the husband's presence.

We believe it is important for nurses to recognize that husbands and wives may be at different stages in their desire to seek help. Some of this may be attributable to gender differences, with females generally more likely than males to utilize social support networks. Women are more than twice as likely as men to speak to someone about their problems. It seems likely, then, that wives would lead the discussion regarding assistance and help their husbands along the process.

Another idea for inviting an anxious or a threatened family member to an interview is to suggest that the person be asked to be present as an observer, just to see what is happening. Also, the person can come whenever he or she is "in the mood" as a historian, an accuracy checker, or a consultant. If these suggestions are followed, it is important to ask the "observer" or "historian" to react at the *end* of the interview to what the family has discussed in the session. Gradually, as the family member continues to observe sessions, he or she often becomes more comfortable and is willing to participate *during* the interview. This may be a particularly useful way of engaging some adolescents. Telling the member not to talk places no direct pressure on that member to participate. Silent members are often closely attuned to the process, and when a sensitive area is broached, they forget their defensive stance and join in the process. Other times, they may remain silent but hear the information.

How to Deal With Family Nonengagement and Referral Sources

If you have difficulty engaging the family on the telephone, you may need to contact the referral source—that is, physicians frequently tell a patient on discharge, "The nurse will be out to check on you and see how you are doing." When you contact the patient, the patient may have forgotten what the physician said, may be confused about the purpose of the visit, or simply may not be interested in being "checked on."

Sometimes in situations of suspected child abuse, the physician may contact the nurse and ask him or her to drop in on the family just to see if there is any abuse. You may then find yourself in an awkward situation, trying to explain the purpose of your visit to a family who may be reluctant to have you come. One way to approach this is to say, "Doctor Fishkin asked me to set up a visit with your family to discuss issues about raising children. Dr. Fishkin feels that most families who have infants and preschoolers who are close in age sometimes find it helpful to talk to a nurse." In approaching the situation this way, you have clearly indicated that it is on Dr. Fishkin's request that you are calling, and you have attempted to normalize the purpose of the interview. If, however, the family is still reluctant to have you visit, initiate contact with the physician and have the physician set the stage for future work with the family. You should not consider this inability to engage a family your fault or the fault of the family, but rather as a problem of inadequate preparation by the referral source.

Several other ideas have emerged over the past few years about dealing with referral sources. We find it best for interviewers to avoid focusing prematurely on family dynamics if the request for the interview comes from another agency or if the interview is compulsory. Treatment failure often ensues because of powerful conflict between the family and the referral source. In such situations, we recommend that the nurse engage the family and conceptualize their work together as collaboration to deal not with family issues per se, but with dynamics between the family and the agency. In this way, the interviewer can join with the family around a problem such as, "That school is always making trouble for us." Thus, the focus of the nurse's work would not be on family dynamics but on work with the family to "get the school off their case."

We believe that the interviewer must identify and grapple with the expectations of the person referring the "problem family" for assessment. Some useful questions to ask include:

- Why is this referral being made to me at this time?
- What is the relationship between the referral source and my agency?
- Who is paying? For whom? For what?
- What are the expectations of the hierarchy within which I work?
- If the referral source is unhappy with the assessment, who will hear about it?
- If I am unhappy about the assessment process, who will hear about it?

In any situation in which nonengagement occurs, the nurse must realize that the reluctance provides important information about the dynamics between the interviewer and the family. The hypothesized reason that a person is not present should be explored at the first interview. For example, we were once asked to consult with the family members of a 59-year-old woman who had terminal cancer. The hospital staff nurse arranged the interview for a time convenient for the husband and adult daughter. However, only the daughter and the mother showed up for the interview. In exploring the reasons that the husband did not attend, we discovered that he was 73 years old and in poor health himself, a fact unknown to the hospital staff. By asking the adult daughter about the impact of her mother's illness, we also discovered information about the father's absence. The daughter wept openly about her mother's impending death. She then stated, "If you think I'm a basket case, you should see my father. He's in worse shape than I am." Thus, in this situation, the husband's absence from the interview provided important information about the family's emotional state. It is important for nurses to understand reluctance as a systems phenomenon rather than an individual issue. In this case, we hypothesized not only that the father was reluctant to attend but also that the adult daughter was trying to protect him.

CONCLUSIONS

In preparing for family interviews, it is important for nurses to first remind themselves of the type of relationship they would like to develop with the client and the purpose of the family meeting and then to generate hypotheses related to this purpose. Box 6–8 outlines areas for nurses to consider in preparing for family interviews. These ideas are the result of striving toward a collaborative relationship between the nurse and the family.

Box 6-8 Helpful Hints for Planning a Family Meeting

Before initiating a family meeting, the nurse needs to:

- Ascertain the purpose and benefit of a family meeting from the family's perspective.
- Explain why a family meeting may be beneficial to the family.
- Determine who in the family agrees that a problem exists, and who might be willing to come to a family meeting.
- Mutually determine with the family when and where a meeting could take place (home, office, school).
- Read literature about working with families experiencing similar health problems to better understand the issues, concerns, and lived experiences of that specific population.
- Begin to formulate hypotheses (explanations about the family's behaviors that connect the family system and the particular problem).
- Prepare linear and circular questions that will elicit relevant data about family structure, development, and function. (See the discussions of CFAM in Chapter 3 and CFIM in Chapter 4 for examples of questions.)

Levac, A.M.C., Wright, L.M., & Leahey, M. (2002). Children and families: Models for assessment and intervention. In J.A. Fox (Ed.): *Primary health care of infants, children, and adolescents* (2nd ed.). St. Louis: Mosby, pp. 10–19. Copyright 2002. Adapted with permission from A.M.C. Levac, L.M. Wright, & M. Leahey.

References

Bell, J.B. (2011). Relationships: The heart of the matter in family nursing. *Journal of Family Nursing, 17*(1), 3–10.

Bell, J.M., & Wright, L.M. (2011). Creating practice knowledge for families experiencing illness suffering: The Illness Beliefs Model. In E. Svavarsdottir & H. Jonsdottir (Eds.): *Family Nursing in Action*. Reykjavik, Iceland: University of Iceland Press, pp. 15–52.

Benzein, E., Johansson, P., Arenstedt, K., et al. (2008). Nurses' attitudes towards families' importance in nursing care – a survey of Swedish nurses. *Journal of Family Nursing, 14*(2), 162-180.

Bergadahl, E., Benzein, E., Ternestedt, B., et al. (2011). Development of nurses' abilities to reflect on how to create good caring relationships with patients in palliative care: An action research approach. *Nursing Inquiry, 18*(2), 111-122.

Burke, S.O., et al. (2001). Effects of stress-point intervention with families of repeatedly hospitalized children. *Journal of Family Nursing, 7*(2), 128–158.

Duran, C.R., et al. (2007). Attitudes toward and beliefs about family presence: A survey of healthcare providers, patients' families, and patients. *American Journal of Critical Care, 16*(3), 270–279.

Fleuridas, C., Nelson, T., & Rosenthal, D. (1986). The evolution of circular questions: Training family therapists. *Journal of Marital and Family Therapy, 12*(2), 113–127.

Foucault, D., Leahey, M., Harper-Jaques, S., et al. (2008). Perceptions of family involvement in mental health care: Through the lens of clients and their families. Presentation at Institute for Family-Centered Care Annual Conference, Calgary, Alberta, Canada.

Hougher Limacher, L., & Wright, L.M. (2006). Exploring the therapeutic intervention of commendations: Insights from research. *Journal of Family Nursing, 12*(3), 307–331.

Hubble, M.A., Duncan, B.L., & Miller, S.D. (1999). Introduction. In M.A. Hubble, B.L. Duncan, & S.D. Miller (Eds.): *The Heart & Soul of Change: What Works in Therapy*. Washington, DC: American Psychological Association, pp. 1–19.

Jonsdottir, H., & Ingadottir, T.S. (2011). Nursing practice partnership with families living with advanced lung disease. In E.K. Svavarsdottir & H. Jonsdottir (Eds.): *Family Nursing in Action*. Reykjavik, University of Iceland Press, pp. 357–375.

Leahey, M., & Harper-Jaques, S. (1996). Family-nurse relationships: Core assumptions and clinical implications. *Journal of Family Nursing, 2*(2), 133–151.

Leahey, M., & Wright, L.M. (1987). Families and chronic illness: Assumptions, assessment, and intervention. In L.M. Wright & M. Leahey (Eds.): *Families and Chronic Illness*. Springhouse, PA: Springhouse, pp. 55–76.

Levac, A.M.C., Wright, L.M., & Leahey, M. (2002). Children and families: Models for assessment and intervention. In J.A. Fox (Ed.): *Primary Health Care of Infants, Children, and Adolescents* (2nd ed.). St. Louis: Mosby, pp. 10–19.

Madsen, W.C. (2007). *Collaborative Therapy With Multi-Stressed Families*. New York: The Guilford Press.

Miller, B.F., Teevan, B., Phillips, R.L., et al. (2011). The importance of time in treating mental health in primary care. *Families, Systems & Health, 29*(2), 144–145.

Miller, S.D., & Duncan, B.L. (2000). Paradigm lost: From model-driven to client-directed, outcome-informed clinical work. *Journal of Systemic Therapies, 19*(1), 20–33.

Sveinbjarnadottir, E.K., Svavarsdottir, E.K., & Saveman, B.I. (2011). Nurses attitudes towards the importance of families in psychiatric care following an educational and training intervention program. *Journal of Psychiatric and Mental Health Nursing*, doi: 10.1111/j.1365-2850.2011.01744.x.

Tapp, D.M. (2000). The ethics of relational stance in family nursing: Resisting the view of "nurse as expert." *Journal of Family Nursing, 6*(1), 69–91.

Walsh, F. (2011). *Strengthening Family Resilience*. 2nd Ed., New York, NY: Guilford Press.

Wright, L.M., & Bell, J.M. (2009). *Belief and Illness: A Model to Invite Healing*. Calgary, AB: 4th Floor Press.

Wright, L.M., & Levac, A.M. (1992). The non-existence of non-compliant families: The influence of Humberto Maturana. *Journal of Advanced Nursing, 17*, 913–917.

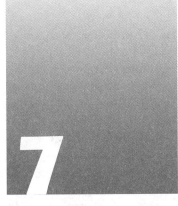

Chapter

How to Conduct Family Interviews

Once a nurse and a family have decided to meet, the nurse can begin to consider how to conduct the meeting. Just as there is an interviewing procedure, there is also a process in initial family interviews. This process provides the nurse with an interview structure and can help to allay the nurse's anxiety.

In this chapter, we present guidelines for each stage of an initial family interview. Afterward, we address the stages involved in the entire interviewing process.

GUIDELINES FOR FAMILY INTERVIEWS

The following stages generally occur in initial interviews:

1. **Engagement stage:** The family is greeted, made comfortable, and the relationship continues.

2. **Assessment stage:**

   ■ *Problem identification,* in which the nurse explores the family's presenting concerns and/or suffering.

   ■ *Relationship between family interaction and health problem,* in which the nurse explores the family's typical responses to the health problem and how the health problem is affecting their family life and relationships.

   ■ *Attempted solutions,* in which the family and nurse talk about the solutions the family has tried and their effects on the presenting issues.

   ■ *Goal exploration,* in which the nurse draws together the information, and the family members specify what goals, changes, or outcomes they are seeking (note: if family members are suffering from the impact of an illness, it is also important to clarify if they desire an alleviation or softening in their suffering in the emotional, physical, and/or spiritual domains).

3. **Intervention stage:** The nurse and family collaborate on areas for desired change.

4. **Termination stage:** The nurse and family conclude the interview.

Engagement Stage

During the engagement, or first stage of the interview, the nurse and family begin to establish a therapeutic relationship. Engagement has several purposes (Box 7–1). The goal is for family members and the nurse to develop a mutual alliance so that they can collaborate on the desired changes. In the beginning, the nurse is often perceived as a stranger, unknown, untrusted, and potentially helpful or unhelpful. Because family members do not know what to expect from the nurse, the nurse must establish a relationship with the members by demonstrating understanding, competence, and caring. Family nursing is relational nursing practice, acknowledging the expertise and knowledge of families.

We encourage nurses to consider the type of relationship that they would like to establish with families. Thorne and Robinson (1989) have described various stages of the evolution of relationships between families experiencing chronic illness and their health-care professionals: naïve trust, disenchantment, and guarded alliance. They propose that naïve trust among the chronically ill, their families, and health-care providers is inevitably shattered in the face of unmet expectations and conflicting perspectives. Anxiety, frustration, and confusion often result in disenchantment. Trust can then be reconstructed on a more guarded basis so that the chronically ill patient, the family, and the nurse can continue to engage in health-care activities. Thorne and Robinson (1989) state that this reconstructed trust is highly selective and is based on revised expectations of the roles of both patient and provider. They suggest that there are four relationship types in guarded alliance: hero worship, resignation, consumerism, and team playing. In hero worship and team playing the trust dimension is high, whereas in resignation and consumerism it is low. Both team playing and consumerism place a high value on competence, whereas hero worship and resignation put a low value on competence. Important guidelines for the engagement of families with children are provided in Box 7–2.

Box 7-1 Purpose of Engagement

- To promote a positive nurse–family relationship by developing an atmosphere of comfort, mutual trust, and cooperation between the nurse and the family
- To recognize that the family members bring strengths and resources to this relationship that may have previously gone unnoticed by health-care professionals
- To prevent potential nurse–family misunderstandings or problems later on in the therapeutic relationship

Levac, A.M.C., Wright, L.M., & Leahey, M. (2002). Children and families: Models for assessment and intervention. In J.A. Fox (Ed.): *Primary Health Care of Infants, Children, and Adolescents* (2nd ed.). St. Louis: Mosby, p. 11. Copyright 2002. Adapted with permission.

Box 7-2	The ABCs of Engaging Families	
A	**B**	**C**
Assume an active, confident approach.	Begin by providing structure to the meeting (time frame, orientation to the context).	Create a context of mutual trust.
Ask purposeful questions that draw forth family assessment data.	Behave in a curious manner, and take an equal interest in all family members, whether present or not.	Clarify expectations about your role with the family.
Address all who are present, including small children.	Build on family strengths by offering commendations to the family.	Collaborate in decision-making, health promotion, and health management.
Adjust the conversation to children's developmental stages.	Bring relevant resources to the meeting (list of agencies, phone numbers, pamphlets).	Cultivate a context of racial and ethnic sensitivity. Commend family members.

Levac, A.M.C., Wright, L.M., & Leahey, M. (2002). Children and families: Models for assessment and intervention. In J.A. Fox (Ed.): *Primary Health Care of Infants, Children, and Adolescents* (2nd ed.). St. Louis: Mosby, p. 11. Copyright 2002. Adapted with permission.

Reciprocal trust is a critical dimension to consider during the engagement phase of family interviewing. The nurse helps the patient and family to feel more confident in their own competence in managing illness. In order to develop a high degree of trust in the nurse, the patient and family are encouraged to explicitly state their expectations for health care. The nurse provides the opportunity for family members to express their desires. If the patient and family are to have a high degree of trust in their own competence, family members and health-care providers must acknowledge the family's resources.

One way of reminding ourselves not to fall into the trap of certainty, judgmentalness, and expertness on the family's situation has been to develop a strong sense of curiosity. When initiating engagement, we assume a position of neutrality or curiosity. Cecchin (1987) draws connections between neutrality or curiosity and hypothesizing. He maintains that curiosity is a delight in the invention and discovery of multiple patterns. "Curiosity helps us to continue looking for different descriptions and explanations, even when we cannot immediately imagine the possibility of another one . . . hypothesizing is connected to curiosity. Hypothesizing has more to do with technique. Curiosity is a stance, whereas hypothesizing is what we do to try to maintain this stance" (p. 411). We believe that curiosity nurtures circularity and is useful in the development of hypotheses. We have found hypothesizing, circularity, and curiosity to be extremely important components of our clinical work.

We agree with Cecchin (1987), who states, "circular questioning can be understood as a method by which a clinician creates curiosity within the family system and therapy system" (p. 412). (See Chapters 2 and 3 for more information about circularity, and see Chapter 6 for additional ideas about hypothesizing.) By using hypothesizing, circularity, and curiosity, nurses become more open to families, and families, in turn, develop more reciprocal trust. The family perceives the nurse as inquisitive when he or she does not take sides with any one member or subgroup. Nurses who are inquisitive are seen as aligned with everyone and no one in particular at the same time. They are seen as nonjudgmental and accepting of everyone.

Increased societal, professional, and personal experiences with fear and suffering have caused nurses to engage clients in more personal, open ways than ever before, especially since September 11, 2001. The societal experiences of large-scale death, both foreign and domestic terrorism (e.g., the Virginia Tech massacre), and revolutions such as the Arab Spring have made nurse relationships with families more human, less clinical, and more transparent. Nurses' own sufferings and losses of family members and friends also enhance this transparency. Therapeutic relationships in recent years have become less formal, more connected as nurses experience similar fears and suffering when crises erupt or illness or loss occurs.

Wright and Bell (2009) pose a reflective question when they ask, "Are clinicians to remain neutral and non-hierarchical when confronted with illegal or dangerous behaviors?" They answer this important question by stating that each family functions in the way that members desire and in a way that they determine most effective. However, being part of a larger system, nurses are bound by moral, ethical, legal, cultural, and societal norms that require them to act in accordance with those norms in regard to illegal or dangerous behavior. Cecchin (1987) assented that, in these situations, "clinicians may need to take a different position—one which is distinct from a non-hierarchical, collaborative stance. Confronted by illegal behavior, a nurse may have to abandon a curious, therapeutic manner and become a social controller" (p. 409) in order to conform to the moral or legal rules and their consequences.

To enhance engagement, the nurse must provide structure, be active and empathic, and involve all members of the family. To provide structure, the nurse might say something such as, "We'll meet now for about 10 minutes so that I can get a better sense of your expectations and any concerns you have about hospitalization. We can then talk about what I might be able to help you with. How does that sound to you?" By stating the structure at the beginning of the meeting, the nurse reduces the family's anxiety about how long they will meet and also gives some direction for the conversation. Sunder's (2011) findings that families found it helpful when the clinician asked questions, gave time, and structured the work further support this idea.

One way in which the nurse can be active during the engagement phase of the interview is to find out who is present. Many times, we have found that "extra" family members attend interviews in the hospital. Leahey, Stout, and Myrah (1991) found that of families invited to meetings on an inpatient mental health unit in a Canadian community hospital, 94% attended. Extra family members attending interviews held constant over a 7-year period. In many cases, family members of whom the nurse was unaware showed up for the family meeting. For example, extended family members or ex-spouses might have been invited by the patient or other family members who believed it was important for them to be present.

Some nurses have found it useful to start an interview by working with the family in constructing a genogram or ecomap (see Chapter 3). Duhamel and Campagna's genograph (2000) is a particularly helpful educational tool that can assist nurses in drawing a genogram and determining what questions to ask. Families generally find that constructing a genogram is an easy way to involve themselves in giving the nurse relevant information. The genogram can be obtained reliably and accurately in a brief interview. Furthermore, genograms obtained by a health-care provider are likely to have more influence on care and health outcomes than those completed by the patient or health assistant and placed on file.

At the start of the interview, the nurse should ask questions of each member. This is particularly important for nurses working with families with adolescents. Engaging adolescents by asking what their favorite computer games or school subjects are and why, whether they play sports, what musical groups they like, and whether they have any special talents and hobbies can sometimes be useful. The purpose of these questions is to start establishing a shared habit (between the nurse and the young person) of discussion and banter about the young person's opinions about personal aspects of their lives. However, we do not recommend that this type of conversation go on for longer than 5 minutes because it seems easier for families to engage around the presenting problem than to chat in a general nature. We believe it is important for the nurse to create an environment where the client expects to get down to business, work on the hard issues, and make the necessary changes to improve their family functioning in the context of illness, loss, or disability.

Nurses should initially attempt to spend an equal amount of time with each family member. We suggest that the nurse ask the same question or a similar one of each member to gather each person's ideas about a particular topic. We believe that when families answer questions, they are not retrieving particular experiences. Rather, in the conversation with the clinician, family members put forth their own storytelling of their unique experiences, suggest beginnings and endings for these experiences, and highlight portions of experiences while diminishing or excluding others.

Examples of questions used to foster a collaborative working relationship and engagement have been offered by Levac, Wright, and Leahey (2002). These provide an implicit message to family members that the practitioner cares about them. They also provide opportunities for the family to exert more power in the conversation, voice concerns, and clarify the working arrangement. Some examples are:

- What was most and least useful in your past relationships with health professionals like me?
- If you become frustrated with our work together, would you be open to having a conversation with me about your concerns?
- On a scale of 1 to 10 (with 1 being very low and 10 being very high), how well do you think I understand your situation?
- In what ways was our discussion useful (or not) to each of you?

Both students and practicing nurses have often asked us for tips on how to deal with verbose clients. Some ideas we have found helpful include:

- Letting the person tell his or her illness story or particular concern.
- Setting the time frame at the beginning such as, "We have 20 minutes to meet. What are the most important things that we need to discuss?"
- Saying, "I know we only have time to skim the surface today in talking about your experiences, so what shall we focus on?"
- Explaining, "I'm not connecting what you're telling me with the reason you've come in today. Could you help me out on this, please?"
- Taking a break to pull your thoughts together or to seek a consult.
- Stopping the discussion and setting limits such as, "We can spend 10 minutes talking about the poor addiction services in our city and 10 minutes on what you said your goals were and how you're addressing them. How does that sound as a plan for today?"
- Using humor and interrupting by saying something such as, "Seems like we could talk all day about this issue, but I'm mindful of the time."
- Determining who is most interested in the client being seen if the client has been referred by another health professional: "The note from your physician indicated she wants you to have . . . Is this your understanding of why you are here today? Did you have another goal for our meeting?"

If the engagement between the nurse and family does not proceed well or if a fit cannot be established, we recommend that the nurse stop and think about the relationship. We have found the following ideas about relationships with families helpful to keep in mind in our clinical practice:

1. Both the health-care provider and patient and/or family members are experts. The patient is expert in the illness experience, and usually, but not always, the health-care provider is expert in the physiology of the disease process, illness management, and softening suffering.

2. The health-care provider will try to facilitate change, but the ultimate agent of change is the patient/family.

3. To construct a workable management plan, the patient/family and the health-care provider's interpretation of the symptoms must both be acknowledged.

The engagement stage is also the phase of the interview in which a context for change is created that constitutes the central and enduring foundations of the therapeutic process (Bell & Wright, 2011; Wright & Bell, 2009). Wright and Bell suggest that all obstacles for change need to be removed during this stage so that a full and meaningful nurse-family engagement may be made. Examples of obstacles to change in working with families include a family member who does not want to be present or who attends the meeting under duress, previous negative experiences with health-care professionals, and unrealistic or unknown expectations of the referring person about treatment.

Most central to this stage, however, is that the family should feel that the nurse is willing to listen and witness their voice, to "do hope," as Weingarten (2000) calls it. But hope does not reside within one individual; it is not solitary. Hope is something we do with others. "It is the responsibility of those who love you to *do hope* with you" (Weingarten, 2000, p. 402). One study sought to understand couples' experiences in nurse-initiated health-promoting conversations about hope and suffering during home-based palliative care. It was revealed that couples found these conversations with nurses to be a healing experience that also enabled them to learn and find new ways for managing daily life (Benzein & Saveman, 2008). Ward and Wampler (2010) suggest distinguishing categories of hope on a continuum from lost hope, ambivalent/low hope, to solid hope.

We find this notion useful in our clinical work. Especially during the engagement phase, nurses should follow the clients' lead, listening for and adopting their language, worldview, goals, ideas about the problem, and legitimizing their illness experiences to foster a trusting relationship nested in hope. We encourage nurses to get to know their clients outside of the influence of the problem and connect with them in their lives. For example, a nurse could appreciate their experience as skilled immigrants who have made tremendous sacrifices to stand up to oppressive regimes, learn a new language, and make a significant move to a new country. She could wonder how this stamina might now serve the family as they stand together against illness.

If the engagement relationship is not going well, we encourage nurses to recognize this difficulty. For example, the nurse could tune into potential difficulties such as the client's repetitions or interruptions. The nurse could acknowledge the difficulties to the patient and say, "I'm having trouble understanding how you'd like me to help." Or, "It doesn't seem that this visit is going the way you had hoped." Or, "I would like to work with you even though we see some things differently."

Assessment Stage

During the assessment stage, the nurse and family explore four areas: problem identification, relationship between family interaction and the health problem, attempted solutions to solving problems, and goals.

Problem Identification: Exploration and Definition

During this phase of the family interview, the nurse asks family members about their main concerns, complaints, or suffering. The nurse could ask, for example, "What is the concern that each family member would most like to see addressed or changed?" A focus on change and expectation for something to happen is important for time-effective therapeutic meetings. Slive and Bobele (2011) have demonstrated this in their landmark work documenting single session walk in therapy. After exploring each family member's perception of the most pressing concern, preferably at the end of the interview (once adequate engagement has occurred), we have found it useful to ask the "why now?" question: "What made you decide to come in today?" We assume the family probably consulted others prior to meeting with the nurse and are curious about why, at this point in time, the client chose to seek help.

Another useful question is the "one-question question" (OQQ) suggested by Wright (1989): "If you could have only one question answered during our work together, what would that one question be?" At the end of the clinical meeting, this is a particularly effective way to elicit the family's deepest concern or greatest area of suffering (Duhamel, Dupuis, & Wright, 2009). It provides a focus for the conversation and generates sharing of new information among family members and between the nurse and the family. For example, the husband of a 44-year-old woman with newly diagnosed multiple myeloma asked, "How can I support my wife and children better during this time?" The teenage daughter asked, "How can I learn more about my mother's illness?" The patient asked, "How long do I have to live?" The young adult son asked, "Should I avoid having my friends come over to the house so that the house can be quieter for my mother when she returns home?" These four very different questions made it clear that each family member had different concerns and issues, expectations for the interview, and expectations for the relationship with the nurse. We are drawn to Madsen's phrase "Honor before helping," in which he reminds us how important it is not to attempt to help a family without its authorization to do so (2007).

It is important to emphasize that an effective interview does not depend on the use of one type of question but on the knowledge of when, how, and to what purpose questions are used with particular family members at particular points in time. (For more information on various types of questions, see Chapters 4 and 8.)

Leahey and Wright (1987) give examples of how to elicit the family's concerns by asking circular questions that focus on the present, past, and future:

Present. The nurse should ask each family member, including the children, to share their knowledge and understanding of the present situation. For example, the community health nurse working with a family with teens could ask such questions as:

■ What is the family's main concern now about Mobina's cyber-bullying?

■ How is this concern a problem for the family now as compared with before?

■ Who agrees with you that this is a problem? Is this a problem that Mobina believes she has control over?

■ What is your explanation for this?

Past. In exploring the past, the nurse can again ask questions pertaining to:

■ *Differences:* How was Mobina's behavior before her cyberbullying was noticed?

■ *Agreement or disagreement:* Who agrees with Dad that this was the main concern when the family lived in Uganda?

■ *Explanation or meaning:* What do you think was the significance of Mobina's decision to stop using the family computer for her messaging?

Future. During the initial interview with a new family, the nurse must learn about the family's own hypotheses or beliefs about the problems. In asking the family to explain the present situation, the nurse should attempt to identify previously unrecognized connections. This might be accomplished by asking such questions as:

■ If Rahim suddenly developed renal disease, how would things be different from the way they are now?

■ Does Rahim agree with you?

■ If this were to happen, how would you explain the change in Mobina's relationship with Mom?

If children or adolescents are reluctant to identify concerns in the family, the nurse may need to ask the children alternative questions. Children may hesitate to disagree with their parents' description of the situation. A nurse can ask a child what he or she would like to see different in the family or how he or she would know if the problems went away. For example, one 8-year-old repeatedly stated that there were no difficulties surrounding his brother's diabetes and his mother's intense involvement with the sick child. However, when the nurse asked a future-oriented question about what differences he would notice in the family if his brother did not have diabetes, the 8-year-old said that he and his mother could go to basketball games after school. At the time of the interview, the mother had stated she was hesitant to leave the house after the boys returned from school for fear that her oldest son, Raja, would have an insulin reaction.

Other ideas for involving children in interviews have also been presented. For example, having paper, markers, and crayons in the office and using strategies such as:

■ Art techniques (e.g., drawing a family picture)

■ Verbal techniques (e.g., the "Columbo" strategy of taking a position of not knowing)

■ Role playing or make-believe

■ Storytelling techniques to allow families to personify, reframe, and externalize problems

- Puppet and doll techniques to ask the family about interactions
- Experiential techniques (e.g., family sculpture or "a can of worms in action")

Relationship differences can be explored by providing props, such as scarves, hats, and glasses, to the children. This role-playing technique using props enables children and adults to display their perceptions. Another idea is to give the child an ordered array of pictures ranging from a frowning face to a smiling face and then ask, "Which one of these is most like how you and your brothers got along this week?" Engaging children through video games offers many other possibilities. Whatever strategy is used to engage young people in conversation, we recommend nurses be aware of the importance of inviting active thinking by children and adolescents versus the expectation of compliance with adult thinking. This is foundational to relational practice.

In exploring the presenting concern, the nurse should obtain a clear and specific definition of the situation. We recommend that nurses pay attention only to the concern as defined by the family, setting aside their own definition of the problem. We believe it is helpful to coevolve a problem description using the family's language and to initiate conversations about family members' preferences. Box 7–3 lists some factors for the nurse to consider when defining the problem.

In our conversations with families, we try to remember that each family expresses its pain and suffering in a unique way. Al-Krenawi (1998) points

---

Box 7-3 Factors to Consider in Defining the Problem

1. Presenting problem
   - Specify
2. Problem identification
   - Who in the family was the first to identify the problem? And then who?
   - When was the problem identified?
   - What were the concurrent life events or stressors at the time of identification of the problem?
   - Who else (family members, friends) agrees that it is a problem? Who disagrees?
   - How does the family understand that this problem developed (beliefs)?
3. Problem evolution
   - What behaviors became problematic?
   - Pattern of development
   - Frequency of problem emergence
   - Time intervals of quiescence
   - Factors aggravating
   - Factors alleviating
   - Who in the family is most and least concerned?

Adapted from Family Nursing Unit records, Faculty of Nursing, University of Calgary.

out that Bedouin Arab patients routinely express their personal or family problems in proverbs. For example, a wife of a husband engaged in polygamy described how her husband's multiple marriages affected her deeply by saying, "My eye is blind and my hand is short." She meant that she felt unable to do anything (p. 73). Another example of how a presenting problem can be described is how some African American couples frequently use metaphors to describe issues. For example, a couple experiencing major disagreement and conflict used the metaphor "a glass wall between us, we can see each other, but we never seem to touch." The nurse can identify conflict among family members about the problem definition if it arises. When differences exist, the nurse should clarify the issues further to help define the problem for which the family is seeking change.

The nurse can also ask questions of each member about his or her own explanation for the current situation. It is important for nurses to attend to *how* clients talk about the concerns that prompted them to show up for a meeting. To bring a family focus to the situation when interviewing an individual, the nurse could ask the following family-oriented questions:

1. Has anyone else in the family had this problem? (This addresses family history.)

2. What do other family members believe caused the problem or could treat the problem? (This explores the individual's explanatory model and health beliefs.)

3. Who in the family is most concerned about the problem? (This helps to understand the relational context of the concern.)

4. Along with your illness and symptoms, have there been any other recent changes in your family? (This addresses family stress and change.)

5. How can your family be helpful to you in dealing with this problem? (This focuses on family support.)

Wright and Bell (2009) believe that exploring the family's illness beliefs in the first meeting and at times of crisis is particularly important. If the family thinks that their beliefs or explanations about the illness are not acknowledged, they may feel marginalized. The nurse can ask them to explain, for example, why they believe this problem exists at this point in time. We believe it is also important to ask if the client and family have any control over the problem. The simplest way to do this is to ask direct, explanation-seeking questions such as, "What do you think is the reason for your son's violence toward his peers? Do you think Salahuddin has any control over the problem?"

Another idea is to ask clients to use their imagination to discuss an explanation. The interviewer can also offer a variety of alternative explanations or "gossip in the presence" by asking triadic questions such as, "Yael, what do you think is Zack's explanation for your mother's depression?" In exploring the family's preexisting explanations, it is essential for the interviewer to be curious and to avoid agreeing or disagreeing with the explanation.

There are several advantages to exploring the family's causal explanations, including improving cooperation between the interviewer and the family, developing systemic empathy with all family members versus selective empathy with one or two, detaching oneself from explanations provided by other professionals, recognizing and avoiding coalitions, loosening firmly held explanations, diluting negative explanations, and developing an ability to speculate with the clients about the effects of believing in one explanation or the other.

The problem-defining process, or "co-evolving the definition," is a critical aspect of family work. Cecchin (1987) warns clinicians to accept neither their own nor the client's definition too quickly, and Maturana and Varela (1992) caution clinicians to adopt an attitude of permanent vigilance against the temptation of certainty. By remaining curious, a clinician has a greater chance of escaping the "sin of certainty," or the sin of being too invested in one's own opinion. As clinicians, nurses need to avoid being preoccupied with their own brightness or ideas. Rather, each nurse should ask, "What does the client need from me? What are the client's beliefs, thoughts, hunches, and theories about the problem? About the extent of their control over the problem? Their solutions?" We try to always "keep the problem on the table" as we engage with families.

Relationship Between Family Interaction and the Health Problem

Once the main problems have been identified, the nurse asks questions about the relationship of family interaction to the health problem. Box 7–4 lists some factors to consider in exploring family interaction related to the presenting problem. The nurse conceptualizes the information that he or she has already gathered from the family in light of the meaning it has for the family and the hypotheses generated before the interview. For example, a home-care nurse talking with parents caring for a technology-dependent child at home might be mindful of the parents' new role as care specialists, the transformation of family space and privacy with the introduction of multiple health-care professionals, and the financial drain on their resources.

Box 7-4	Factors to Consider in Exploring Family Interaction Related to the Problem

- Current manifestations of the problem.
- Typical responses of family members and others to the problem.
- Other current associated problems, challenges, or concerns.
- How the problem influences family functioning.
- What family members appreciate about how they have coped with this challenging situation.
- How family members understand that they have not been successful in conquering this problem (beliefs).

Adapted from Family Nursing Unit records, Faculty of Nursing, University of Calgary.

The nurse then begins to develop additional questions that focus on interactional behaviors dealing with the three time frames of present, past, and future. Within each time frame, the nurse once again explores differences, agreements and disagreements, and explanations or meanings. It is important to emphasize that the purpose of asking these questions is not merely to gather data—that is, by asking circular questions, the nurse generates new ideas and explanations for himself or herself and the family to consider.

Present. In exploring the present situation, the nurse could ask, "Who does what, when? Then what happens? Who is the first to notice that something has been done?" The nurse should steer away from asking about traits that are supposedly intrinsic to a person, for example, being shy. Rather, the nurse might ask, "When does Ari *act* shy?" or "To whom does he *show* shyness?" Then, "What does Jennifer do when Ari shows shyness?" The nurse can inquire about differences between individuals: "Who is better at getting Grandmother to make her meals, Shanghi or Puichun?" The nurse can also inquire about differences between relationships: "Do your ex-husband and José fight more or less than your ex-husband and Nadiya?" In working with families with chronic or life-threatening illness, the nurse should explore differences before or after important events or milestones. For example, the nurse could ask, "Do you worry more, less, or the same about your wife's health since her emergency surgery?"

In addition to exploring areas of difference, the nurse can inquire about areas of agreement or disagreement: "Who agrees with you that Brandon is most likely to forget to give your mother her eyedrops three times per day? Who disagrees with you?" The nurse should explore the family's explanation for the sequence of interaction: "How do you understand Brandon's tendency to be most forgetful about the eyedrops? Are there times when he does remember? What seems to be different about the times when he remembers?"

Past. In exploring the past, the nurse should use similar types of questions to explore:

Differences: "How was Brandon's caregiving different before he had high-speed Internet? How does that differ from now?"

Agreement or disagreement: "Who agrees with Murdock that Dad was more involved in Genevieve's exercise program?"

Explanation or meaning: "What does it mean to you that, after all this time, things between your wife and her mother have not changed?"

In addition to exploring how the family saw the problem in the past, we have found it extremely useful to explore how they have seen changes in the problem. Change in the problem situation frequently occurs before the first meeting with the interviewer. If prompted, families can often recall and describe such changes. It is important to note that, in many cases, the family must be prompted to emerge from their problem-saturated view of the situation. For example, a man may tell the nurse at the community mental health center that his male partner drinks very heavily and has done this "until recently." If the nurse is attuned to inquiring about pretreatment changes, he or she will ask questions about the differences that the man has noticed recently. For example, the nurse might inquire, "Is his recent behavior the kind of change you would like to continue to have happen?" The idea of noticing exceptions to problems is one that we have used frequently in our clinical work, and we are indebted to de Shazer (1991) and White (1991) for emphasizing it.

Future. By focusing on the future and how the family would like things to be, nurses instill hope for more adaptive interaction regarding the presenting concern. They also co-construct a reality between family members and themselves for a system in which the problem has dissolved. The nurse can ask questions pertaining to:

Differences: "How would it be different if your grandfather did not side with your mother against your father in managing Paola's Crohn's disease?"

Agreement or disagreement: "Do you think your mother would agree that, if your grandfather stayed out of the discussions, things would be better?"

Explanation or meaning: "Dad, if your wife stopped phoning her father for advice about Paola's Crohn's disease, what would that mean to you?"

We believe it is especially important to ask future-oriented questions when working with families dealing with hereditary disorders such as Huntington's disease. For at-risk individuals, the possibility of detecting the disease-provoking gene exists, but no treatment is available. It is not so much the test result itself that may be disrupting to family life transitions but instead the changed expectations and possibilities for the future.

During this part of the interview, the nurse attempts to gain a systemic view of the situation and a description of the cycle of repeated interactions. These interactions may be between family members or between family members and the nurse. We stress that it is not important for the nurse to understand or agree with the problem but instead to be curious about the family's description of its positive and negative impact. We are drawn to the idea of using appreciative inquiry, a line of questioning that elicits and builds on appreciated practices and engages family members in discussion with each other about what works for them.

Such questions invite members to distinguish, understand, and amplify the appreciated life-sustaining forces within their family. In this way, families can take a "both/and" position. For example, they can relate the challenges of trying to raise a child with Down syndrome and discuss how raising this child has brought the family closer together and helped them pool their collective strengths and be a stronger family unit. Striking examples of how families have pooled their strengths to cope with a dying family member's illness have been recounted on numerous blogs and on Facebook.

During this phase of the interview, the nurse should be able to describe the sequence of the problem's development over time, the current contextual problem interaction, whether the family believes it has some control over the problem, the times when the problem does not show itself, and what the family members appreciate about their personal and cooperative efforts to work together.

All of the scenarios previously described relate to clients who believe there indeed is a problem, who believe they have some control over it, and who want to see it changed. But, what of those clients who don't see themselves as having a problem and yet are referred to the nurse? They may be mandated for treatment or present under duress. For example, a 16-year-old boy verbally abused an elderly woman in his high school and then pushed her off the elevator. When the principal asked what happened, he said, "Oh, it's nothing. We got into an argument because I didn't let her get away with that 'age stuff' and let her on the elevator first. It's no big deal." His grandmother whom he lived with stood by helplessly as the principal talked.

In situations where clients and helpers have different agendas for a meeting and different definitions of the problem, we believe it's important for the nurse not to inadvertently rigidify the interaction—that is, by insisting too early that it *is definitely* a problem, the nurse can invite a rigid no-problem response from the client. We do not use the word *denial,* as this generally just fosters an antagonistic relationship over the question of who is "right." Although we sometimes find ourselves tempted to give advice and confront the situation head-on, we have found this typically invites defensiveness and promotes shame. (Additional ideas on how not to give advice prematurely are given in Chapter 11.)

Attempted Solutions to Solving Problems

During this next phase of the assessment, the nurse explores the family's attempted solutions to the problem. Box 7–5 lists some factors to consider when exploring the family's attempted solutions. The process can begin with general questions related to the problem. For example, "What improvements have you noticed since you first contacted our clinic?" This type of question conveys the idea to families that they have the strengths and resources to change, and it assumes that changes have already occurred, which can help set in motion a positive self-fulfilling prophecy for them. Another example might be, "How have you tried to obtain information from physicians and nurses about Mandeep's condition in previous hospitalizations?"

More specific questions should then be used to identify the least and most effective solutions for achieving what the family desires. The nurse can ask when these solutions were used. For example, "What was least helpful in trying to get information from the nurses about Surjit's resuscitation? What was most effective?" The nurse can ask if any successful elements in the solutions are still being used, and if not, why. Similar types of sequences of

---

Box 7-5	Factors to Consider in Exploring the Family's Attempted Solution

- How has the family tried to resolve the problem?
- Who tried?
- With whom?
- What were the results?
- What were the events precipitating the search for professional help?
- Who is most in favor of agency help? Most opposed?
- What are the client's thoughts about the nurse's role in the change process?
- What was the sequence of events resulting in actual contact with the agency?

Adapted from Family Nursing Unit records, Faculty of Nursing, University of Calgary.

---

interaction questions that focus on difference, agreement or disagreement, and explanation or meaning can be used to explore the family's attempted solutions to the presenting concerns.

In our work with families, we have frequently been told that no solutions have been attempted or that "nothing has worked." In these circumstances, we sometimes ask, "How come things aren't worse? What are you doing to keep this situation from getting worse?" Then we amplify these problem-solving strategies by asking about their frequency, effectiveness, and so forth. We also try to expand our view of typical solutions to include complementary and alternative medical and health approaches.

We also find it useful to draw on the concept of resilience in these situations. In talking with families about their resilience, we use such terms as *endurance, withstanding, adaptation, coping,* and *survival* and try to draw forth other qualities surfacing in the face of hardship or adversity. We talk about the ability to "bounce back" or make up for losses. We believe resilience is forged *through* adversity, not *despite* it. Bouncing back is not the same as "breezing through" a crisis. Resilience involves multiple recursive processes over time. It is this layering and recursiveness that we inquire about when we ask families about their coping and attempted solutions.

In working with families dealing with life-threatening or chronic illness, the nurse should be aware of additional "helping agencies" involved in health-care delivery. We have found it important to ask questions such as, "Have any other agencies attempted to help you with this problem? What has been the most useful advice that you have received? Did you follow this advice? What has been the least helpful advice?" It is useful to explore the differing ideas espoused by the helping systems. If there is unclear leadership or a confused hierarchy within the helping systems, the family can be placed in a conflictual situation that is similar to that of a child whose parents continually disagree. Confusion among helping agencies can exacerbate the family's concerns. In this way, the attempted solution (assistance by helping agencies) can become an entirely new problem for both the family and other agencies. It is important for the nurse to be aware of whether this situation exists before attempting to intervene.

Having consolidated a shared view of the problem and elicited some relevant solutions, the nurse can simply state to the family that she or he would like to work with them to achieve their goals. This small but profound acknowledgment is an opportunity for the nurse to show compassion to the client and enter into a deeper relationship and collaboration.

Goal Exploration

At some point during the interview, the nurse and family establish what goals or outcomes the family expects as a result of change. Box 7–6 lists some factors for nurses to consider when exploring goals. Families are pragmatic: They are seeking practical results when they come to a health-care provider; they are "in pain" or "suffering," and their desire is to get rid of a problem. The problem may be between themselves as family members or between the family and the nurse (e.g., the family desires practical information about the acceptable level of physical activity after a myocardial infarction [MI], and the nurse has not provided such concrete information). Family members may expect a large change (e.g., "My brother Sheldon will be able to walk without the aid of a cane") or a small but significant change (e.g., "We will be able to leave our handicapped daughter, Kayla, with a babysitter for 1 hour a week").

In many cases, a small change is sufficient. We believe that a small change in a person's behavior can have profound and far-reaching effects on the behavior of all persons involved. Experienced nurses are aware that small changes lead to further progress.

Goals describe what will be present or what will be happening when the complaint or concern is absent. We believe that unidimensional behavioral goal statements such as "I will be eating less" are not as desirable as multidimensional, interactional, and situational goal statements that describe the "who, what, when, where, and how" of the solution. Such a multidimensional goal statement might be, "I will be eating a small, balanced meal in the evening at the dinner table with my partner and our children; the television and computer will be off, and we will be talking to each other."

There are many ways in which the nurse can clarify the family's goals with future or hypothetical questions such as, "What would your parents do differently if they did not stay at home every evening with Snanna?" The nurse can explore future or hypothetical areas of difference (e.g., "How

---

Box 7-6	Factors to Consider When Exploring Goals

• What general changes does the family believe would improve the problem?
• What specific changes?
• What are the expectations of how the agency may facilitate change in the problem?

Adapted from Family Nursing Unit records, Faculty of Nursing, University of Calgary.

would your parents' relationship be different if your dad allowed your uncle to take care of Snanna one evening a week?"), areas of agreement or disagreement (e.g., "Do you think your dad would agree that your parents would probably have little to talk about if they went out one evening a week?"), and explanation or meaning (e.g., "Tell me more about why you believe your parents would have a lot to talk about when they went out that one evening a week. What would that mean to you?").

We find it useful sometimes to combine past and future questions. For example, "If you were to tell me next week (or month or year) that you had done X, what could I find in your past history that would have allowed me to predict that you would have done X?" The questions capitalize on the "possibility to probability" phenomena at the same time as inviting a richer account of the history of the new/old story.

We have found it particularly useful in our clinical work to ask the "miracle question" (de Shazer, 1988) to elicit the family's goals; de Shazer (1991) describes the question in this way:

> Suppose that one night there is a miracle and while you are sleeping the problem . . . is solved: How would you know? What would be different?
>
> What will you notice different the next morning that will tell you there has been a miracle? What will your spouse notice? (p. 113)

The miracle question elicits interactional information. The person is asked to imagine someone else's ideas as well as his or her own. The framework of the miracle question (and others of this type) allows family members to bypass their causal explanations. They do not have to imagine how they will get rid of the problem but instead can focus on results. Thus, the goals developed from the miracle question are not limited to just getting rid of the problem or complaint. Clients often are able to construct answers to this "miracle question" quite concretely and specifically. For example, "Easy, I'll be able to say no to cocaine," or "She'll see me smile more and come home from work with less tension."

McConkey (2002) suggests strategies for solution-focused meetings that we believe are particularly useful if a family is angry and the nurse is feeling defensive. The nurse can shift the meeting from the problem picture to the future solution picture by engaging in conversation such as this:

> Obviously, you want things to be better for your child and so do I. (Validating the parent)
>
> In order to make the most of this meeting, I'm going to ask you an unusual question. (Bridging statement)
>
> How will you know by the time you leave here today, that this meeting has been helpful? (Shifting to the future)
>
> When things are better, what will your son be doing? What will I be doing? What will you be doing? (Including all the stakeholders in the solution picture) (p. 192)

Nurses working with families of a patient who has a chronic or life-threatening illness commonly find family members quite vague about the changes they expect. For example, "We would like Attila to feel good about himself even though he has a colostomy." Experienced clinical nurses know that "feeling good about oneself" is very difficult to describe or measure. In this example, we recommend that the nurse ask the family to describe the smallest concrete change that Attila could make to show that he "feels good about himself." By asking for this degree of specificity about desired change early in the nurse–family relationship, we believe it is more likely that the family and nurse can accomplish the desired change.

GUIDELINES FOR THE REMAINING INTERVIEWING PROCESS

Once the nurse has completed the initial interviews or assessment, he or she can consider the entire interviewing process. The stages of the interviewing process generally include:

1. Engagement
2. Assessment
3. Intervention
4. Termination

Planning and Dealing With Complexity

After an initial assessment is completed, a beginning nurse interviewer frequently worries about whether to intervene with a family. The following questions often arise: Am I the appropriate person to offer intervention? Is the situation too complex? Do I have sufficient skills, or should another professional, such as a social worker, psychologist, or family therapist, be called in?

Does every family that is assessed need further intervention? This is not to say that interventions begin only at the intervention stage. Rather, they are part of the total interview process from engagement to closure. For example, just by asking the family to come together for an interview, the nurse has intervened. Each time the nurse asks a circular question, he or she influences the family, generates new information, and intervenes.

For nurses, the decision to offer interventions, refer the family to others, or discharge them is a complex one. Several factors need to be examined before making the choice: the level of the family's functioning, the level of the nurse's competence, and the work context.

Level of the Family's Functioning
The nurse should recognize the complexity of the family situation. Some clinicians have advocated that treatment begin if the referring problem has been detected early and clearly defined procedures for management have been published. Most nurses would agree with this position but would find

it very idealistic. Community health nurses and mental health nurses, in particular, often work with families who are not referred early. Some of these families present with several complex physical and emotional problems and are frequently involved in one crisis after another. These families offer specific challenges for nurses.

Our recommendation is that nurses carefully assess the family's level of functioning and its desire to work on specific issues, such as management of hemiplegia after a stroke, impact of cystic fibrosis on the family, negotiation of services for elderly family members, or caring for a child with special needs. If the family is at all amenable to working on such an issue, it is incumbent on the nurse either to offer intervention or to help them get appropriate assistance by referring them to others. Guidelines for the referral process are provided in Chapter 12.

The nurse must consider ethical issues in deciding who should be treated. With the popularization of counseling, a surface inspection would seem to indicate that everyone is in need of psychotherapy in one form or another. The childless couple, the family with young infants, the family with adolescents, the single-parent family, and the aging family can all be considered candidates for psychotherapeutic aid. Many people lead psychologically constricted and difficult lives, but should they be "treated"? This is a troublesome question for helping professionals.

Our recommendation is that nurses ethically weigh two opposing positions when they decide to intervene with, refer, or discharge a family. One position states that if a person is potentially dangerous to self or others, that person must receive intervention. On an individual level, a suicidal or homicidal patient is such an example. On a larger system level, a family in which there is physical, sexual, or emotional abuse or violence is an example. On a community level, a person who is threatening to the community and mentally unstable is an example.

Single-parent adoptive families as well as lesbian, gay, bisexual couples or committed families are entitled to be considered various family forms versus alternatives to "normal" families. It is our hope that nurses will ethically and wisely consider the family's level of functioning and their own legal responsibilities. This is a necessary step before deciding to offer further treatment. This weighing of alternatives can be particularly challenging for nurses when dealing with client confidentiality, crisis situations, and non-emancipated minors. For example, a 16-year-old girl overdosed with 30 tablets of naproxen and was brought to the emergency room by her boyfriend. She refused to talk about what had happened and repeatedly said she did not want to talk with her parents who were in the waiting room; however, she texted her girlfriend from her bed in the emergency room to say that she had overdosed. The nurse read the text message and had to weigh several options in deciding how to proceed with care. In Chapter 12, we present some ideas that we have used when we have decided not to offer additional treatment to families.

Another ethical consideration for a nurse to weigh is the balance between his or her own beliefs about a client and his or her respect for the client's situation. This is especially important with regard to issues such as sexual orientation, culture, religion, and ethnic self-determination. For example, we believe that when discussing decision-making at the end of life, nurses should recognize and honor that people who are dying are still living and have the right to be in control of their lives. A real (unflinching) and ethical relationship between the patient, the staff, and the family should be maintained and valued as end-of-life issues are decided. This is particularly salient when the nurse may be unfamiliar with the views of Native American groups such as the Navajo, who hold strong beliefs about spirituality, healing, rituals concerning the end of life, and death practices.

The contrasts between the beliefs of the dominant health-care system and the views of various religious groups, such as, for example, those who practice the Islamic and Hindu religions, need to be explored. With regard to homosexuality, Green (2003) has persuasively argued the firm value of respecting a client's choices and not trying to "make them" into who they are not. We believe that nurses should be able to support a client along whatever sexual-orientation path he or she ultimately takes. Respect for the client's and family's sense of integrity and interpersonal relationships is the most central goal.

To avoid ethnocentrism and paternalism, some nurses have embraced certain politically correct ideas with enthusiasm. We advocate that nurses engage in critical thinking about responsible practice, safeguard human dignity, and not blindly follow injunctions to be politically correct. Nurses are responsible for their own choices in exercising independent professional judgment and moral agency. We have found it useful in our clinical work with families to be collaborative, open, and direct with them in discussing ethical dilemmas involving them.

The Nurse's Level of Competence

When choosing to work with a family, nurses should consider their personal and professional capacity. If the nurse has experienced a recent death of a family member, he or she may not be able to facilitate grieving in family members. Likewise, a nurse with strong views that people who are on disability are shirkers would be best advised not to attempt work with such families. We do not subscribe to the view that a nurse has to have personally dealt with a situation (e.g., raising teenagers) to help a family. Most noteworthy in a nurse is clinical competence and compassion. However, we do believe that the nurse should attempt to be well informed and not just offer advice that might or might not be helpful. We believe that nurses should consider scope of practice as the care for which they are competent, educated, and authorized to provide. On a professional level, the nurse needs to evaluate his or her competence by asking self-reflective questions such as, "Am I at the beginning or the advanced level of family interviewing skill?" and

"Can I obtain supervision to aid in dealing with families who present with complex issues?" Each nurse should examine these questions and their answers before making a decision about intervening with a given family.

The genetic revolution is an explosive area of knowledge for nurses. Situations resulting from the application of the abundant knowledge gained from the Human Genome Project (HGP) require decisions for which there most likely will be limited precedent. Nurses and families alike struggle with uncertainty and ambiguity as new discoveries are made in the HGP (VanRiper, 2011). Now is an exciting and meaningful time for nurses to work alongside families dealing with new information about risk, risk expression, and treatment options.

Work Context

Considerable controversy is sometimes raised about the issue of who is competent to assist clients. This controversy involves issues of definition and professionalism. How a "family problem" and a "medical problem" are defined in a particular work setting can fuel the controversy. For example, if a nurse is working with a patient who has had a stroke and invites the relatives to come for an educational class, is the nurse treating a family or a medical problem? We take the approach that the definition of the problem is less important than the solution—that is, if the whole family is involved, the definition of the problem is a question of semantics.

The issue of professional territoriality is a very thorny one with no pat answers. Sometimes the patient sees the psychologist for psychodiagnostic testing and sees the social worker to deal with the family and outside agencies. The role of the nurse with the family in this situation can become controversial. If the nurse does a family assessment and decides to intervene with the family, is the nurse usurping the social worker's position? Or, perhaps, is the nurse usurping the physician's position by making the decision to intervene?

One way around these dilemmas is for the nurse to consider assuming various roles in his or her work with families. For example, the nurse can serve as mediator, patient and family advocate, capacity builder for family health, empowerer, alliance builder, guide, navigator, and so forth.

There are no simple answers to complex professional and territorial issues. We urge nurses to work cooperatively to ensure the best family care possible. In general, we believe the best person to intervene in a situation is the one with the most ready access to the system level in which the problems manifest themselves. However, we believe that, in the past, nurses have been too quick to turn over family care to other professionals. Nurses are now reclaiming their important role in providing relational, family-centered care.

Changes in health-care reimbursement have required all nurses and health-care providers to examine and adapt their practices to account for the provision of timely, efficient, and cost-effective services. Managed care in its many varieties, health insurance reform, increased focus on primary care, and other complex issues have changed the face of nursing practice. The coming together of the consumer movement, health economics, and technology has huge implications for practice. Nurses have to do more than just heal their patients. Day after day, they must also attend to the socioeconomic and political context of health care and to the survival of their careers. We believe that it is vital for nurses to find ways to thrive professionally and for families to receive optimal care. Strategies to address bureaucratic disentitlement of cultural, ethnic, racial, and other minority groups must be put forth. Models for access to health care for economically disadvantaged families need further refinement and implementation.

Accountability structures and practices need to recognize the centrality of structured power differences in our society. We believe that, as nurses work with diverse families and are increasingly transparent in this work, they will find ways to positively influence their employment contexts.

Intervention Stage

Once the nurse has decided to intervene with the family, we recommend that he or she review the CFIM (see Chapter 4). This model, which stimulates ideas about change, can help the nurse design interventions to work with the family to address the particular domain of family functioning affected: cognitive, affective, or behavioral. Helpful hints about intervention are offered in Box 7–7.

In choosing interventions, we encourage nurses to attend to several factors to enhance the likelihood that the interventions will focus on change in the desired domain of family functioning. Interventions, offered within a collaborative relationship, are not a demand but rather an invitation to change. Some factors to consider when devising interventions are outlined in Box 7–8. First, the intervention should be related to the problem that the

---

Box 7-7	Helpful Hints About Interventions

- Interventions are the core of clinical work with families.
- They should be devised with sensitivity to the family's ethnic and religious background.
- They can only be *offered to* families. The nurse cannot direct change but can create a context for change to occur.
- They are offered in the context of collaborative conversations as the nurse and family together devise solutions to find the most useful fit.
- When the nurse's ideas are not a good fit for the family, the practitioner should be open to offering other ideas rather than becoming blameful of self or the family because the intervention was not chosen.

Levac, A.M.C., Wright, L.M., & Leahey, M. (2002). Children and families: Models for assessment and intervention. In J.A. Fox (Ed.): *Primary Health Care of Infants, Children, and Adolescents* (2nd ed.). St. Louis: Mosby, p. 18. Copyright 2002. Adapted with permission.

Box 7-8 Factors to Consider When Devising Interventions

• What is the agreed-upon problem to change?
• At what domain of family functioning is the intervention aimed?
• How does the intervention match the family's style of relating?
• How is the intervention linked to the family's strengths and previous useful solution strategies?
• How is the intervention consistent with the family's ethnic and religious beliefs?
• How is the intervention new or different for the family?

---

nurse and the family have contracted to change. Second, the intervention should be derived from the nurse's hypothesis about the problem, what the family says the problem means to them, and their beliefs about the problem (Wright & Bell, 2009). Third, the intervention should match the family's style of relating. (We have found in our own clinical work that we are sometimes biased toward one particular domain of family functioning, such as cognitive or affective, and that we have thus erred in devising interventions that we are most comfortable with rather than ones that the family may find most useful.) Fourth, the interventions should be linked to the family's strengths. We believe that families have inherent resources and that the nurse's responsibility is to encourage families to use these resources in new ways to tackle the problem. Fifth, the interventions should take into consideration the family's beliefs, which are influenced by ethnicity, spirituality, race, class, gender, and sexual orientation. Sixth, the nurse should devise a few interventions so that nurse and family can consider their relative merits—for example, are these ideas new to the family, or are they more of the same types of solutions that the family has already tried?

We do not believe that there is one "right" intervention. Rather, there are only "useful" or "effective" interventions. In our experience, we have found that a nurse sometimes reaches an impasse, with a family not changing, when the nurse persists in either using the same intervention repeatedly or switching interventions too rapidly. Sometimes we find that clients fail to notice responses containing possible solutions. The same can be said of nurses. Interventions are successful when constraints are lifted and important aspects of life change are noticed. The result is a clearer image of how things can be different in the future.

We have also found that sometimes the nurse is too constrained and fails to consider alternate system levels for intervention. For example, if a family does not want to hear or discuss the possibility of older adults having sexual activity at a residential care center, then the nurse may design an intervention not with the family but rather with the care center. Such an intervention with a residential care center could be to plan an in-service around the topic of HIV and older adults. The outcome is that condoms are available in the center and clients have the information they need to keep themselves safe.

With the availability of computers, smartphones, tablets, e-readers, instant messaging, Twitter, and Facebook, we believe that nurses have become increasingly creative in finding electronic means to facilitate intervention. For example, telephone-based skill building can help dementia caregivers' sense of social support, reduce their depressive symptoms, and improve their life satisfaction in the midst of caregiving. Campbell-Grossman and colleagues (2009) found that providing social support to single, low-income African American mothers via e-mail was effective. Just as the use of computers, e-mail, chat rooms, Listservs, blogs, and smartphones for business and education has had dramatic effects on family interaction, we believe their use in health care has also profoundly affected nurse–family interaction.

Once the nurse has devised an intervention, he or she must attend to the executive skills (see Chapters 5 and 10) required to deliver it. Part of the success of any intervention is the manner in which it is offered. The family must feel confident that the intervention will promote change. The nurse also needs to show that he or she has confidence in the intervention or task requested and believes that it will benefit the family.

However, interventions need to be tailored to each family; therefore, the preamble or preface to the actual intervention will vary. For example, if family members are feeling very hopeless and frustrated with a particular problem, the nurse may say, "I know this might seem like a hard thing that I'm going to ask you to do, but I know your family is capable of . . ." On the other hand, if the nurse is making a request of family members who tend to be quite formal with one another, then the nurse might preface it with, "What I'm going to ask you to do may make you feel a little foolish or silly at first, but you'll notice that, as you do it a few times, you will become more comfortable."

A good example of a generic intervention is the "What are you prepared to do?" question. The term *prepared* suggests a voluntary decision to participate in the change process.

When giving a particular assignment for a family to do between sessions, the nurse should try to include all family members. The nurse must review the particular assignment with family members to ensure they understand what is being requested. Reviewing the assignment is a good idea, whether it is carried out within the interview or between interviews. If assignments or experiments are given between sessions, the nurse should always ask for a report at the next interview. If the family has not completed or only partially completed the assignment, the reason should be explored.

We do not subscribe to the view that families are noncompliant or resistant if they do not follow our requests. Rather, we become curious about their decision to choose an alternate course and try to learn from their response. We believe that family interviewing is a circular process. The nurse intervenes, and the family responds in its unique way. The nurse then responds to this response and the process continues. See Chapter 2 for more ideas about circularity.

During the intervention stage, the nurse must be aware of the element of time. How useful or effective an intervention is can be evaluated only after the intervention has been implemented. With some interventions, change may be noted immediately. However, more commonly, changes will not be noticed for a lengthy period. Just as most problems occur over time, problems also need an appropriate length of time to be resolved. It is impossible to state how long one should wait to ascertain if a particular intervention has been effective, but changes within family systems need to filter through the various system levels. Families themselves offer useful observations and feedback about what interventions are most useful. Robinson and Wright (1995), in discussing a study conducted by Robinson, cite that families identified interventions within two stages of the therapeutic change process that they thought were critical to healing: creating the circumstances for change and moving beyond and overcoming problems. (For further elaboration on these stages, see Chapter 1.) More information about devising interventions is provided in Chapters 4, 8, 9, 10, and 12.

Termination Stage

The last stage of the interviewing process is known as *termination* or *closure*. It is critically important for the nurse to conceptualize how to end treatment with the family to enhance the likelihood that changes will be maintained. In Chapter 5, we outlined the conceptual, perceptual, and executive skills useful for the termination stage. In Chapter 12 we address in depth the process of termination and focus on how to evaluate outcomes.

CLINICAL CASE EXAMPLE

The following is an example of how a nurse conducted family interviews using the guidelines we have given in Chapters 6 and 7. An example of a 15-minute interview is given in Chapter 9.

Pre-Interview

Developing Hypotheses

A home health agency received a referral on the Auerswald family for home nursing services, physiotherapy, nutrition counseling, and mental health counseling. Heinz Auerswald, 51, was a paraplegic and in a wheelchair because of a multiple trauma suffered in an industrial accident. He was unemployed. Eva Auerswald, 49, a homemaker, was the primary caregiver. She was reported to be depressed. The home-care nurse hypothesized that Mrs. Auerswald's depression could be related to feeling overresponsible for caring for her husband. The nurse wondered if the husband's role and beliefs might be perpetuating this. She was also curious to know what other social and professional support systems were involved and what their beliefs were about the family's health problems. During the course of the family interview, the nurse gained much evidence from both the husband and wife to confirm the usefulness of her initial hypothesis. She used this hypothesis to provide a framework for her conversation with the couple.

Relation to CFAM. The nurse generated her hypothesis based on knowledge of and clinical experience with other families in similar situations and with similar ethnic backgrounds. The nurse also based it on the structural category of CFAM (internal and external family structure, ethnicity, gender), the developmental category (middle-aged families), and the functional category (roles, power or influence, circular communication, beliefs).

Arranging the Interview
The wife stated that she did not want to discuss her depression with the nurse while her husband was awake. For the first home visit, the nurse requested that the husband and wife be interviewed together. The couple agreed to this.

Relation to CFAM. The nurse thought about family roles and gender. She speculated that Eva may be protecting her husband, Heinz, from her problem. In terms of the CFAM category of verbal communication, the nurse speculated that clear and direct communication between Heinz and Eva might be absent or infrequent.

Interview

Engagement
The genogram data revealed that:

- The husband and wife are alone in the city; extended families and children live in other cities and visit infrequently.
- Eva had been married previously and had stayed with her first husband for 18 years, although he physically abused her. She thought it was her responsibility to protect her children.
- This was the husband's first marriage.

Relation to CFAM. The preceding information added some support for the nurse's initial hypothesis in terms of Eva's beliefs about responsibility and an isolated family structure.

Assessment
Problem Definition. Eva described the problem as, "Heinz has had such a hard tragedy, but now I'm the one who is depressed. It doesn't make sense." Mr. Auerswald described the problem as Eva is "worrying too much."

Relationship Between Family Interaction and Health Problem. By asking circular questions, the nurse discovered that Eva had not allowed herself a break from caregiving for 2 years. Heinz encouraged her to "go out and meet people," but she stated that she was fearful he might be too lonely if she met other people. Mr. Auerswald stated that this would not be a problem for him. They both reported that Eva had recently become depressed. She cried frequently and had difficulty sleeping.

Mrs. Auerswald takes excellent physical care of Heinz and bathes him daily. He is appreciative of all her nursing care. She feels guilty about asking for help from his parents.

Attempted Solutions. Eva had recently visited her family doctor, who prescribed an antidepressant for her. She had requested home-care services once before, but she said that because "their schedule is unreliable [and she] never know[s] when they are coming," she had discontinued treatment with the nurses. On the advice of her physician, Mrs. Auerswald agreed to try home care again.

Relation to CFAM. The nurse noted that the Auerswalds' problem-solving approaches involved either self-sufficiency or professional resources outside the family. They sought help from the family doctor and from the home-care agency only infrequently, and they were reluctant to call on extended family for assistance.

Goals. Eva's desire was to "not feel depressed, [to] feel good about myself." The smallest significant change that she was able to describe was to be able to "go out one afternoon a week without feeling guilty." Heinz was in agreement with his wife's goals.

Intervention
Consideration of CFIM. Having developed a collaborative relationship with the couple and a workable hypothesis that fit the data from the family assessment, the nurse began to consider interventions with Mr. and Mrs. Auerswald in the cognitive, affective, and behavioral domains of family functioning. The focus of intervention was Eva's depression.

Interventions and Outcome. Knowing that Mrs. Auerswald had stayed in a physically abusive first marriage for 18 years to protect her children, the nurse asked questions about beliefs and feelings of responsibility. The nurse encouraged change in Eva's beliefs by asking both husband and wife behavioral effect, triadic, and hypothetical questions about responsibility. She asked the couple to engage in behavioral experiments to try new ways of being self-responsible. Both Mr. and Mrs. Auerswald challenged their own beliefs about depression being a solely biological problem and began to take more responsibility for their own lives. Heinz stated that he wanted a bath only three times per week. Eva requested caregiving help from her mother-in-law and was able to leave her husband alone for 2 hours, three times per week while she played cards with friends. The couple reported significant improvement in her depression. The home-care agency continued to provide nursing and physical therapy services for the family. The nurse and home health aide focused on supporting the couple's new beliefs about responsibility.

CONCLUSIONS

Guidelines for particular stages of family interviews for nurses to consider during an initial interview and during the whole process of interviewing have been delineated. We recommend that nurses use these guidelines as ideas and suggestions for how to maximize the effectiveness of their time with families. It is not uncommon to move back and forth between the stages of a family interview to obtain more clarity or additional assessment about the concerns. Sometimes it is even necessary to return to the engagement guidelines to strengthen the therapeutic relationship before further intervention ideas can be offered. Thus, there should be fluidity between these stages so that they remain truly guidelines rather than a rigid prescription for how to conduct a family interview. We also caution nurses to remember the uniqueness of every family situation and encourage them to use these guidelines with sensitivity to each clinical situation, being mindful of the family's cultural, religious, spiritual, and ethnic heritage.

References

Al-Krenawi, A. (1998). Family therapy with a multiparental/multispousal family. *Family Process, 37*(1), 65–81.

Bell, J.M., & Wright, L.M. (2011). The illness beliefs model: Creating practice knowledge in family systems nursing for families experiencing illness. In E.K. Svavarsdottir & H. Jonsdottir (Eds.): *Family Nursing in Action*. Reykjavik, Iceland. University of Iceland Press, pp. 15–52.

Benzein, E. & Saveman, B-I. (2008). Health promoting conversations about hope and suffering with couples in palliative care. *International Journal of Palliative Nursing, 14*(9), 439-445.

Campbell-Grossman, C.K., Hudson, D.B., Keating-Lefler, R., et al. (2009). The provision of social support to single, low-income, African-American mothers via email messages. *Journal of Family Nursing, 15*(2), 220–236.

Cecchin, G. (1987). Hypothesizing, circularity, and neutrality revisited: An invitation to curiosity. *Family Process, 26*(4), 405–413.

deShazer, S. (1988). *Clues; Investigating Solutions in Brief Therapy*. New York: Norton.

De Shazer, S. (1991). *Putting Difference to Work*. New York: Norton.

Duhamel, F., & Campagna, L. (2000). Family genograph. Montreal: Universite de Montreal, Faculty of Nursing. Available from *www.familynursingresources.com*.

Duhamel, F., Dupuis, F., & Wright, L. (2009). Families' and nurses' responses to the "one question question": Reflections for clinical practice, education, and research in family nursing. *Journal of Family Nursing, 15*(4), 461–485.

Green, R.J. (2003). When therapists do not want their clients to be homosexual: A response to Rosik's article. *Journal of Marital and Family Therapy, 29*(1), 29–38.

Leahey, M., Stout, L., & Myrah, I. (1991). Family systems nursing: How do you practice it in an active community hospital? *Canadian Nurse, 87*(2), 31–33.

Leahey, M., & Wright, L.M. (1987). Families and chronic illness: Assumptions, assessment and intervention. In L.M. Wright & M. Leahey (Eds.): *Families and Chronic Illness*. Springhouse, PA: Springhouse Corp, pp. 55–76.

Levac, A.M.C., Wright, L.M., & Leahey, M. (2002). Children and families: Models for assessment and intervention. In J.A. Fox (Ed.): *Primary Health Care of Infants, Children, and Adolescents* (2nd ed.). St. Louis: Mosby, pp. 10–19.

Madsen, W.C. (2007). *Collaborative Therapy With Multi-Stressed Families* (2nd ed.). New York: Guilford Press.

Maturana, H.R., & Varela, F. (1992). *The Tree of Knowledge: The Biological Roots of Human Understanding*. Boston: Shambhala Publications.

McConkey, N. (2002). *Solving School Problems: Solution Focused Strategies for Principals, Teachers, and Counsellors*. Alberta, Canada: Solution Talk.

Robinson, C.A., & Wright, L.M. (1995). Family nursing interventions: What families say makes a difference. *Journal of Family Nursing, 1*(3), 327–345.

Slive, A., & Bobele, M. (Eds.). (2011). *When One Hour Is All You Have: Effective Therapy for Walk-in Clients*. Phoenix, AZ: Zeig, Tucker, & Theisen.

Sunder, R. (2011). Collaboration: Family and therapist perspectives of helpful therapy. *Journal of Marital & Family Therapy, 37*(2), 236–249.

Thorne, S.E., & Robinson, C.A. (1989). Guarded alliance: Health care relationships in chronic illness. *Image: Journal of Nursing Scholarship, 21*(3), 153–157.

VanRiper, M. (2011). Family nursing and genomics in the 21st century. In E.K. Svavarsdottir & H. Jonsdottir (Eds.): *Family Nursing in Action*. Reykjavik, Iceland. University of Iceland Press, pp. 69–84.

Ward, D.B. & Wampler, K.S. (2010). Moving up the continuum of hope: Developing a theory of hope and understanding its influence in couples therapy. *Journal of Marital and Family Therapy, 36*(2), 212–228.

Weingarten, K. (2000). Witnessing, wonder, and hope. *Family Process, 39*(4), 389–402.

White, M. (1991). Deconstruction and therapy. *Dulwich Centre Newsletter, 3,* 21–40.

Wright, L.M. (1989). When clients ask questions: Enriching the therapeutic conversation. *Family Therapy Networker, 13*(6), 15–16.

Wright, L.M., & Bell, J.M. (2009). *Beliefs and Illness: A Model to Invite Healing*. Calgary, AB: 4th Floor Press.

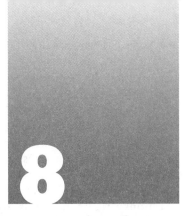

Chapter **8**

How to Use Questions in Family Interviewing

Throughout our book we have discussed the usefulness of asking questions in family interviewing. We believe questions are useful for family assessment, and they are one of the most helpful family interventions nurses can offer. We have found the research of Healing and Bavelas (2011) to be encouraging in this regard. Their "controlled experiment confirmed that interview questions on the same topic but with a different focus can affect the interviewee, producing different attributions and even different behaviors" (p. 43). This is an important finding for clinical work.

Through the use of clinical examples, we demonstrate and reveal how questions are used in relational practice. These clinical interviews appear in our DVD *How to Use Questions in Family Interviewing* (Wright & Leahey, 2006; available at www.familynursingresources.com). We will discuss the application of questions in various clinical settings and contexts to:

- Engage all family members and focus the meeting
- Assess the impact of the problem or illness on the family
- Elicit problem-solving skills, coping strategies, and strengths
- Intervene and invite change
- Request feedback about the meeting

QUESTIONS IN CONTEXT

First, we discuss a few ideas about asking questions in the context of clinical practice, specifically in the context of a therapeutic conversation between a nurse and a family. We believe that useful or helpful questions have the potential to provide information to *both* the family and the nurse, invite family members to reflect on their illness experience, and can be potentially healing when the nurse asks them in a manner of sincere inquiry or curiosity. Questions are not effective in and of themselves; rather, it is only through a therapeutic conversation that questions help nurses be effective. (See Chapter 7 for more ideas about therapeutic conversation.) Questions also enhance a nurse's understanding of family members' experience with a particular illness or problem. Answers to questions can help the nurse and the family appreciate the family's coping strategies, unique strengths, and resources. These types of conversations are very different from ones that a family may have with an intake worker or data clerk.

There are numerous and various types of questions, such as difference questions, triadic questions, hypothetical questions, and behavioral-effect questions (see Chapter 4). In this chapter, we offer a simple dichotomy of questions that a nurse can ask: assessment and interventive questions:

- Assessment or linear questions are meant to inform the nurse; these are often investigative questions, such as asking a family member to describe the illness experience or problem. We have frequently found that just telling the story can be therapeutic. For example, talking about developmental transitions, such as the birth of a child or the placement of a parent in a nursing home, can draw forth remembrances of strength and meaning that may have been overlooked or forgotten.

- Interventional, or circular, questions are meant to invite a reflection and effect change; these questions may encourage family members to see their problems in a new way and subsequently to see new solutions. Some clinicians and authors recognize how questions can introduce alternative possibilities, theories, beliefs, and views, simply in their posing (Katie, 2003; McGee, Del Vento, & Bavelas, 2005; Wright & Bell, 2009).

The important difference between these two categories of questions is in their *intent*. Thus, as the family's answers provide information for both the family and the nurse, the nurse's questions may provide information for the family.

It can be helpful for the nurse at the start of the family meeting to explain to the members that she will be asking various kinds of questions to obtain a thorough understanding of their situation. Also, it gives the family an opportunity to familiarize themselves with the nurse. In a social conversation, it is often considered rude to interrupt someone to ask a question while he or she is speaking. However, in a time-limited family interview, it could be considered rude not to obtain each family member's perception of the health concern. Sometimes interrupting one family member to include the perspective of another is most appropriate.

It is also appropriate in therapeutic conversation for nurses to understand they are not invading a family's privacy by asking questions. In training our students to overcome such a mental barrier, we have found it helpful to teach them to say to clients, "I don't know you very well, so can I trust that if I ask you something too sensitive, or something you would prefer not to talk about, that you will let me know?" In this way, the student obtains the family's permission to have a wide-ranging discussion. If conflict among family members erupts as a result of the nurse's questions, we encourage our students not to be frightened or intimidated by this. Rather, the nurse could say, for example, "Is this typically what happens when the two of you do not agree on an issue?" The nurse's tone is also important when asking questions so as not to convey judgment or criticism but rather to convey a message of the nurse's desire to seek a sincere understanding of the illness or issue and invite the family to a reflection that hopefully would result in a new perspective and new behaviors. (See Chapter 7 for additional ideas about engagement and assessment.)

In summary, useful, effective, and time-efficient questions are part of relational practice in that they aid in relationship building and collaboration between nurses and families. Most important, questions can be very effective in creating a safe context for the family to describe their illness experience and hopefully glean ideas for how to soften or diminish their suffering. Through the asking of interventive questions as well as other useful interventions, the nurse can invite, encourage, and support families to change.

Example 1: Engage All Family Members and Focus the Meeting

In this first example, Dr. Lorraine Wright is meeting with a couple, Nicholas and Bev. Nicholas had a heart attack recently, and this is a follow-up clinic visit. Lorraine asks the "one question question": "What one question would you most like to have answered during our meeting together?" The *one question question* is a term that Lorraine coined (Wright, 1989), and themes of answers to this question have been explored in a study by Duhamel, Dupuis, and Wright (2009). This question emphasizes a *specific* concern and also asks the couple to prioritize their concerns; she asks what they would *most* like to have answered. The question also includes a time frame (i.e., "during our meeting together").

In this first clinical vignette, Lorraine asks the one question question of both Nicholas and Bev. She does not ask Bev to comment on Nicholas's answer. Rather, she engages *each* family member and elicits their primary concern. Lorraine paraphrases and clarifies each person's response so that both she and the person are in agreement about what has been said. The following is an example of relational practice, the nurse and the client collaborating in setting the focus for the meeting:

> **Dr. Wright:** I'm wondering, then, in the brief time we have, is there any particular question you would most like to have answered during our meeting today?
>
> **Husband:** I'd like for her (*looking at his wife*) to deal differently with her anxiety. Me . . . I'm fine.
>
> **Wife:** Hmm . . . Oh yes, he wants me to go on tranquilizers. So . . . sure . . . (*Turning away*)

> **Dr. Wright:** (*Looking at the husband*) So you want to know how to help your wife deal with her anxiety?
>
> **Husband:** Oh yeah . . .
>
> **Dr. Wright:** And for you, Bev, what is the one question you would most like to get answered?
>
> **Wife:** I would like to get him to start exercising more, watch his diet, spend some time with the family, and stop worrying so much about work. . . .
>
> **Husband:** (*Looking down*)
>
> **Dr. Wright:** Is there one question you'd like, Bev . . .
>
> **Wife:** Well, how can we get him to change his lifestyle?
>
> **Dr. Wright:** Okay . . .

In reading the transcript of the actual interview, did you notice how the nurse, Lorraine, persisted in obtaining an answer from Bev? Gentle persistence can be an important skill in establishing a focus.

There are many other kinds of questions that could also be used in focusing a conversation. For example, a nurse could ask, "What would you like to see happen today so that you would know our meeting has been helpful for you?" We want to emphasize that there is no single, "correct" question to ask. Rather, by engaging in purposeful conversation with patients and their families, nurses will choose and select the most helpful questions in the context of each particular family along with their unique concerns and issues.

Example 2: Use Questions to Assess the Impact of the Problem/Illness on the Family

Asking questions about the impact of the illness or problem is essential to understanding the effect, impact, and changes caused by illness in family members' lives and relationships. By inquiring in this manner, we are giving the family an opportunity to talk about their illness experience or illness story. Families have reported to us that often telling their illness story or narrative was helpful in their emotional, physical, or spiritual healing as the illness is understood, listened to, acknowledged, and witnessed. Too often families have not been given this opportunity to tell their illness story through useful and skillful questions posed by a caring nurse.

In the next clinical vignette, Dr. Maureen Leahey is meeting with a middle-aged couple that is experiencing multiple chronic illnesses. In particular, Phyllis is coping with osteoarthritis and uses a scooter for mobility. Both Ken and Phyllis are 59 years old. They have two sons: the eldest, age 26, is married while the youngest, age 22, lives in the family home.

In this interview, Dr. Leahey explores the impact of osteoarthritis on the couple. Notice how initially the husband says it has not had an impact on them but then does talk about the impact of his wife's pain upon him. Phyllis commends her husband for his support and assistance with household chores but then offers, with sadness, her decision to leave the teaching profession, which she loved, as her energy is being depleted by her illness. Phyllis believes she needs to save her energy for her family but openly admits that it is a huge adjustment to being a full-time homemaker.

This one question about the impact of the illness upon them as a couple opened up a very useful discussion about how osteoarthritis has dramatically changed their lives, careers, and relationships and offered a window into their suffering, coping, and healing experiences.

> **Dr. Leahey:** What has been the impact of these illnesses on the two of you?
>
> **Husband:** I don't know if there has really been an impact . . . I know that I feel at times . . . I wish I could take some of the pain away. It is very hard on me to see . . . especially someone I love so much, suffering with pain.
>
> **Wife:** (*Looking at husband*)
>
> **Dr. Leahey:** (*Nodding*)
>
> **Husband:** And it's a continual, chronic pain . . .
>
> **Dr. Leahey:** Yes. (*Nodding*)
>
> **Husband:** But I try to be as supportive as I possibly can, but . . .
>
> **Wife:** He is just so helpful and so wonderful . . . When I think about the impact . . . I was a teacher, an elementary teacher, and when my arthritis got to bother me so badly, I decided to take a leave of absence because at school, I had to be cheerful and bubbly. I had to put myself forward, but when I came home I was not (*Turning toward husband and laughing*) quite as bubbly. I thought this is not really fair to my own children. So I thought if I am at home, I will be able to do more for them with less effort. So actually, it did impact our lives because I stopped teaching . . . and when I was teaching, I was really quite independent, I think . . .
>
> **Husband:** (*Nodding*) You were . . . It took you a long time to adjust . . .
>
> **Wife:** It did. Away from school, from being a teacher at school to just being at home, it was really difficult for me, but Ken adjusted really quickly with helping me with things I needed help with. Also, our boys, I think, were very aware of the change in our family . . . how things changed, because truly they were different.
>
> **Dr. Leahey:** It sounds like the two of you made tremendous changes.

Other kinds of interventive questions that can assess the impact of an illness are:

- What changes, if any, have there been in your life since you were diagnosed with serious illness?
- What has been the effect of this illness on your family? Your sexual relations? Your work life?

These types of questions address the suffering the family may be enduring and the systemic effects of that suffering. We find it helpful to remember that talking can be healing, and these kinds of questions have the potential for simultaneously assessing and intervening. If the couple in the preceding example expressed a desire to work on changing or modifying a particular coping strategy, Dr. Leahey could then have asked them a variety of other questions to foster change. Some examples might include:

- What has been most helpful for you in adjusting? What do you think your sons noticed?
- What has been least helpful?
- What advice have you been given by family members? Friends? Health-care providers? Did you try it? What did you discover?
- What ideas for change have you been considering? What would be a first step in trying out these ideas? Who would support you in this change? Who might not support you? How might you resist the temptation to fall back into old habits? How might you reward yourself for developing new habits?

You can see that these kinds of questions about possible ideas and ways to change are ones that invite families to reflect on what has and has not been useful in the past and to develop new ideas for the future.

Example 3: Use Questions to Elicit Problem-Solving Skills, Coping Strategies, and Strengths

Families coping with chronic or life-threatening illness or psychosocial problems can commonly feel defeated, hopeless, or failing in their efforts to overcome the illness or live alongside it. Asking questions about the family's problem-solving abilities and their coping strategies and strengths not only serves as assessment but also can be considered interventive.

Exploring these areas of problem-solving skills and coping strategies can remind families of often forgotten or suppressed skills and strengths. Through interventive questioning, families can rediscover and reclaim their own abilities to solve problems and bring back to their hearts and minds their inherent strengths. McGoldrick, Carter, and Garcia-Preto (2011, p. 451) offer some questions to help clients look beyond the stress of their current situation and access the strengths of their heritage. For example, the nurse could ask:

- "How might your grandfather, who dreamed of your immigration but never made it himself, think about the problem you are having with your children?"

- "Your great-grandmother immigrated at age 21 and became a piece-worker in a sweat shop but managed to support her six children and had great strength. What do you think were her dreams for you, her daughter's daughter's daughter? What do you think she would want you to do now about your current problem?"

Following is a vignette of a biracial family with young children: Chris, age 36; Carleen, age 28; Reuben, age 5; Mariah, age 2; and Rebecca, age 9 months. Chris, an immigrant from Zimbabwe, is employed full-time; Carleen, who grew up in a small, rural town in western Canada, is the resident manager in their building. The health concern for this family is the mother's thyroid condition.

In the first section of the example, the husband and father, Chris, comments on the many changes in his life with three preschoolers, in addition to his working full-time and taking evening courses. Notice how Lorraine empathizes with the many demands upon Chris but then asks the couple an interventive question: "What have you learned that works to assist you with all of these demands"?

This interventive question invites Carleen to talk about how things are more organized for her family when she mobilizes resources such as friends to assist them. This solution gives her an opportunity to do her own work as resident manager plus gives her husband more time for his studies.

> **Husband:** The accounting program is very demanding time-wise . . . and then the kids . . . I'm finding it . . . I am having a hard time finding time to study because we have three of them . . . to feed them, get them ready for bed sometimes and then to help clean up the house. By the time . . . I am so tired . . .
>
> **Wife:** (*Looking over at him*)
>
> **Dr. Wright:** Well, sure . . . you are pooped yourself.
>
> **Husband:** I do not put in as much time as I should into studying. This has been one of the biggest changes from my point of view.
>
> **Dr. Wright:** So many demands upon yourself . . . and so what have you learned to handle this? What have you learned that works, does not work?
>
> **Husband:** Mmm . . .

> **Wife:** If I can get things ready, have them all fed, have the place cleaned, have my work done . . .' cause often when he comes home I have to go out and do some of my work. I have friends who help me out and I help them out. We babysit for each other.
>
> **Dr. Wright:** Oh really . . . that is good . . .
>
> **Wife:** That allows me to get work done during the day.
>
> **Dr. Wright:** That's a good idea . . . a good arrangement.
>
> **Wife:** It gives me more time in the evening.

Notice that, after Carleen shared her thoughts about "what works" in the family to assist with all of their demands, Dr. Wright commended the couple for their very good idea of friends taking turns caring for each other's children.

In this next section of the vignette, Dr. Wright normalizes the difficulty of time pressures for mothers and fathers; she asks if Carleen has been able to work out finding any time for herself. An important conversation unfolds with Carleen illustrating her problem-solving skills. She talks about involving her son to watch the youngest child while she does yoga in their home. This sparks the father to remember how he gives his wife some time for herself when he takes all three children to the park. Once again, Dr. Wright is able to commend the family for these efforts.

> **Dr. Wright:** *(To wife)* Have you been able to find any time for yourself?
>
> **Wife:** Yeah, I have. I try to get up before the kids . . . that does not always work, though. This one *(Turning toward 5-year-old Reuben)* gets up, and then the baby is up . . . I'll go downstairs and I'll do yoga, and Reuben will just watch me. Or I'll do aerobics . . .
>
> **Dr. Wright:** *(Looking at Reuben)* So you watch Mommy do yoga . . . Do you ever join in and do it with her?
>
> **Reuben:** *(Looking at Dr. Wright)* . . . when the baby's awake . . . watching her . . .
>
> **Wife:** He watches the baby.
>
> **Dr. Wright:** Very nice.
>
> **Husband:** Sometimes what I do is take the kids out to the park so she can have the day to herself. I still try to do it, but some days she'd rather be doing her work.

Asking about a family's problem-solving skills, coping, and strengths can set the stage for further interventions, if needed. For example, if Carleen had stated she wanted to increase her problem-solving skills, Lorraine could have pursued this with her. For instance, they could have discussed possible play groups in the area, available community resources, and so forth. Other questions that could be asked to bring forth a family's problem-solving skills and strengths include:

- Asking the husband in his wife's presence: "What do you think your devotion and caring for your wife during her illness does for your marriage?"
- Asking the teenagers in a family meeting: "What do you think other families could learn from your family about coping with a chronic illness?"

Example 4: Use Questions as Interventions and to Invite Change

The intervention process represents the core of clinical practice with families. Myriad interventions are possible, but nurses need to tailor their interventions to each family they encounter. Openness to certain interventions is profoundly influenced by the relationship between the nurse and the family and the nurse's ability to help the family reflect on their health problems.

Questions in and of themselves can provide new information and answers for the family; thus, they become interventions. Interventive questions can encourage family members to view their problems or illness experience in a new way or to change their beliefs and subsequently discover new solutions.

The next clinical example is with a couple, Al and Benz. She is a documented Chinese immigrant, and this is her first marriage. Al is a native Canadian, and this is his second marriage. Benz is close to being discharged from the hospital following surgery for breast cancer. The first interventive question in this clinical vignette is, "Who between the two of you was the most upset with the news of the diagnosis?" This leads to a very poignant therapeutic conversation about Benz's future.

> **Dr. Wright:** (*Looking at the wife*) Have there been any other kinds of cancer in your family?
>
> **Wife:** No . . . we are all pretty healthy.
>
> **Dr. Wright:** (*Looking at the husband*) . . . and what about for you, Al, has there been any history of cancer in your family?
>
> **Husband:** No . . . I cannot think of any . . . I had an aunt and uncle who got lung cancer. Both were heavy smokers.
>
> **Dr. Wright:** So this was something very new for both of you dealing with cancer. And who would you say, between the

two of you, was most upset about this diagnosis and news when you got it?

Husband: Oh, Benz was, I think.

Wife: I would say so, too. I cried and cried. I just could not handle it.

Dr. Wright: Yes . . .

Husband: . . . and I just don't see what a lot of crying accomplishes. I think you have to really think positively and know in your heart that you can beat this thing.

Dr. Wright: That's how you've been trying to encourage Benz?

Wife: Yeah, he kept telling me that. I just felt I needed to cry. That's the only thing I needed to do . . .

Dr. Wright: Yes . . .

Husband: Well, a certain amount of this is understandable, and I have tried to be sympathetic, but you have got to get onto the positive thinking path and really believe you're going to beat this thing.

Dr. Wright: (*Nodding*)

Husband: I really do believe that. I really do believe that.

Dr. Wright: (*Looking at husband*) . . . You do. (*Looking at wife*) And what are your thoughts for the future? Because I've met other women with breast cancer that worry . . . What are your thoughts?

Wife: Some days I am pretty good about it. I am in good hands; my doctor is good. And some days, I just do not know. It fluctuates. Some days are good and some are bad.

Dr. Wright: So some days you are more optimistic about your future and other days you . . .

Wife: I think the worst.

Dr Wright: And what do you think about when you think the worst?

Wife: That Al and our child, Bryan, would be alone without me. I care about them so much.

Husband: And this is the kind of thinking I try to discourage. I do not think it is good.

Dr. Wright: So when you hear your wife talking this way and I am not here, do you try to cheer her up and get her off of this topic?

Husband: Oh yeah. I allow her a little bit of it. She has to express herself and express her feelings, but once she has got that out, she has to get back to being hopeful.

Dr. Wright: (*Looking to wife*) And do you like that approach Al takes? He tries to get you off of this topic and to think optimistically. Or do you want to be able to say more about the other side, the "worry side" . . .

Wife: Well, I know he is being kind and wants me to do well. But sometimes, that is just the way I feel. Maybe if he would just listen to me . . .

In this therapeutic conversation, Benz was very concerned about her prognosis. Dr. Wright had asked about Benz's beliefs about her prognosis when she said to Benz, "What are your thoughts about your future?"

These are not easy conversations when a nurse "speaks the unspeakable" by introducing a conversation about their beliefs about prognosis (Wright & Bell, 2009). Knowing the family's beliefs about various aspects of their illness assists the nurse in knowing if their beliefs are constraining or facilitating. We believe that nurses have a socially sanctioned role and thus can talk about such delicate and intimate topics with families. In our clinical experience, we have found that families rarely mind any question if it is asked in a kind, nonjudgmental, purposeful, and thoughtful manner. We have encouraged our students to be curious and pursue hard topics with families. If the nurse working with the family cannot address potentially difficult areas with them, then we encourage the nurse to transfer the family to another nurse if possible or request that another nurse continue the conversation.

Dr. Wright's question invited a very useful disclosure about this couple's differences in beliefs about how to cope with worries and face the future. Benz wanted to talk about her fears for the future, whereas Al preferred to deal with worry by being optimistic. Instead of Lorraine taking sides with either Al or Benz about the best way to handle fears, she asked Benz, "Do you like this approach (her husband's optimism), or do you want to say more about the 'worry side'?"

This simple, but powerful, interventive question had the potential for inviting healing change in one or both spouses. Benz offered very clearly that she would prefer that her husband listen to her. It is very understandable that Al wanted to cheer her up, but it was not Benz's preferred way for her husband to comfort her.

In this clinical example, interventive questions invited family members to explore and reflect on their beliefs about the illness experience, the prognosis, and how best to manage their illness. Reflections are invited through very deliberate, thoughtful, and purposeful interventive questions.

Examples of other interventive questions are:

- ■ How do you make sense of your suffering?
- ■ In 6 months from now, how do you think your family will have adjusted to this illness?

In our therapeutic conversations with families, we hope that healing will be enhanced as new illness beliefs, thoughts, ideas, or solutions come forth, are pondered, and acted upon. As family members consider how to best live their lives with illness, change may occur.

Example 5: Use Questions to Request Feedback About the Family Meeting

We seek to ask questions that are in keeping with our philosophy of fostering collaborative relationships between nurses and families. These kinds of questions imply to family members that their satisfaction with the meeting, or lack thereof, matters and that we want to improve our care to families. Collaborative questions also give the family the chance to voice concerns about what specifically was helpful to them.

In the following vignette, at the end of the meeting with Al and Benz, Dr. Wright asks if the conversation has been helpful to them. Benz gives a short answer and comments on the relationship with Lorraine by saying, "You are kind."

But notice how Lorraine's question invites much more pondering from Al. He reflects back on Benz's suggestion about wanting him to listen more. This is a lovely example of how an interventive question invited a reflection and how Al decides on his *own* that he could make a behavioral change that would be more his wife's preferred way to be comforted. This is always the most desirable and sustaining kind of change—that is, when a family member initiates the change rather than being instructed to do so.

> **Dr. Wright:** (*Looking at the couple*) Well, just before we end, was there anything about this conversation that has been useful or helpful for you or not helpful?
>
> **Wife:** . . . I think you are very kind.
>
> **Dr. Wright:** (*Nodding to the wife and then looking to the husband*) Anything that was helpful for you, Al?
>
> **Husband:** Yeah . . . it made me think. It made me think. Perhaps I need to listen a little bit more and not be so free with the advice.
>
> **Dr. Wright:** (*Looking at the wife*) I think it is wonderful to have a husband who wants to cheer you up and make you feel better . . .

Wife: I'm lucky.

Dr. Wright: But there are times when you want him to hear you out about what you are thinking and feeling.

Other questions that can invite feedback about the usefulness of the therapeutic conversations that nurses have with families are:

- In what ways was our discussion useful to each of you, or not useful?
- On a scale of 1 to 10 (with 1 being very low and 10 being very high), how well do you think I understood your situation?
- Is there anything you were hoping for in this meeting that did not happen?

Of course, families do not always convey positive feelings about the meeting with the nurse. If the family expresses dissatisfaction or discontent, we encourage the nurse to explore their reasons for being dissatisfied and accept the feedback nondefensively. The nurse can thank the family for their insights and ask their suggestions for how she could be more helpful to other families. If the nurse takes a sincere "one-down" position when receiving feedback, it encourages the family to maintain a collaborative relationship. It also permits the nurse to reflect on her practice and potentially alter her actions for future family meetings.

CONCLUSIONS

We hope this chapter has given you ideas on how to use questions in family interviewing—questions that invite possibilities for healing and change. Of course, there is an unending number of questions that nurses could ask families. But we hope that this sample roadmap for the interview will assist you to be more selective, skilled, and time-efficient when asking your questions. We hope you will find that asking families questions will give you an increased understanding and appreciation of their illness experience or concerns and will open possibilities to soften suffering and invite more hope and healing.

References

Duhamel, F., Dupuis, F., & Wright, L.M. (2009). Families' and nurses' responses to the "one question question": Reflections for clinical practice, education, and research in family nursing. *Journal of Family Nursing, 15*(4), 4–485.

Healing, S., & Bavelas, J.B. (2011). Can questions lead to change? An analogue experiment. *Journal of Systemic Therapies, 30*(4), 30–48.

Katie, B. (2003). *Loving What Is: Four Questions That Can Change Your Life.* New York: Three Rivers Press.

McGee, D., Del Vento, A., & Bavelas, J.B. (2005). An interactional model of questions as therapeutic interventions. *Journal of Marital and Family Therapy, 31*(4), 371–384.

McGoldrick, M., Carter, B., & Garcia-Preto, N. (Eds.). (2011). A multicultural life cycle framework for clinical assessment. In M. McGoldrick, B. Carter, & N. Garcia-Preto. (Eds.). *The Expanded Family Life Cycle: Individual, Family, and Social Perspectives* (4th ed.). Boston, MA: Allyn & Bacon, pp. 447–455.

Wright, L.M. (1989). When clients ask questions: Enriching the therapeutic conversation. *Family Therapy Networker, 13*(6), 15–16.

Wright, L.M., & Bell, J.M. (2009). *Belief and Illness: A Model to Invite Healing.* Calgary, AB: 4th Floor Press.

Wright, L.M., & Leahey, M. (Producers). (2006). *How to Use Questions in Family Interviewing.* [DVD]. Calgary, Canada. Available at www.familynursingresources.com

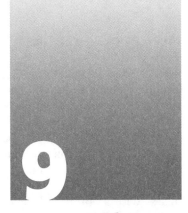

Chapter **9**

How to Do a 15-Minute (or Shorter) Family Interview

Family nursing *can* be effectively, skillfully, and meaningfully practiced in just 15 minutes or less. We have listened to and read in professional journals the many stories and reports by nurses of how these ideas have been implemented into their practice and thus how their practice with patients and families has changed in rewarding ways (Goudreau, Duhamel, & Ricard, 2006; LeGrow & Rossen, 2005; Moules & Johnstone, 2010). Bell (2012) offered a compelling idea that the 15-minute family interview is one of the most "sticky" ideas in family nursing. By "sticky" she is referring to ideas that are unexpectedly introduced, credible, efficient, and subsequently have had enthusiastic worldwide implementation in family nursing teaching, research, and practice.

One of our goals in developing these ideas was to address head-on the perception among nurses that they lack the time to involve families in their practice, and this effort seemed to resonate with many nurses. To further assist nurse educators and nursing students with implementing these ideas in practice, we produced an educational DVD titled *How to Do a 15-Minute (or Less) Family Interview* (see Family Nursing Resources at www.family nursingresources.com to view video vignettes of actual family interviews; Wright and Leahey, 2000).

"I don't have time to do family interviews" is the most common reason nurses offer for not routinely involving families in their practice. In numerous undergraduate and graduate nursing courses, professional workshops, and presentations, we have encountered this statement as the resounding reason for the exclusion of family members from health care. With major changes in the delivery of health-care services through managed care, emphasis on providing more care in the community, budgetary constraints, increased acuity, and staff cutbacks, time is of the essence in nursing practice. However, it is our belief that families need not be banned or marginalized from health care. To involve families, and especially in a time-limited conversation, nurses need to possess sound knowledge of family assessment and intervention models, interviewing skills, and questions. We have witnessed and conducted interviews to know that family nursing knowledge can be applied effectively even in very brief family meetings. We also claim that a 15-minute, or even shorter, family interview can be purposeful, effective, informative, and even healing. Any involvement of family members, regardless of the length of time, is better than no involvement.

But what is time? And what exactly can be accomplished in 15 minutes or less with a family? We have noticed that much of nursing practice time is socially and culturally coordinated, highly ritualized, and therefore honored. Nurses clearly articulate the start and end of their shifts, their schedules, and so forth. We propose that ritualizing and coordinating meeting time with families, even if it is only 15 minutes, can also become part of nursing practice.

However, for nurses' behaviors to change, they must first alter or modify their beliefs about involving families in health care. We have discovered that, when nurses do not include family members in their practice, some very constraining beliefs usually exist (Wright & Bell, 2009). Some of these beliefs are:

- "If I talk to family members, I will not have time to complete my other nursing responsibilities."
- "If I talk to family members, I may open up a can of worms, and I will have no time to deal with it."
- "It is not my job to talk with families; that is for social workers and psychologists."
- "I cannot possibly help families in the brief time I will be caring for them."
- "If the family becomes angry, what would I do?"
- "What if they ask me a question and I do not have the answer? What would I do? It is better not to start a conversation."

Another constraining belief that nurses and other health-care professionals often have is that nothing meaningful can be accomplished in one meeting with a client. Slive and Bobele (2011) challenge this belief in their landmark book documenting clinical success with clients who use walk-in single-session therapy. The significance of having an opportunity to converse with a professional at the time most meaningful to the family cannot be overestimated. Research on time-effective single session therapy has demonstrated its effectiveness and client satisfaction with the outcome (Green, Correia, Bobele, et al, 2011).

In South Calgary Health Center, Calgary, Canada, where Dr. Leahey and colleagues initiated a single-session walk-in mental health clinic in 2004, evaluation studies demonstrated ease of access for clients, with 65% being seen on average within 13 minutes of handing in their forms to the admitting clerk; clients' mean presession distress levels (7.9) dropped significantly to 5.4 postsession (Harper-Jaques & Leahey, 2011). Of the 240 clients who answered a written questionnaire about overall satisfaction with the service,

94% stated they were satisfied or delighted (Harper-Jaques & Leahey, 2011). The value of having a meaningful conversation with a health professional stands out as significant.

Uncovering these constraining beliefs makes it more comprehensible why nurses may shy away from routinely involving families in nursing practice. We postulate that if nurses were to embrace only one belief, that "illness is a family affair" (Wright & Bell, 2009), it would change the face of nursing practice. Nurses would then be more eager to know how to involve and assist family members in the care of loved ones. They would appreciate that everyone in a family experiences an illness and that no one family member "has" diabetes, multiple sclerosis, or cancer. By embracing this belief, they would realize that, from initial symptoms through diagnosis and treatment, all family members are influenced by and influence the illness. They would also come to realize that our privileged conversations with patients and their families about their illness experiences can contribute dramatically to healing and the softening or alleviation of suffering (Wright, 2005; Wright & Bell, 2009). Our evidence for this belief comes from our clinical and personal conversations as well as from reading numerous blogs and books about illness narratives.

We also believe that nurses will increase their caring for and involvement of families in their practice, regardless of the practice context, if such behavior is strongly supported and advocated by health-care administrators (Leahey & Harper-Jaques, 2010; Leahey & Svavarsdottir, 2009). One powerful and visual way for health-care administrators to show their commitment to family-centered care is to involve nurses in the creation, development, and implementation of family-friendly policies and services (International Council of Nurses, 2002). Examples of family-friendly policies and actions at the larger system level could include having family members as advisory board or task force members, focus group participants, program evaluators, and participants in quality and safety initiatives. Ensuring that parking is available at health-care facilities for families with limited income is another strategy.

At the department or unit level, examples can include providing family-friendly visiting hours and space, such as a play area for children; offering a quiet room for retreat or for family discussion of difficult situations or moments; and lobbying for routinely providing family nursing therapeutic conversations when families are suffering. Inviting family members to participate in new staff orientation or volunteering to orient new families to the inpatient unit and mentor other families are additional options. Nurses can invite families to patient conferences, accompany patients to tests, support patients during procedures, assist patients with personal care, and so forth. A combination of administrative support, family-friendly facilities, and nurses who have the commitment, knowledge, and skills to routinely involve families in their practice is necessary for nurses to be able to maximize their time with families.

Following are some specific ideas for conducting a 15-minute (or shorter) family interview. These ideas are the condensed version of the core elements previously presented in Chapters 5 through 7 about conducting family interviews. The ideas honor the theoretical underpinnings of the Calgary Family Assessment Model (CFAM; see Chapter 3) and the Calgary Family Intervention Model (CFIM; see Chapter 4) and highlight some of the most critical elements of these models.

KEY INGREDIENTS

What are the key ingredients of a healing, productive, and effective 15-minute family interview? From our observations and experience, they are therapeutic conversations, manners, a family genogram (and in some situations an ecomap), therapeutic questions, and commendations. Of course, all of these elements can be involved only within the context of a therapeutic relationship between the nurse and family.

Research on and clinical evidence for the usefulness of the 15-minute family interview are now appearing in family nursing's primary journal, the *Journal of Family Nursing*. Holtslander (2005) described how the 15-minute family interview was successfully applied to the needs of families in a postpartum unit. Martinez, D'Artois, & Rennick (2007) conducted research to explore nurses' perceptions of the impact of the 15-minute interview on the hospital admission process and on their family nursing practice. They found that practicing pediatric hospital nurses perceived the genogram, therapeutic questions, and commendations as having a positive impact on their ability to conduct family assessments and family interventions. These nurses concluded that a 15-minute interview should be routinely incorporated into practice at the time of a child's admission.

Key Ingredient 1: Therapeutic Conversations

All human interaction takes place in conversations. Each conversation in which nurses participate effects change in their own and in patients' and family members' biopsychosocial-spiritual structures. No conversation that a nurse has with a patient or family member is trivial (Wright & Bell, 2009). Nurses are always engaged in therapeutic conversations with their clients without perhaps thinking of them as such.

The conversation in a brief family interview is therapeutic because from the start it is purposeful and time-limited, as are the relationships. Therapeutic conversations between a nurse and a family can be as short as one sentence or as long as time allows. All conversations between nurses and families, regardless of time, have the potential for healing through the very act of bringing the family together (Hougher Limacher & Wright, 2003, 2006; McLeod, 2003; Robinson & Wright, 1995; Wright & Bell, 2009). One study evaluated the usefulness of short therapeutic conversations with families (15 to 50 minutes with an average of 30 minutes) with a child/adolescent experiencing chronic illness. The study yielded both expected and unexpected results (Svavarsdottir, Tryggvadottir, & Sigurdardottir, in press).

A positive, expected result was that parents in the experimental group perceived significantly higher family support after the intervention, compared with the parents in the control group. An unexpected result was that these same parents in the experimental group perceived significantly lower expressive family functioning (e.g., emotional communication, collaboration, problem-solving, and verbal communication) after the intervention of a short therapeutic conversation.

The researchers offer possible explanations for the lower expressive family functioning following the therapeutic conversation intervention. One might be that parents with children with acute illnesses were generally younger and may not have had the instrumental or emotional resources to adequately cope with this illness crisis. Another explanation might be that the parents may have trusted the nurse more during and after receiving the therapeutic conversation intervention and therefore offered more of their "real" experience of family functioning in the context of illness. These results point the direction that additional studies will need to examine further what happens "inside" the intervention and in the nurse-family relationship.

It is not only the length of the conversation or time that makes the most difference but also the opportunity for patients and family members to be acknowledged and affirmed in their illness experience that has tremendous healing potential (Bell & Wright, 2011; Hougher Limacher, 2003; Hougher Limacher & Wright, 2003, 2006; Moules, 2002; Moules & Johnstone, 2010; Wright & Bell, 2009). Nurses are socially empowered and privileged to bring forth either health or pathology in their conversations with families.

Another pretest/post-test research study that illustrates the possibility for healing within families was conducted in four acute psychiatric units with patients and family members (Sveinbjarnardottir, Svavarsdottir, & Wright, [in press]). The experimental group received two to five short therapeutic conversations. A control group of patients and families received traditional nursing care. The family members in the group who received the short therapeutic conversation intervention perceived higher cognitive and emotional support than those receiving traditional care. As more research studies examine the short therapeutic family interviews, they will add to the knowledge base about the effectiveness of short interviews and thus what needs to be implemented into practice.

The art of listening is also paramount. The need to communicate what it is like to live in our individual, separate worlds of experience, particularly within the world of illness, is a powerful need in human relationships (Wright, 2005). Frank (1998) suggests that listening to families' illness stories is not only an art but also an ethical practice. Nurses commonly believe that listening also entails an obligation to do something to "fix" whatever concerns or problems are raised. However, in many cases, the most therapeutic move, intervention, or action the nurse can perform is showing compassion and offering commendations (Bell & Wright, 2011;

Bohn, Wright, & Moules, 2003; Hougher Limacher, 2003, 2008; Hougher Limacher & Wright, 2003; Moules, 2002; Moules & Johnstone, 2010; Wright & Bell, 2009).

It is the integration of task-oriented patient care with interactive, purposeful conversation that distinguishes a time-effective 15-minute (or shorter) interview. The nurse makes information giving and patient involvement in decision-making integral parts of the delivery process. He or she takes advantage of opportunities and searches for ways to engage in purposeful, healing conversations with families. These practices differ from social conversations and can include basic ideas such as:

- Families are *routinely* invited to accompany the patient to the unit, clinic, or hospital.
- Families are *routinely* included in the admission procedure.
- Families are *routinely* invited to ask questions during the patient orientation.
- Nurses acknowledge the patient's and family's expertise in managing health problems by asking about routines at home.
- Nurses encourage patients to practice how they will handle different interactions in the future, such as telling family members and others that they cannot eat certain foods.
- Nurses *routinely* consult families and patients about *their* ideas for treatment and discharge.

Key Ingredient 2: Manners

Good manners have always been the core of common, everyday social behavior and interaction. However, in the last two decades in North America, social behavior has dramatically shifted from formal to casual social interaction; some would say it has even progressed to being rude or occasionally abusive. Style of dress has been altered from "Sunday Best" to "Casual Friday." Martin and Kamen's (2005) *Miss Manners' Guide to Excruciatingly Correct Behavior* offers their perspective and humor on manners. Miss Manners, as Martin is known, comments on what is missing in social interactions and thus what is missing in society. Manners are simple acts of courtesy, politeness, respect, and kindness. Culture as a whole seems to be undergoing an erosion of manners and thus civility. This erosion has spilled over into the nursing profession.

Nursing has not been immune to the changes in social behavior. In some situations, we can argue that formal nursing behaviors (such as dressing in starched uniforms and caps) perhaps inhibited our relations with clients and families. Countless nurses still maintain respectful, polite, and thoughtful relations with their clients. However, we have witnessed and listened to far too many professional and personal encounters between nurses, patients, and families in which manners were absent.

One of the most glaring examples of the absence of manners in nursing is in the basic social act of an introduction. Numerous stories have been told of nurses who do not introduce themselves to their patients, let alone the patients' family members. For example, Pablo, a 23-year-old Hispanic man, was seen in an outpatient clinic in a large metropolitan hospital after open-heart surgery. He reported that the nurse did not introduce herself but began touching his body and adjusting his intravenous PICC line without telling him what she was doing or why. He found this experience very invasive, frightening, and rude.

This clinical anecdote is consistent with what nurses have told us about nurse-family relationships in the intensive care unit. We believe that one of the nursing strategies that inhibits the establishment of therapeutic relationships is depersonalization of the patient and family. Examples include not referring to the patient by name, labeling the patient or family difficult, providing care without encouraging participation by the patient or family, and not talking or making eye contact.

Therefore, introduction is obviously an essential ingredient of a successful family interview and relational family nursing practice. However, introductions by nurses have changed from overly formal to overly casual. Just a few years ago, nurses might introduce themselves as "Miss Garcia," whereas now a more typical introduction is "Hello, my name is Sasha, and I'm your nurse today." Any introduction is better than no introduction, but as one client remarked to us, "Nurses don't introduce themselves any differently from a waiter who says, 'Hi, my name is Josh, and I'm your waiter tonight.'" We encourage nurses always to introduce themselves by their full names, except in unique circumstances when there might be concerns for safety.

An equally serious omission is the lack of introduction by nurses to their patients' family members. What inhibits or prevents nurses in hospitals, community health clinics, and home care from introducing themselves to the people at a patient's bedside? What prevents nurses from inquiring about their relationships to the patient? Worse yet, what precludes nurses from making eye contact with family members or friends, one of the most expected social norms in our North American culture? We have discussed this phenomenon with our nursing students and professional nurses. It has been revealed to us that the belief of "lack of time" constrains many nurses from talking with anyone but their patients for fear that family members or close friends may "ask questions" or "require time from me that I just don't have." We would like to counter this belief by suggesting that, in the end, nurses would *save* time if they would use a few manners with family members or friends. Nurses who did so would not be pursued at even more inopportune times by family members or friends inquiring about their loved ones. Nurses who have involved family members in their practice have reported that they have enjoyed greater rather than less job satisfaction (Leahey, et al, 1995).

Good manners also instill trust in family members. Examples of good manners that invite a trusting relationship are:

1. Always call patients and family members by name.

2. Always tell the patient and family members your name.

3. Explain your role for that shift or meeting or any encounter with the patient and/or family.

4. Explain a procedure before coming into the room with the equipment to do it.

5. If you tell the patient or a family member that you will be back at a certain time, attempt to keep to that time or provide an explanation about why it didn't occur.

Key Ingredient 3: Family Genograms and Ecomaps

Nurses need to make it a priority to draw a quick genogram (and sometimes, if indicated, an ecomap) for *all* families, but particularly for families who will likely be part of their care for more than a day. Extensive details for the collection of genogram and ecomap information were given in Chapter 3 in the discussion about the "structural assessment" category of the CFAM. In a brief interview, the collection of genogram and ecomap information needs to be brief also. This information can be gleaned from family members in a couple of minutes.

The most essential information to obtain includes data about ages, occupation or school grade, religion, ethnic background, immigration date, and current health status of each family member. Begin by asking "easy" questions (e.g., ages, current health) of the household family members. Drawing out information relating to, for example, siblings' divorces or grandchildren is not necessary or time-efficient unless this information immediately relates to the family and health problem. Once the genogram information is obtained, if indicated, expand the data collection to obtain external family structure information in the form of an ecomap. It may be useful to ask questions such as, "Who outside of your immediate family is an important resource to you or is a stress for you?" and "How many professionals are involved in treating your husband's current heart problems?" Obtaining structural assessment data through the genogram and ecomap also serves as a quick engagement strategy because families are usually very pleased that a nurse is asking about their entire family rather than just the person experiencing the illness. It quickly acknowledges to the family the nurse's underlying belief that illness is a family affair.

Ideally, the genogram should become part of any documentation about the family and patient. In one cardiac unit, genogram information is collected on admission, and the genogram is hung at the patient's bedside. Emergency telephone numbers for family members are listed on the genogram. In this way, the genogram acts as a continuous visual reminder for all health-care professionals involved with the patient to "think family."

Key Ingredient 4: Therapeutic Questions

Therapeutic questions are a key, defining element in a therapeutic conversation. Many ideas about and examples of linear, circular, and interventive questions were given in the presentation of the CFIM (see Chapter 4) and in the discussion of family nursing skills (see Chapter 5) and were given in the vignettes demonstrating the use of questions (see Chapter 8). When nurses attempt to have a very brief family meeting, they can ask key questions of family members to involve them in family health care. We encourage nurses to think of at least three key questions that they will routinely ask all families.

Of course, these questions need to fit the context in which the nurse encounters families. For example, the questions that a nurse may ask family members in an emergency or oncology unit in a hospital might differ from the questions that a nurse might routinely ask family members in an outpatient diabetic clinic for children or in primary care. However, some basic themes need to be addressed, such as the sharing of information, expectations of hospitalization, clinic or home-care visits, challenges, sufferings, and the most pressing concerns or problems. The following are some examples of questions that address these particular topics:

- How can we be most helpful to you and your family (or friends) during your hospitalization? (Clarifies expectations and increases collaboration.)
- What has been most and least helpful to you in past hospitalizations or clinic visits? (Identifies past strengths and problems to avoid and successes to repeat.)
- What is the greatest challenge facing your family during this hospitalization, discharge, or clinic visit? (Indicates actual or potential suffering, roles, and beliefs.)
- With which of your family members or friends would you like us to share information? With which ones would you like us not to share information? (Indicates alliances, resources, and possible conflictual relationships.)
- What do you need to best prepare you or your family member for discharge? (Assists with early discharge planning.)
- Who do you believe is suffering the most in your family during this hospitalization, clinic visit, or home-care visit? (Identifies the family member who has the greatest need for support and intervention [Wright, 2005].)
- What is the one question you would most like to have answered during our meeting right now? I may not be able to answer this question at the moment, but I will do my best or will try to find the answer for you. (Identifies most pressing issue or concern [Duhamel, Dupuis, & Wright, 2009; Wright, 1989].)

- How have I been most helpful to you in this family meeting? How could we improve? (Shows a willingness to learn from families and to work collaboratively.)

Key Ingredient 5: Commending Family and Individual Strengths

The important intervention of offering commendations (Bell & Wright, 2011; Hougher Limacher, 2003, 2008; Hougher Limacher & Wright, 2006; Moules & Johnstone, 2010; Wright, 2005; Wright & Bell, 2009) was fully discussed in the presentation of the CFIM (see Chapter 4). In each session, we routinely commend families on the strengths observed during the interview. In a brief family interview of 15 minutes or less, we endorse the practice of offering at least one or two commendations to family members of individual or family strengths, resources, or competencies that the nurse directly observed or gathered from another source. Remember that commendations are observations of behavior that occur across time. Therefore, the nurse is looking for patterns rather than a one-time occurrence that is more likely going to elicit only a compliment. An example of a commendation is "Your family is showing much courage in living with your wife's cancer for 5 years." A compliment would be "Your son is so gentle despite feeling so ill today."

Families coping with chronic, life-threatening, or psychosocial problems commonly feel defeated, hopeless, or failing in their efforts to overcome the illnesses or live with them. In our clinical experience, we have found that most families who are experiencing illness, disability, or trauma also suffer from "commendation-deficit disorder." Therefore, nurses can never offer too many commendations.

Immediate and long-term positive reactions to commendations indicate that they are powerful, effective, and enduring therapeutic interventions (Bell & Wright, 2011; Bohn, Wright, & Moules, 2003; Hougher Limacher, 2003, 2008; Hougher Limacher & Wright, 2003, 2006; Moules, 2002; Moules & Johnstone, 2010; Wright & Bell, 2009). Robinson's (1998) study explored the processes and outcomes of nursing interventions with families experiencing difficulties with chronic illness. The families reported the clinical nursing team's "orientation to strengths, resources, and possibilities to be an extremely important facet of the process" (p. 284). Hougher Limacher's 2003 study, which specifically focused on understanding more about the intervention of commendations, lends even further validation to the power of commendations. Families who internalize commendations offered by nurses appear more receptive and trusting of the nurse–family relationship and tend to readily take up ideas, opinions, and advice that are offered.

By commending families' resources, competencies, and strengths, nurses offer family members a new view of themselves. When nurses change the view families have of themselves, families are commonly able to look at their health problem differently and thus move toward more effective solutions to reduce any potential or actual suffering.

PERSONAL EXAMPLE OF INVOLVING FAMILY IN NURSING PRACTICE

To illustrate how involving family members in health care can be effective and healing—or ineffective and resulting in a needless increase of suffering—Dr. Wright offers a personal story to illustrate the best and worst of family nursing. These experiences occurred during two very brief interactions with nurses in the emergency unit of a large city hospital while Dr. Wright accompanied her mother for a possible admission:

Over the last 5 years of my mother's life, she experienced several major exacerbations of multiple sclerosis (MS), with frequent hospitalizations. Each exacerbation left my mother more physically disabled. The extreme exacerbations of the last year of her life left her a quadriplegic. With each exacerbation, she never returned to the level of either physical or cognitive functioning that she previously enjoyed. Despite all of these setbacks, there was tremendous courage on the part of both my mother and my father. Amazingly, my mother's moments of complaining, sadness, or grief were minimal, which of course buffered other family members' suffering. I saw my father become a very caring caregiver and "nurse" while his own life became very constrained.

On one of my mother's admissions to the hospital, I encountered two very brief but powerful conversations with nurses in the emergency department (ED). One I prefer to call "Naughty Nurse" and the other "Angel Nurse." Both of these nurses had a profound impact on my emotional suffering. Both of these nurses interacted with me for a very brief time, not more than 5 minutes each.

Before our arrival at the hospital ED, I spent a few very exhausting hours with my mother. My father, mother, and I were enjoying a day at our cottage about an hour out of the city. As the afternoon unfolded, it became apparent that my mother was becoming more wobbly when walking (at that time she was still able to walk a few steps with assistance). As we were packing to leave, she became unable to bear weight. With great difficulty, my father and I lifted her into her wheelchair and headed down the ramp of our cottage to the car. The greater challenge lay ahead of us: to get her from the wheelchair into the car. It took all of our strength and ingenuity to accomplish this task, with my mother, of course, frightened that we would drop her. After some 30 minutes and lots of perspiration, we realized our goal, with my mother safely in the car. On the way into the city, we made a mutual decision to take her to the hospital where she had been admitted on previous occasions to have her assessed for possible admission. We all believed that she was having another severe exacerbation.

When we arrived at the ED, I was very relieved. It had been a very worrisome and arduous few hours. I now looked forward to my mother's receiving nursing and medical assessment and treatment to assist her and us. My father waited with her in the car at the curb of the ED while I entered to seek assistance to lift my mother out of the car. On arriving at the nursing station, I encountered Naughty Nurse. I explained the current situation to her and requested assistance to lift my mother out of the car and into the ED. Naughty Nurse responded in a curt, mistrusting tone by saying, "How did you get her into the car?" This initial brief interaction was shocking to me; it was accusatory, blaming, and mistrusting of one another. No therapeutic relationship was being developed. This nurse's response invited me to counter with an equally rude, impolite response. I said, "With great [difficulty], so we will need help to lift her out of the car." Our conversation now escalated in terms of accusations and recriminations as Naughty Nurse retorted, "Well, I can't lift her out of the car." I suggested that perhaps one of her male colleagues could assist us. As Naughty Nurse and a male colleague approached the car to assist my mother, they did not introduce themselves to my mother nor did they discontinue their conversation with each other. This was an extreme example of what family nursing should not be. By now, I was very distressed and upset about our treatment by this particular nurse. Of course, she was completely unaware that, in my professional life, I teach, practice, research, and write about family nursing.

However, all was not lost. Within a short while, we were placed in a room in the ED, and after a brief wait, "Angel Nurse" appeared. First, she introduced herself to my mother, explained that she would be taking her blood pressure and temperature and that blood work had been ordered. Angel Nurse competently and kindly attended to my mother, inquiring about both her medical history and her illness experiences with MS. In a very impressive manner, she reassured my mother that she would probably be admitted for another round of intravenous steroids and that everything would be done to keep her comfortable.

Then she came to me, reached out her hand to shake mine, introduced herself, and warmly inquired about the nature of my relationship to the patient. I was softened by this nurse's kind and competent approach. I offered the information that I was the patient's daughter and that I was visiting from another city. Then the nurse offered a possible hypothesis in the form of a statement: "This must be very upsetting for you." In that one sentence, this nurse assessed and acknowledged my suffering. Angel Nurse provided comfort and understanding through her very brief interaction with me in probably less than 2 minutes. However, in just those 2 minutes, she had involved me in her practice and some of my emotional suffering had healed.

Later, on reflection, I realized that my reaction to this nurse's encounter with me was to make every effort to assist her in caring for my mother because I could see that she was overloaded with patients in the ED. Angel Nurse's particular nursing approach had encouraged me to want to be more helpful to her. Kindness invites kindness; accusations invite accusations.

In this very brief interaction, Angel Nurse had entered into a therapeutic conversation with me, my mother, and my father. She also showed good manners by shaking my hand, introducing herself, eliciting some genogram information, and validating my suffering. Perhaps not all the key ingredients that we have suggested for a brief family interview are evident in this interaction with Angel Nurse; however, it exemplifies how the context and the appropriateness of the situation determine how much family members can be involved. This nurse beautifully demonstrated that family nursing can be done, even in busy EDs, in just 2 minutes and still effect healing.

PROFESSIONAL EXAMPLE OF A BRIEF FAMILY INTERVIEW WITHOUT FAMILY MEMBERS PRESENT

Dr. Leahey offers an example of a situation she was involved in while consulting with staff nurses on a medical unit:

> Greta, a 32-year-old woman, was admitted to a medical unit with a questionable diagnosis of influenza. Her weight had dropped to 82 pounds, a loss of 10 pounds in the week before admission.

Greta also had a genetic disease involving weakness and wasting of skeletal muscles. The nursing staff perceived her to be angry and abrupt; they also wondered what the medical problem was. They felt sorry for Greta and thought of her as "very dependent." A brief interview was scheduled to explore Greta's expectations, beliefs, and resources. Her family was invited to the meeting, which was held on the unit, but they did not come.

In a 15-minute interview with Greta alone, the nurse initially drew a quick genogram. She learned that Greta lived with her two younger brothers and their mother, all of whom had what Greta called "the disease" (wasting of the muscles). She was the only family member who was able to drive, and this was why the others did not attend the meeting. (This was new information for the nurse.)

The nurse then asked Greta about her expectations for the hospitalization and how the nurses could be most helpful. Greta responded to the circular questions by saying that she would know how the staff would care for her "by how they talk with me and other patients, show me respect and trust, and treat me independently." She stated that she needed to be strong to care for her brothers and mother, "who depend on me."

The nurse asked Greta what hopes and expectations the other family members had for Greta's hospitalization. She replied that, when her mother had previously been hospitalized, the staff had "pushed her to eat." Greta found this very disrespectful. The nurse asked how the current staff was treating Greta's reluctance to eat. Greta described that they offered her food choices and reported that she found this quite satisfactory. The interview concluded with the nurse inviting Greta to talk more with her if she had any concerns about her care.

From this interview, the nurse revised her opinion of Greta being "very dependent" to thinking of her as someone who needed to be commended for her independence and caregiving. She now saw Greta as a "strong person" and passed this message on to her nursing colleagues.

A few days after the 15-minute interview, Greta commented to the nurse during morning care, "Remember when you told me to tell you if something wasn't going right?" She then related that the evening staff was "pushing me to eat and not respecting my choices." She had lost 1 pound. The nurse listened and remembered that, in the morning report, Greta was talked about as being "manipulative." The staff members were concerned with her weight loss and therefore "pushed her" to eat more. In turn, Greta ate less. The nurse conceptualized the problem as a vicious circular interaction (see Chapter 3) between the patient and the evening staff. She decided to intervene by:

- Inviting the dietitian to talk with the staff regarding food groups and choices

- Putting a note in the record system that Greta could "eat on demand"

- Encouraging individual members of the nursing staff to give Greta more choices of various types of food

> The outcome of this brief, family-oriented interview and interventions was that Greta gained some weight over the course of hospitalization. The other staff nurses said that they felt "less responsible for making Greta eat" and more responsible for offering her choices and promoting her independence. Most significant to the primary nurse was the intervention used in the unit documentation system in which she identified the problem, provided a rationale, and recommended direction for other staff members.

From our perspective, an important outcome was that Greta's skills and competencies to manage and live with her chronic illness were reinforced. She went home stronger, both physically and emotionally. In addition, she was able to assist herself and other family members with ongoing health issues. This 15-minute interview also indicates how nurses can include other family members in the therapeutic conversation even if the members are not present. Involving family members in relational nursing practice includes inquiring about them whether they are present or not.

CONCLUSION

In conclusion, an overall framework for ritualizing a 15-minute (or shorter) family interview is:

1. Begin a therapeutic conversation with a particular purpose in mind that can be accomplished in 15 minutes or less.

2. Use manners to engage or reengage. Introduce yourself by offering your name and role. Orient family members to the purpose of a brief family interview.

3. Assess key areas of internal and external structure and function—obtain genogram information and key external support data.

4. Ask three key questions of family members.

5. Commend the family on one or two strengths.

6. Evaluate usefulness and conclude.

We generally find this framework to be a useful guide when conducting 15-minute (or shorter) family interviews. However, these key ingredients of a brief family interview need to be adapted according to the competence of the nurse, the practice context in which nurses and families encounter one another, and the appropriateness and purpose of the family meeting. We are confident that, if the interview is suitably implemented, both nurses and families will be satisfied with the usefulness of a brief family interview. Short therapeutic conversations are not intended, nor is it possible to resolve all of the issues that may be of concern to a family experiencing illness. Brief meetings are intended to address the most pressing and immediate concerns of families and to empower nurses so they can soften and/or relieve families' physical, emotional, and spiritual suffering in just 15 minutes (or even in one sentence) in the micro-context of a therapeutic conversation!

References

Bell, J.M. (2012). Making ideas "stick": The 15-minute family interview [Editorial]. *Journal of Family Nursing, 18*(2), 171-174.

Bell, J.M., & Wright, L.M. (2011). Creating practice knowledge for families experiencing illness suffering: The Illness Beliefs Model. In E. Svavarsdottir & H. Jonsdottir (Eds.): *Family Nursing in Action.* Reykjavik, Iceland: University of Iceland Press, pp. 15–52.

Bohn, U., Wright, L.M., & Moules, N.J. (2003). A family systems nursing interview following a myocardial infarction: The power of commendations. *Journal of Family Nursing, 9*(2), 151–165.

Duhamel, F., Dupuis, F., & Wright, L.M. (2009). Families' and nurses' responses to the "one question question": Reflections for clinical practice, education, and research in family nursing. *Journal of Family Nursing, 15*(4), 461–485.

Frank, A.W. (1998). Just listening: Narrative and deep illness. *Families, Systems and Health, 16*(3), 197–212.

Goudreau, J., Duhamel, F., & Ricard, N. (2006). The impact of a family systems nursing educational program on the practice of psychiatric nurses: A pilot study. *Journal of Family Nursing, 12*(3), 292–306.

Green, K., Correia, T., Bobele, M., et al. (2011). The research case for walk-in single sessions. In A. Slive & M. Bobele (Eds.): *When One Hour Is All You Have: Effective Therapy for Walk-in Clients.* Phoenix, AZ: Zeig, Tucker & Theisen, pp. 23–36.

Harper-Jaques, S., & Leahey, M. (2011). From imagination to reality: Mental health walk-in at South Calgary health centre. In A. Slive & M. Bobele (Eds.): *When One Hour Is All You Have: Effective Therapy for Walk-in Clients.* Phoenix, AZ: Zeig, Tucker & Theisen, pp. 167–184.

Holtslander, L. (2005). Clinical application of the 15-minute family interview: Addressing the needs of postpartum families. *Journal of Family Nursing, 11*(2), 5–18.

Hougher Limacher, L. (2003). *Commendations: The Healing Potential of One Family Systems Nursing Intervention* [Unpublished doctoral thesis]. Calgary, Alberta, Canada: University of Calgary.

Houger Limacher, L. (2008). Locating relationships at the heart of commending practices. *Journal of Systemic Therapies, 27*(4), 90–105.

Hougher Limacher, L., & Wright, L.M. (2003). Commendations: Listening to the silent side of a family intervention. *Journal of Family Nursing, 9*(2), 130–135.

Hougher Limacher, L., & Wright, L.M. (2006). Exploring the therapeutic family intervention of commendations: Insights from research. *Journal of Family Nursing, 12*(8), 307–331.

International Council of Nurses. (2002). Nurses always there for you: Caring for families. *Information and Action Tool Kit.* Geneva: Switzerland.

Leahey, M., et al. (1995). The impact of a family systems nursing approach: Nurses' perceptions. *Journal of Continuing Education in Nursing, 26*(5), 219–225.

Leahey, M., & Harper-Jaques, S. (2010). Integrating family nursing into a mental health urgent care practice framework: Ladders for learning. *Journal of Family Nursing, 16*(2), 196–212.

Leahey, M., & Svavarsdottir, E.K. (2009). Implementing family nursing: How do we translate knowledge into clinical practice? *Journal of Family Nursing, 15*(4), 445–460.

Martin, J., & Kamen, J. (2005). *Miss Manners' Guide to Excruciatingly Correct Behavior, Freshly Updated.* New York: WW Norton.

LeGrow, K., & Rossen, B.E. (2005). Development of professional practice based on a Family Systems Nursing Framework: Nurses' and families' experiences. *Journal of Family Nursing, 11*, 38–58.

Martinez, A., D'Artois, D., & Rennick, J.E. (2007). Does the 15 minute (or less) family interview influence nursing practice? *Journal of Family Nursing, 13*(2), 1–22.

McLeod, D.L. (2003). *Opening Space for the Spiritual: Therapeutic Conversations With Families Living With Serious Illness* [Unpublished doctoral thesis]. University of Calgary, Alberta, Canada.

Moules, N.J. (2002). Nursing on paper: Therapeutic letters in nursing practice. *Nursing Inquiry, 9*(2), 104–113.

Moules, N., & Johnstone, H. (2010). Commendations, conversations, and life-changing realizations: Teaching and practicing family nursing. *Journal of Family Nursing, 16*(2), 146–160.

Robinson, C.A. (1998). Women, families, chronic illness, and nursing interventions: From burden to balance. *Journal of Family Nursing, 4*(3), 271–290.

Robinson, C.A., & Wright, L.M. (1995). Family nursing interventions: What families say makes a difference. *Journal of Family Nursing, 1*(3), 327–345.

Slive, A., & Bobele, M. (Eds.). (2011). *When One Hour Is All You Have: Effective Therapy for Walk-in Clients.* Phoenix, AZ: Zeig, Tucker & Theisen.

Svavarsdottir, E.K., Tryggvadottir, G.B., & Sigurdardottir, A.O. (In press). Does a short-term therapeutic conversation intervention benefit families of children or adolescents within a hospital setting? *Journal of Family Nursing.*

Sveinbjarnardottir, E.K., Svavarsdottir, E.K., & Wright, L.M. (In press). What are the benefits of a short therapeutic conversation intervention with acute psychiatric patients and their families? A controlled before and after study. *International Journal of Nursing Studies.*

Wright, L.M. (1989). When clients ask questions: Enriching the therapeutic conversation. *Family Therapy Networker, 13*(6), 15–16.

Wright, L.M. (2005). *Spirituality, Suffering, and Illness: Ideas for Healing*. Philadelphia: F.A. Davis.

Wright, L.M., & Bell, J.M. (2009). *Beliefs and Illness: A Model to Invite Healing*. Calgary, AB: 4th Floor Press.

Wright, L.M., & Leahey, M. (Producers). (2000). *How to Do a 15 Minute (or Less) Family Interview*. [DVD]. Calgary, Canada. Available at www.familynursingresources.com.

Wright, L.M., & Leahey, M. (Producers). (2006). *How to Use Questions in Family Interviewing*. [DVD]. Calgary, Canada. Available at www.familynursingresources.com.

Chapter **10**

How to Move Beyond Basic Family Nursing Skills

Researchers and clinicians have identified the needs of family members when illness arises. Family interventions that enhance the possibility of support and healing with serious illness have also been well documented (see Chapters 4, 5, and 8). Yet, there still remains a gap between knowledge and relational practice. The circularity between knowledge and practice remains underappreciated. Graham and colleagues (2006) articulated the value of two cycles in thinking circularly about knowledge exchange. The first cycle involves inquiry, synthesis, and development of tools. The second cycle involves action and leads to application of knowledge through problem identification, selection of knowledge, implementation of change, and evaluation of outcomes. Knowledge exchange between nurses and families involves skills, basic and advanced, that enhance and promote healing.

A major challenge in determining core competencies for family work is to distinguish what can be called "general skills and knowledge"—which are needed by all nurses working with clients—from unique, advanced practice skills and knowledge, particularly those of family nurses. Another challenge is to delineate sufficient competencies to cover the range of practice settings and yet not specify so many that the practitioner is overwhelmed.

In Chapter 5 we discussed basic essential skills and stages in family nursing interviews. In this chapter we discuss the more advanced skills that we have identified and labeled as vital in interviewing families in various settings. Two clinical vignettes are offered to highlight advanced practice skills. In particular, we present sample skills for interviewing families of the elderly at times of transition and advanced skills for interviewing an individual to gain a family perspective on chronic illness. We also offer tips for advanced practice with these populations and delineate advanced micro-skills. Ideas for how to integrate family nursing into various practice contexts will also be offered. The two educational family nursing DVDs that we have produced that are most relevant to this chapter are *Tips and Microskills for Interviewing Families of the Elderly* (Wright & Leahey, 2010b) and *Interviewing an Individual to Gain a Family Perspective With Chronic Illness: A Clinical Demonstration* (Wright & Leahey, 2010a). See the section following the Index for a full description of each DVD and ordering information.

FAMILY NURSING SKILLS IN CONTEXT

The importance of specifically tailoring family nursing interviewing skills to the relational practice context cannot be overstressed. We have found in our review of the literature that the contextual and clinical competence application is often overlooked. Leahey and Svavarsdottir (2009) advocate that knowledge translation and exchange is a shared responsibility requiring the involvement of researchers with potential knowledge users such as practicing nurses. Astedt-Kurki and Kaunonen (2011) recommend making family nursing more visible through intervention studies involving skilled nurses.

However, awareness of research findings does not necessarily mean adoption. Rather, interventions must be adapted to local settings that are inevitably varied, complex, and idiosyncratic. Duhamel (2010), who developed a Center of Excellence in Family Nursing at the University of Montreal, advocates "engaged scholarship" to create knowledge and application into practice in unique clinical settings. Svavarsdottir and Sigurdardottir (2011) have provided excellent examples of knowledge exchange in pediatric settings. In an ambitious and innovative project, Moules and colleagues (2011) have undertaken a program connecting family research in pediatric oncology to practice; they are devising interventions in an effort to reduce family suffering in the experience of childhood cancer.

The new knowledge created must be useful for nurses and families in the unique relational practice setting. McLeod, Tapp, Moules, and Campbell (2010) found that the skill of addressing specific family concerns in the oncology unit was particularly helpful. Gathering family members and opening space for conversation allowed the nurse to feel he or she "knew" the families. Coming to know the families as individuals with histories was an important skill identified by the researchers. Vandall-Walker, Jensen, and Oberle (2007) found that in the ICU, skills identified as important in this setting included engaging with family members, sustaining them, and disengaging from them.

Leahey and Harper-Jaques (2010) created a method for integrating family nursing into practice settings and used a mental health urgent care context in a Canadian community health center as an example (Southern et al, 2007). Leahey and Harper-Jaques (2010) developed a grid and listed the main four elements of clinical practice in the setting: mental health/psychiatric assessment, physical health assessment, family nursing, and integrated behavioral health care. Alongside these practice framework elements, they listed Benner's (2001) skill levels from novice to advanced beginner to competent to proficient to expert. See Table 10–1 for mental health urgent care practice framework elements and ladders.

Table 10-1	Mental Health Urgent Care Practice Framework Elements and Ladders			
LADDERS	MENTAL HEALTH/ PSYCHIATRIC ASSESSMENT	PHYSICAL NURSING ASSESSMENT	FAMILY NURSING	INTEGRATED BEHAVIORAL HEALTH
1 Novice				
2 Advanced/Beginner				
3 Competent				
4 Proficient				
5 Expert				

Leahey, M., & Harper-Jaques, S. (2010). Integrating family nursing into a mental health urgent care practice framework: Ladders for learning. *Journal of Family Nursing, 16*(2), 200. Copyright 2010 by Maureen Leahey and Sandy Harper-Jaques. Reprinted by permission of SAGE Publications.

Staff had identified the need for a practice framework specific to their setting and participated in generating the skills relevant for each section of the grid. Through team discussion, observation of clinical work, reviews of the literature, clinical documentation audits, supervision, and feedback from clients and families, family nursing practice took hold in the setting. Family nursing grew to be seen as an integral part of practice rather than as an "add on" or "one more thing to do." The value of this tool is that it can be adapted to various settings by tailoring the practice framework elements and specifying the unique family nursing skills for the context.

Duhamel and Dupuis (2011) believe that utilizing family systems nursing knowledge in clinical practice requires more administrative and educational support than is usually offered. They advocate a circular process among education, research, and practice, especially favoring the idea of having facilitators or coaches in the clinical setting to advance practice skills and implementation. The work of Litchfield (2011) in New Zealand similarly supports the value of a mentor and the inclusivity of stakeholders.

BEYOND BASIC SKILLS

Differentiating basic and advanced skills in family nursing is a challenge. Education can be thought of as a differentiation point with higher nursing education implying advanced skill level. Moules, Bell, Paton, and Morck (2012) stress that "teaching graduate family nursing students the important and delicate practice of entering into and mitigating families' illness suffering signifies an educational practice that is rigorous, intense, and contextual, yet not articulated as expounded knowledge" (p. 1). More conceptual knowledge aims to lead to more advanced skill level, but as Chesla (2008) points out, awareness of information does not necessarily lead to implementation or executive skills.

Experience can be another delineator of levels. For example, the novice interviewer typically talks with the family to obtain information *for the nurse,* whereas the more experienced nurse invites the family to ask questions and designs interventions *for the family's needs.* This is an important distinction. The more proficient nurse demonstrates curiosity about the family's needs, styles of coping, and so forth, in an effort to maximize the family's and nurse's ability to care for their loved one. In this situation, the nurse and family collaborate on a plan of care instead of the nurse controlling and directing the interview process with less regard to the needs and concerns of the family.

Another way to conceptualize expert or advanced practice skills is the "10,000-hour rule" popularized by social science commentator Malcolm Gladwell (2008). He claims that to be an expert and successful in any field requires 10,000 hours of deliberate practice. The 10,000-hour rule is usually attributed to the research done by Anders Ericsson (2006). He and his team divided students into three groups ranked by excellence at the Berlin Academy of Music and then correlated achievement with hours of practice. They discovered that the elite had all put in about 10,000 hours of practice, the good 8,000 hours, and the average 4,000 hours. This rule was then applied to other disciplines, and Ericsson found that it proved valid.

More recently, Ericsson's work on deliberate practice has been geared toward application in established domains of expertise, such as nursing and medicine (Ericsson, Whyte, & Ward, 2007). It is our belief that the 10,000-hour rule could be one useful guideline to determine when nurses have become expert in their clinical skills when working with families.

Recognition and the ability to make relevant observations are factors in increasing perceptual skill development. Benner's ladders (2001) are another way of differentiating various skills by the changes in familiarity, integration, flexibility, and efficiency that accompany each skill level. We believe that whatever method one chooses to differentiate basic and advanced skills is less important than the compassionate application of these skills with unique families in specific relational practice contexts.

CLINICAL VIGNETTES

Number 1: Interviewing Families of the Elderly at Time of Transition

Setting, Family Composition, and Purpose of the Interview

Dr. Leahey interviews two siblings whose mother is entering a long-term care facility. The two senior children being interviewed are Ross, age 72, and Myrna, age 70. They have two younger sisters, ages 69 and 60, who live in different cities. Ross is retired and separated from his wife. He has four children and four grandchildren.

Myrna is a widow with two sons and four grandchildren, and she continues to work three days a week. Ross and Myrna's father died 15 years ago, and their mother has recently been admitted to the care facility. Myrna and Ross have a photo of their mother at her 99th birthday party.

The purpose of this clinical vignette is to offer tips for collaborating with senior children at the time of their elderly parents' transition to a care facility and to demonstrate the advanced micro-skills for quickly engaging with family members, obtaining a brief relevant history, discussing caregiver impact and burden, and responding to senior children's suggestions about their parents' care.

Clinical Skills:

- Engagement
- Creating welcoming context for collaboration
- Involving all family members
- Obtaining brief relevant history by co-constructing an illness narrative versus a medical narrative

> **Dr. Leahey:** First of all, let me introduce myself. I'm Maureen. Glad to meet you. Myrna is it?
>
> **Myrna:** Yes, it is.
>
> **Dr. Leahey:** And Ross? Glad to meet you, hi. So thanks very much for coming in this afternoon. I understand that this is the third facility that your mom has been in. And so one of the routine practices that we have here is that when our clients have been in other facilities, we like to meet with the family as soon as possible.
>
> Maybe one way we could start is for me to ask you, how did it come to be that your mom came to this facility?
>
> **Ross:** Do you want to start, Myrna?
>
> **Myrna:** Mom has lived at home until this year. She's been very independent, and she feels independent, but that's partly because the family's protecting her. But she was getting to a point where she really couldn't look after herself. She was getting quite forgetful, and we had several caretakers at different times in the home, but they didn't seem to work out. Things would go fine for a little while, and then Mom would not like something they did. So we went through a succession of those people but decided that we just really couldn't keep Mom in her home. So we have talked about it for years and finally really encouraged her last year that we just had to find a place for her and started looking.
>
> **Dr. Leahey:** So what—

Ross: And it was trying because she's so independent. She's a tough old Norwegian, and independence is most important to her, so she was very resistant. We eventually did get her to look at two or three facilities, and she kind of gave in to it in a way. She was in her own home, multi-level, a lot of steps and preparing her own meals. She was not eating properly. We had to do something, so we did find a seniors' residence. That was the first place that she moved into.

Dr. Leahey: Yes.

Ross: And she was...started to have some falls, so they...at one point they thought she had broken some bones and she had to be admitted to the hospital. In the hospital she was assessed and told that she could not go back to her—

Myrna: Assisted living.

Ross: Her assisted living.

Dr. Leahey: Okay. So this has been a long haul for your family in getting your mom to this facility.

Ross: Very, very long.

Clinical Skill:

- Eliciting impact of illness on family members

Dr. Leahey: What do you think has been the impact of that on you, Ross?

Ross: Oh, the impact? I went through 14 years of always being there and available, and it just got more intense as time went on. The impact? By the time when we finally got her into a facility last August until December, I lost 18 pounds. I mean, my weight was dropping. It was really, really a big thing because when she was in the assisted living, I'd be getting phone calls every day. What do you want to do about this? What are you going to do about that?

Dr. Leahey: You look sad just talking about it. It's okay with me if you cry.

Ross: Oh, I'm not going to cry.

Dr. Leahey: Okay.

Ross: It's . . . but it is a fact of life and this is—

Dr. Leahey: Yes.

Ross: Unfortunately the way it went.

Dr. Leahey: And what do you think the impact has been on Myrna of looking after your mom?

Ross: She'll have to answer that. (Smiles and nods.)

Myrna: I think it's...there's been a much less impact on me partly because Ross has taken the major role. Having worked and not being available has made me less accessible to care.

Ross: It's that, but the other fact is that Mother is from a—

Myrna: A patriarchal viewpoint.

Ross: She has a patriarchal viewpoint that the girls cannot do the job as well as a man, and that's unfortunate because they can do better than I could probably. But it always has to be me who makes the final decision.

Clinical Skills:

- Demonstrating curiosity
- Inquiring about the biopsychosocial spiritual factors when asking about the impact of stress on family members.

Dr. Leahey: Do you have some health problems, Myrna?

Myrna: I do. I was diagnosed with Parkinson's almost seven years ago, and one of my main symptoms is tiredness. So I just find it hard to cope with any extra requests or demands of Mom. I think it's kind of settled down now. We've each got kind of our own jobs and that's what we do.

Dr. Leahey: And how did you manage as a group of siblings to figure out your own jobs?

Ross: It just fell into place.

Dr. Leahey: Fell into place?

Ross: I mean, we each have our own strengths.

Dr. Leahey: Yes.

Ross: And we are close and we just . . . we back each other up, and if we need help in an area, we ask the others for help or thoughts. It's cooperation. That's the big thing.

Dr. Leahey: And how about for you, Ross? Do you have any health problems?

Ross: No, my health is pretty good basically.

Myrna: Although your blood pressure has—

Ross: Well, that was the other thing. My blood pressure shot up last fall, too, because of all the extreme stress that we were going through. But it's under control.

Clinical Skill:

■ Asking for other family members' noticings or ideas

> **Dr. Leahey:** What impact would you say your sons would have noticed, Myrna, on you?
>
> **Myrna:** I think they're aware that it creates a strain for me, but day to day I don't think it really affects our relationship. I think they are more concerned about me than they are about their grandmother.
>
> **Dr. Leahey:** And what do you think they're most concerned about you?
>
> **Myrna:** Tiring out. Just, you know the Parkinson symptoms increasing, but I think they feel that Grandma is now in place.
>
> **Ross:** She's being looked after.
>
> **Dr. Leahey:** She's being looked after?
>
> **Myrna:** Yeah.
>
> **Ross:** It's not a concern.
>
> **Myrna:** Yeah.

Clinical Skills:

■ Summarizing

■ Using client's language

■ Commending

■ Asking for others' advice to client

> **Dr. Leahey:** It sounds like your mother has been very fortunate to have the two of you and your sisters who have looked after her as well as you have. And sometimes it sounds like at the expense of your own health. I mean your blood pressure, your weight loss, the tiredness and stress on your Parkinson's. And if your boys were here, what advice might they want to give to you, Myrna, about your health?
>
> **Myrna:** That I shouldn't stress myself. I should take it easy. They really are very sensitive about it.
>
> **Dr. Leahey:** And would you take their advice?
>
> **Myrna:** I think I do. Yeah.
>
> **Dr. Leahey:** What do you think? Does she take it enough?
>
> **Ross:** I don't know.
>
> **Myrna:** They don't put a lot of demands on me.

Clinical Skill:

■ Inviting conversation about various family members' beliefs and coping styles

> **Dr. Leahey:** One of the things I did want to ask you is, if your mom were here with us today, what might she say has been the most challenging part of coming into this facility?
>
> **Myrna:** I think leaving her home.
>
> **Dr. Leahey:** Leaving her home. And what do you think, Ross?
>
> **Ross:** Well, leaving her home is a very big thing to her. I'd say it was her anchor. Also leaving her cat.
>
> **Myrna:** Yeah.
>
> **Dr. Leahey:** Oh.
>
> **Ross:** And her pet was a very big thing in her life.
>
> **Myrna:** And actually that was one of the ways we were able to move her initially because they allowed pets where she moved, so she could take her cat.
>
> **Dr. Leahey:** I see. And is her cat still alive?
>
> **Ross:** It was this morning. *(Laughs)*
>
> **Dr. Leahey:** Okay, good. *(Smiles)*
>
> **Myrna:** Ross inherited the cat.
>
> **Dr. Leahey:** And you know that you can bring the cat into the facility here?
>
> **Ross:** Yes, we're aware and we have plans to do that. We also realize that the shots have to be up to date and that's taken care of.
>
> **Dr. Leahey:** Good, and your mom, does your mom know that the cat can come and visit her?
>
> **Ross:** Yes.
>
> **Dr. Leahey:** Okay.
>
> **Myrna:** She asks about the cat all the time.
>
> **Dr. Leahey:** Okay.
>
> **Myrna:** More so than the family members.
>
> **Dr. Leahey:** And how's that for the family members?
>
> **Myrna:** It's fine.
>
> **Ross:** We understand. She's focused on certain things, more things that have immediate meaning to her.

Clinical Skill:

■ Asking clients what others might appreciate about them

> **Dr. Leahey:** So if your mom were here with us now, what might she say that she most appreciates about the two of you?
>
> **Ross:** I don't know. Probably looking after her affairs.
>
> **Dr. Leahey:** Looking after her affairs.
>
> **Ross:** Yeah. Being the house and her monetary things.
>
> **Myrna:** Well, it's an interesting question because sometimes I wonder if Mom appreciates what we're doing for her, really truly appreciates. There's not a lot of, well, she'll say thank you for doing this or that, but there's...to me there's not a sense of real appreciation.
>
> **Ross:** I don't think she grasps the amount of effort that is involved, and to her, well, it's just you do it and that's the way it is.
>
> **Myrna:** She knows. She gets upset if we don't visit every day, but she doesn't appreciate what that does to our lives.
>
> **Ross:** She's become quite self-centered.
>
> **Myrna:** Which I think is normal.
>
> **Dr. Leahey:** So that can be very hard when you're caregiving as much as you have been to feel like your mom, although appreciative, is not really aware of the impact that it has on your lives. How do you both cope with that?
>
> **Ross:** Well, I understand that her health is deteriorating. Her mental abilities are deteriorating and that just goes with age. We'll all reach that point and just try and understand that this is not the person you knew and they can't help it.
>
> **Dr. Leahey:** So that's your belief—she can't help it and—
>
> **Ross:** For the most part. Sometimes she uses it, but for the most part, yeah.
>
> **Dr. Leahey:** And how about for you, Myrna?
>
> **Myrna:** I think I have the same attitude. It really hurts when she uses it or goes off into a tantrum, which is unfair really.
>
> **Dr. Leahey:** Yes.
>
> **Myrna:** But you very quickly come around to the realization that's how she's feeling and that's the only way she can demonstrate it. I mean, I try to put myself in her place and it must be horrible. I don't know what you wake up every morning looking forward to, so I can certainly understand

some of her comments and criticisms. But I think she's getting much better.

Clinical Skill:

- Eliciting "unspoken" information

> **Dr. Leahey:** Would there be anything that we should know about your mom that maybe she wouldn't tell us that would make it easier for us to care for her or to be helpful to her?
>
> **Ross:** I can't think of anything. Well maybe one thing is that she still insists on her independence. She doesn't like people doing everything for her. I think she would still like to make more choices than are available to her such as seating at meals, choice in meals, times for bathing, things like that. And you know how much help does she need dressing or how much does she want to do herself?
>
> **Dr. Leahey:** Thank you, and I'll make sure to put that with a big star on her care plan.

Clinical Skill:

- Eliciting family expectations for collaborative care and responding to expectations

> **Dr. Leahey:** When you think about what we could do in this facility to both help your mom and help the two of you and your sister, Linda, what comes to mind?
>
> **Ross:** Well, I think I feel our major role is to advocate and be aware of what's going on and to work with the staff to try and work around problems that might occur or suggestions how they could better help her and it just, interaction between the staff and ourselves.
>
> **Dr. Leahey:** We do welcome people's ideas, and it sounds like you've been through a hard time particularly in the last year.
>
> **Ross:** We have.
>
> **Dr. Leahey:** Yes. You're obviously very caring and think about your mom in many different ways like her privacy, her independence, her socialization, her food. Nice. Is there anything else you can think of how we could work with you to make your mom's last years as comfortable as possible?
>
> **Myrna:** I think the open communication is the most important thing, that we feel comfortable being able to make suggestions.
>
> **Dr. Leahey:** Okay.

Myrna: And that works the other way, that you're keeping us up to date on changes in Mom.

Dr. Leahey: So some reciprocity there that you would tell us things you notice and that we would tell you. Some people like to have periodic meetings.

Ross: That was my next point.

Dr. Leahey: Do you like that? Some other families say "no news is good news." What's your preference?

Ross: No, I don't take that attitude at all. I would welcome periodic meetings.

Dr. Leahey: Okay.

Ross: Not just for the sake of having a meeting but because there's purpose in it that it will be beneficial for all those involved.

Dr. Leahey: Okay, good.

Clinical Skills Summary:

Some tips and micro-skills for working with elderly persons and their families include:

- Draw forth the family's illness experience
- Ask difference questions such as, "What do you think your sons are *most* concerned about you?"
- Inquire what absent family members might say about the situation being discussed
- Ask about the biopsychosocial-spiritual domains and identify family and individual strengths

In the preceding vignette, Maureen demonstrated the following clinical skills:

- Empathized with the siblings about the stress of the last year
- Commended their caring for their mother
- Pursued with them what they would find most helpful
- Asked open-ended questions to elicit their desires
- Offered practical, concrete suggestions such as family meetings
- Wove commendations throughout the interview

All these are more advanced micro-skills that a nurse interviewer can compress and use in a thoughtful, purposeful, time-effective interview. Two interventions have shown to be particularly powerful in promoting hope. Weaving commendations throughout the interview we have found to be a very helpful and healing practice. Inviting reflections about what family members appreciate about each other can also be a powerful intervention that invites more confidence and competence in the family and thus leaves the family more hopeful about their abilities to manage in the future.

Number 2: Interviewing an Individual to Gain a Family Perspective on Chronic Illness

Setting, Family Composition, and Purpose of the Interview

Dr. Wright interviews Ralph, age 55. He came to the outpatient clinic looking for more coping strategies to deal with his longstanding chronic pain related to his disability. Ralph has been married for 37 years and has two children, ages 31 and 29. Ralph is self-employed in a mobile knife-sharpening business, and his wife is the bookkeeper in the family business. She is also employed full-time as a paralegal.

What do health professionals do if family members cannot or will not attend a meeting so that a family perspective can be obtained? What if the context in which the health professional works does not lend itself to involving other family members? Yes, it is possible to "bring family members into the room," even if only meeting with an individual.

In these excerpts from a clinical interview, Dr. Wright explores how a chronic illness impacts a middle-aged man's life and relationships. The interview is brief, time-limited, and effective. The purpose is to recognize that illness is a family affair and that all family members are affected by and can influence an illness, demonstrate the skills for gaining a family perspective when interviewing an individual, assess the impact of chronic illness on one's life and relationships, assess solutions and coping strategies, and intervene by offering commendations and planning a ritual.

We begin with the first excerpt of the therapeutic conversation, which has been transcribed verbatim. Dr. Wright asks, "What are you most hoping can happen from this meeting?" This is an example of collaborative interaction where Ralph and Lorraine jointly set the goals.

Clinical Skills:

- Recognize that illness is a family affair and that all family members are affected by and can influence an illness
- Gain a family perspective when interviewing an individual
- Assess the impact of chronic illness on one's life and relationships
- Assess solutions and coping strategies
- Intervene by offering commendations
- Plan a ritual

> **Dr. Wright:** I'm wondering what are you most hoping can happen at the Center and during our meeting together? What are you most interested in?

Ralph: Basically coping mechanisms.

Dr. Wright: Coping mechanisms.

Ralph: To help cope with the pain.

Dr. Wright: To cope with pain, yes?

Ralph: Right. Because of the fact that I have some permanent spinal cord damage?

Dr. Wright: Yes.

Ralph: From my accident.

In this next segment, Dr. Wright inquires about the family's problem-solving strategies.

Clinical Skill:

■ Exploring usefulness/not usefulness of other helpers

Dr. Wright: And so your wife went to the pain clinic?

Ralph: Yes, she went to see the pain psychologist.

Dr. Wright: Right, and was that helpful to her?

Ralph: It was, because it helped to direct our conversations. If I was having a bad day and started to react to everybody around me because I was having a bad day, then it helped her because then she was able to look at me and say, "Is this the pain talking or are you having other issues?"

Dr. Wright: Oh, okay.

Ralph: A lot of times when people are arguing or people are short with their kids or whatever it's because they're in pain and it's a reaction to the action.

Dr. Wright: Do you ever find, though, that it's useful to use your pain as an excuse or an out if you are—

Ralph: Actually—

Dr. Wright: —getting into trouble with your wife or your kids?

Ralph: No, I don't.

Dr. Wright: No? Just say, "Oh, that's the pain talking. It's not really me?" Or...?

Ralph: Actually, I don't personally know.

Dr. Wright: Okay, and so have you and your wife been seen now together as a couple or did she just go?

Ralph: No, we went together and she also went to private sessions. I went to private sessions, too, and then we were seen by the pain psychologist together.

Clinical Skill:

■ Inquiring about the best/worst advice client received

> **Dr. Wright:** Okay, and what was the best and worst advice that was offered to you?
>
> **Ralph:** The world doesn't stop just because you're in pain.
>
> **Dr. Wright:** That was the best advice? Yes?
>
> **Ralph:** That was the best advice.
>
> **Dr. Wright:** Okay. And the worst advice?
>
> **Ralph:** One of the other best advices was if you don't control it, it will control you. That was the second part of that.
>
> **Dr. Wright:** Okay. So if you don't control it—
>
> **Ralph:** It will control you.
>
> **Dr. Wright:** Will control you. And what was the worst advice you received?
>
> **Ralph:** Don't worry. Things will get better.
>
> **Dr. Wright:** Ah.
>
> **Ralph:** Because by expecting things to get better when a person is in chronic pain. It is far better for them to learn how to deal with the situation they're in rather than hoping that it's going to get better or expecting it to get better.

Clinical Skills:

■ Inquiring about the impact of illness on family members
■ Asking difference questions

> **Dr. Wright:** Right. So who do you think the pain has been a bigger problem for over the years? You or your wife?
>
> **Ralph:** Oh, it's definitely been a larger problem for me.
>
> **Dr. Wright:** A larger problem for you. And what's your wife—
>
> **Ralph:** But it definitely has had an impact. It's had an impact on not only my wife but my children as well. For instance—
>
> **Dr. Wright:** Yes. Tell me about that.
>
> **Ralph:** They were 5 and 7 years old when I broke my neck. So I wasn't able to have them sit on my knee.
>
> **Dr. Wright:** Okay.
>
> **Ralph:** It took me a long time to learn how to walk. So—

> **Dr. Wright:** So they only really remember you as a dad with pain or—
>
> **Ralph:** Yes.
>
> **Dr. Wright:**...disabilities or problems, challenges all the time.

Comments

In reading the transcript of this interview, did you notice how Dr. Wright explored Ralph's understanding of the effect of chronic pain on his wife and children? And then how she was curious about the best and worst advice he had been offered? This is very helpful in being able to sidestep errors or mistakes that Dr. Wright could make by offering similar recommendations that were not found to be helpful in the past.

Clinical Skills:

- Naming the illness
- Using client's language

> **Dr. Wright:** What do you call it? Do you call it a disability? Do you call it an accident? How do you refer to it?
>
> **Ralph:** It's...I just . . . I have a permanent disability.
>
> **Dr. Wright:** Permanent disability.
>
> **Ralph:** I consider it to be a permanent disability.
>
> **Dr. Wright:** That's how you refer to it?
>
> **Ralph:** And that's it.
>
> **Dr. Wright:** Okay.
>
> **Ralph:** But it is, actually. It's helped me put life into perspective in that I control how I react to things. And it has helped me by all of the different reading that I've done.
>
> **Dr. Wright:** Okay.

Comments

In this next section of the vignette, Dr. Wright explores the influence of chronic pain on Ralph's life and the pain's influence on him. This line of questioning is called *relative influence questioning,* and we wish to credit the late and brilliant Michael White (1989) of Australia for this very useful way of questioning.

Clinical Skill:

- Relative Influence Questioning

> **Dr. Wright:** What, at this moment today, what percent of the time does pain rule your life and what percent of the time do you think that you have control over the pain?

Ralph: I . . .

Dr. Wright: What percent do you control now?

Ralph: I have to be able to control the pain at least 75 percent of the time.

Dr. Wright: Seventy-five, okay.

Ralph: Because of the permanent spinal cord damage, I have problems in that I spasm.

Dr. Wright: Okay.

Ralph: I have to take an antispasmodic, and there are problems with having permanent spinal cord damage. I've taken a lot of medication, and now the medications have created different problems.

Dr. Wright: Like?

Ralph: Like problems with my liver, problems with my kidneys.

Dr. Wright: Oh, dear.

Ralph: And so consequently there are other things to deal with.

Dr. Wright: So 25 percent of the time the pain controls you.

Ralph: Yes, which is why I have to get up and I have to actually do things in order to control the pain so that I can continue on with my life.

Dr. Wright: So when you say today that you've come to this pain center and you are wanting to have more coping strategies, what percent are you trying to get to manage?

Dr. Wright: Like, what would be your ideal percent that you would say, wow.

Ralph: It would be nice to be 90 percent.

Dr. Wright: 90 percent.

Ralph: I mean, I am not looking for a fairy godmother or some...I don't expect . . .

Dr. Wright: Okay, to wave her magic wand over you and—

Ralph: A magic wand and everything is going to be fine.

Dr. Wright: And the pain is gone forever, yeah.

Ralph: Coping strategies so that I can learn more how to cope so that I don't . . . so I can get on more with a normal life, whatever that might be.

Dr. Wright: Okay. So you really are only asking to have coping strategies for 15 percent more?

Ralph: That's right.

Dr. Wright: That's amazing. So you're willing to live with at least 10 percent pain 24/7. Yes?

Ralph: I have to be realistic.

Clinical Skill:

- Asking the "one question question"

Dr. Wright: Okay. So in our meeting together today, if there was just one question that you could have answered today, what would that one question be around your situation? What you've been dealing with?

Ralph: Actually, I would say that how to help me help myself.

Dr. Wright: How can you help yourself?

Ralph: Is there something that could be pointed out or something that could be better? Because everybody has a different perspective.

Dr. Wright: Yes.

Ralph: Sometimes I don't see certain things because I'm too close to it.

Comments

In this segment, Ralph's response to Dr. Wright's question again demonstrated his openness to new ideas for problem-solving. In this next excerpt, Dr. Wright asks about Ralph's family and the influence of his beliefs on his situation.

Clinical Skill:

- Asking a difference question to bring family members into the room

Dr. Wright: And is there anything differently that your family could be doing to help you to do more of or less of?

Ralph: Actually, I'm very fortunate.

Dr. Wright: Yes.

Ralph: I think that my family has learned to cope very well. It's made them more forgiving, made them more open to dealing with their problems and dealing with other people's problems.

Dr. Wright: Okay. So there's been some good it sounds like that's come out of this.

Ralph: Oh, definitely a lot of good that's come out of it.

Skill

■ Asking about the influence of spirituality and beliefs

> **Dr. Wright:** And what about for you personally? What good has come out of it?
>
> **Ralph:** There has been a lot of good that's come out of it.
>
> **Dr. Wright:** Really. Can you give me a couple of examples?
>
> **Ralph:** Well, when I broke my neck, I was 245 pounds. I had a 21-inch neck and 56 inches across the shoulders and a 52-inch chest. And I used to throw around quarters of beef that weighed up to 300 pounds.
>
> **Dr. Wright:** My.
>
> **Ralph:** And I thought that I was invincible. And then God stepped in and said, "Oops."
>
> **Dr. Wright:** So you have some beliefs about faith or God that had—
>
> **Ralph:** Yes.
>
> **Dr. Wright:** —a part in all of this?
>
> **Ralph:** Actually, God does not make junk. What you do with it after that is up to you.
>
> **Dr. Wright:** So did you pray about your situation when—
>
> **Ralph:** Oh, many times.
>
> **Dr. Wright:** Yes? And what did you pray for when you were injured like that?
>
> **Ralph:** Help.
>
> **Dr. Wright:** Help.
>
> **Ralph:** Actually, that's all a person can do.
>
> **Dr. Wright:** So, Ralph, I just wanted to follow up a little bit more about your faith and your beliefs. Was that helpful to you in being able to cope with the pain or not?
>
> **Ralph:** Actually, I think that I had an uncle once tell me that God doesn't give you any more than you cannot handle with his help.
>
> **Dr. Wright:** And did you adopt that belief?
>
> **Ralph:** And the largest obstacle to that?
>
> **Dr. Wright:** Yes.
>
> **Ralph:** Is asking for that help.
>
> **Dr. Wright:** Okay.
>
> **Ralph:** People have to actually ask. And that's—

Dr. Wright: And were you able to come to that point?

Ralph: Oh definitely. Yes.

Dr. Wright: Okay.

Ralph: And that's God no matter how you perceive him to be. Anybody who doesn't believe that there isn't a higher being really should look within themselves.

Clinical Skill:

■ Inquiring about client's ideas about family members' beliefs about the client

Dr. Wright: Well, I love that you've touched on your beliefs just now and I'm wondering if your children were here, what do you think they would tell me about you and how you've managed this disability all these years? What do you think their comment would be?

Ralph: Actually, I really and truly think that my daughter became a paramedic to help others.

Dr. Wright: Is that right? That's been one of the influences on her?

Ralph: Yes, because she realized that people do get hurt and need help. And my son is very . . . he's a gentle giant. He's six foot one, 230 pounds, and very kind.

Dr. Wright: Oh. So you think the influence of your disability has been that it's invited kindness in your son and your daughter's desire to help people?

Ralph: Yes. I really do.

Dr. Wright: Okay.

Ralph: I think they realize that things happen to people.

Dr. Wright: Yes.

Dr. Wright: And what would they say about you, how you've managed it?

Ralph: They probably think that I've done very well.

Dr. Wright: Okay. So they'd give you a pretty good grade, would they?

Ralph: I would hope so.

Dr. Wright: Yes?

Ralph: Yes.

Dr. Wright: What kind of grade do you think they would give you?

Ralph: I think it would be pretty high.

Dr. Wright: Wow, okay. And your wife, if she was here, what would she say the biggest influence upon her has been?

Ralph: I think it's made us closer, a lot closer.

Dr. Wright: It's made you closer?

Ralph: Yes.

Dr. Wright: Okay. Emotionally close or physically close?

Ralph: Emotionally and physically.

Dr. Wright: And physically? 'Cause one—

Ralph: Emotionally definitely because of the fact that we've had to deal with so much.

Dr. Wright: Okay, 'cause one very personal thing I was going to ask you, because of all your surgeries and back problems and pain, has that interfered with your being able to enjoy sexual relations?

Ralph: It has.

Dr. Wright: Yes?

Ralph: To a certain degree. A lot of the medications I have to be on, anti-inflammatories and muscle relaxants—

Dr. Wright: Yes.

Ralph: And when you're dealing with muscle relaxants ...*(Smiles)*

Dr. Wright: Yes, but you found a way?

Ralph: Oh, definitely.

Dr. Wright: Yes.

Ralph: Yeah, it's a very important part.

Dr. Wright: Yes, absolutely.

Ralph: And not only that, I...we...believe that a good marriage doesn't just happen.

Dr. Wright: How would your wife say that you have evolved over these 20 years or what do you think her description of you would be?

Ralph: Actually, probably sometimes she thinks I'm a little bit too positive.

Dr. Wright: Too positive, oh? Okay. So she and I might share some of that because that was a bit of my worry earlier.

Ralph: Yeah.

Dr. Wright: Okay. So just to go back to your wife for a moment, what did you say was the biggest influence on her, the biggest challenge for her with your chronic pain?

Ralph: Actually, I would say probably in the early years it was staying positive.

Dr. Wright: Staying positive about what aspect?

Ralph: About the situation. For instance—

Dr. Wright: That you were going to get better or that you would . . . what?

Ralph: Well, I mean it was not an easy path. She had to take on the major breadwinner. There was a lot of things that happened.

Clinical Skill:

■ Demonstrating curiosity

Dr. Wright: Okay. Wow, so it impacted every area of your life it sounds like.

Ralph: It did.

Dr. Wright: Financially?

Ralph: Financially, emotionally, physically.

Dr. Wright: So your wife had to become the breadwinner?

Ralph: Mmm-hmm.

Dr. Wright: Changed the roles in your family?

Ralph: Definitely.

Dr. Wright: Wow, so it didn't leave any aspect of your life—

Ralph: Everything has changed.

Dr. Wright: —untouched.

Ralph: Everything has changed.

Dr. Wright: So for your wife in those early years, when you're saying staying positive, I'm still trying to understand staying positive about?

Ralph: That things were going to work out.

Dr. Wright: That things would work out.

Ralph: That eventually, that things would eventually get better.

Dr. Wright: Okay, and is she—

Ralph: And staying positive for me because she didn't want to drag me down because she figured that I already had enough—

Dr. Wright: Yes.

Ralph: —to deal with.

Comments

Let us review what we have just read. Dr. Wright asked the "one question question" (Duhamel, Dupuis, & Wright, 2009; Wright, 1989) "If there were just one question that you would like to have answered today, what might that be?" The "one question question" is an interventive question that assists individuals and the nurse to focus on the issue of most concern. It helps to identify where the greatest concerns, problems, or suffering lie. Duhamel, Dupuis, and Wright (2009) have documented the usefulness of the 'one question question' and illustrate how frequently nurses and families differ in their perspective of what is important in a therapeutic conversation.

Also in the last segment Dr. Wright explored Ralph's religious and spiritual beliefs after he spontaneously told her about the influence of God in his life. Dr. Wright used this opening in the therapeutic conversation about spirituality to also explore if Ralph has prayed about his condition and, if so, what he prays for. In our experience, persons with illness often reach out for comfort, hope, and/or guidance in their lives, and prayer is one alternative of fulfilling that need.

Afterward, Dr. Wright again brought the family into the meeting by asking, if present, what family members would say about Ralph's progress throughout the years. These questions were to assess the influence the family members have had on the ill person. Dr. Wright concludes the session with some very specific interventions. First, she offers Ralph commendations about his strengths and resources that he has utilized to cope and heal from his condition such as his wisdom, his positive approach, and the success he has had on influencing his chronic pain. Finally, she offers a very specific intervention in the form of a prescribed ritual. She suggests taking a holiday from pain talk.

Clinical Skill:

■ Offering interventions of prescribing a ritual, and commendations

> **Dr. Wright:** I've . . . not extensively but I have worked with a number of people who have experienced chronic pain for a variety of things—accidents, illnesses. And it is one of the most difficult things to deal with in terms of how it affects your life and often demoralizes a person and can invite depression. It can invite such terrible suffering. And when you were answering me earlier when I was asking you about what's one question that you might want to have answered today and you said learn more coping strategies. I'd just like to throw out one idea that I have utilized with some clients and families.
>
> **Ralph:** Okay.
>
> **Dr. Wright:** You've been at this so long. You only want to improve 15 more percent. You've already done 75 percent.

Maybe you've done some of these strategies, but one of the ones that some couples and individuals have told me that has worked for them is to have moments when they refuse to talk about pain. So they take a holiday from talking about pain. So if somebody asks them, "How are you doing?" even if they're having pain, they say, "No, this is my time when I don't talk about it."

Dr. Wright: It's the knowing when I can talk about it and when I don't have to discuss it that's important. Some people say if I could just talk about it to my wife or to my husband for 15 or 20 minutes a day and just say what kind of a day it has been, that would be good. And then to take a holiday from pain.

Ralph: Give yourself permission to do that.

Dr. Wright: Permission to do it.

Ralph: Give yourself permission to do that. That's right, yeah.

Dr. Wright: Exactly, to be able to choose when to talk about it and when not to talk. To have moments when you absolutely put a moratorium on talking about pain because pain has a way of—

Ralph: And when somebody asks how you're feeling, you tell them, "With my hands like everybody else."

Dr. Wright: Yeah, yes. So I don't know. That's just one little tip.

Ralph: Yes. I appreciate that.

Dr. Wright: One little hot tip for you. And so I just want to say to you I just think your own wisdom in all of this is so marvelous! It is your own willingness to learn, your willingness to be open to so many ideas from improving your marriage, to improving your health and trying to cope with this disability that is so impressive to me. Now you're at this pain center. You've got a remarkable story.

Ralph: Literally if you do not control it, it will control you. And that's all I try to do is to have the ability to control it better and that's all.

Dr. Wright: Well, I think that the fact you are controlling it 75 percent is just really remarkable and really incredible.

Ralph: Thank you.

Dr. Wright: Because there is many things in our lives, say that people struggle with, whether it is diabetes or whatever health problems they may have that they wish they could be at 75 percent, especially with people experiencing chronic pain. I have met many people, like I said, and some of them would just be thrilled if they could get to 30 percent that they could control and you're up to 75.

Ralph: I'm working on it.

Dr. Wright: So . . .

Ralph: But you have to work at it.

Dr. Wright: But I think you are very clever not to expect to be a hundred percent pain free, that you—

Ralph: That's never going to happen.

Dr. Wright: No, that you always will allow the pain to be in your life about 10 percent. Because if you wanted to be pain free and you always worked toward that, it can be a great disappointment when you are not reaching that goal all the time.

Ralph: And I think realistically you have to look at the fact that it is not going to happen.

Dr. Wright: Yeah.

Ralph: And be happy where you are.

CONCLUSIONS

Moving beyond basic family nursing skills requires increased knowledge, increased clinical practice, and greater attention to the uniqueness of each practice context. It also involves an appreciation of the circularity between knowledge and practice. Entering into therapeutic conversations with families can increase our understanding and knowledge about families while simultaneously offering interventions to promote health and/or to address concerns or soften suffering. Our research efforts can augment the efficacy of our interventions with families, and this new knowledge is extended back into practice. Thus, both clinical practice and research operate in a continuous feedback loop for one another with promising benefits for both families and nurses. Experienced nurses realize that it is always an interactional process of "evidenced based practice" and "practice based evidence" that enhances the care offered to families.

We hope that by presenting these clinical vignettes that you can appreciate how family nursing skills, whether basic or advanced, are not cookie-cutter clinical skills but rather are fluid, relevant, and tailored to each family in each unique interview and relationship situation with a competent and compassionate nurse.

References

Astedt-Kurki, P., & Kaunonen, M. (2011). Family nursing interventions in Finland: Benefits for families. In E.K. Svavarsdottir & H. Jonsdottir, (Eds.): *Family Nursing in Action*. Reykjavik, University of Iceland Press, pp. 115–132.

Benner, P. (2001). *From Novice to Expert: Excellence and Power in Clinical Nursing Practice*. New Jersey: Prentice-Hall.

Chesla, C. (2008). Translational research: Essential contributions from interpretive nursing science. *Research in Nursing & Health, 31*(4), 381–390.

Duhamel, F. (2010). Implementing family nursing: How do we translate knowledge into clinical practice? Part II: The evolution of 20 years of teaching, research, and practice to a center of excellence in family nursing. *Journal of Family Nursing, 16*(1), 8–25.

Duhamel, F., & Dupuis, F. (2011). Toward a trilogy model of family systems nursing. Knowledge utilization: Fostering circularity between practice, education and research. In E.K. Svavarsdottir & H. Jonsdottir (Eds.): *Family Nursing in Action*. Reykjavik, Iceland. University of Iceland Press, pp. 53–68.

Duhamel, F., Dupuis, F., & Wright, L. (2009). Families' and nurses' responses to the "one question question": Reflections for clinical practice, education, and research in family nursing. *Journal of Family Nursing, 15*(4), 461–485.

Ericsson, K.A. (2006). The influence of experience and deliberate practice on the development of superior expert performance. In K.A. Ericsson, N. Charness, P. Feltovich, and R.R. Hoffman, (Eds.): *Cambridge Handbook of Expertise and Expert Performance*. Cambridge, UK: Cambridge University Press, pp. 685–706.

Ericsson, K.A., Whyte, J., & Ward, P. (2007). Expert performance in nursing: Reviewing research on expertise in nursing within the framework of the expert-performance approach. *Advances in Nursing Science, 30*(1), E58–E71.

Gladwell, M. (2008). *Outliers: The Story of Success*. New York: Penguin Books.

Graham, I.D., Logan, J., Harrison, M.B., et al. (2006). Lost in knowledge translation: time for a map? *Journal of Continuing Education in the Health Professions, 26*(1), 13–24.

Leahey, M., & Harper-Jaques, S. (2010). Integrating family nursing into a mental health urgent care practice framework: Ladders for learning. *Journal of Family Nursing, 16*(2), 196–212.

Leahey, M., & Svavarsdottir, E. (2009). Implementing family nursing: How do we translate knowledge into clinical practice? *Journal of Family Nursing, 15*(4), 445–460.

Litchfield, M.C. (2011). Family nursing: A practice and systemic approach to innovation in health care. In E.K. Svavarsdottir & H. Jonsdottir (Eds.): *Family Nursing in Action*. Reykjavik, University of Iceland Press, pp. 285–308.

McLeod, D.L., Tapp, D.M., Moules, N.J., et al. (2010). Knowing the family: Interpretations of family nursing in oncology and palliative care. *European Journal of Oncology Nursing, 14*(2), 93–100.

Moules, N.J., Bell, J.M., Paton, B.I., et al. (2012). Examining pedagogical practices in family systems nursing: Intentionality, complexity, and doing well by families. *Journal of Family Nursing, 18*(2), 261–295.

Moules, N.J., Laing, C., Morck, A., et al. (2011). Family research in pediatric oncology —Connecting research and practice. In E.K. Svavarsdottir & H. Jonsdottir (Eds.): *Family Nursing in Action*. Reykjavik, Iceland: University of Iceland Press, pp. 271–284.

Southern, L., Leahey, M., Harper-Jaques, S., et al. (2007). Integrating mental health into urgent care in a community mental health centre. *Canadian Nurse, 130*(1), 29–34.

Svavarsdottir, E.K., & Sigurdardottir, A.O. (2011). Implementing family nursing in general pediatric nursing practice: The circularity between knowledge translation and clinical practice. In E.K. Svavarsdottir & H. Jonsdottir (Eds.): *Family Nursing in Action*. Reykjavik, Iceland: University of Iceland Press, pp. 161–184.

Vandall-Walker, V., Jensen, L., & Oberle, K. (2007). Nursing support for family members of critically ill adults. *Qualitative Health Research, 17*(9), 1207–1218.

White, M. (1989). The externalization of the problem and the re-authoring of lives and relationships. In M. White (Ed.): *Selected Papers*. Adelaide, Australia. Dulwich Centre Publications, pp. 5–28.

Wright, L.M. (1989). When clients ask questions: Enriching the therapeutic conversation. *Family Therapy Networker, 13*(6), 15–16.

Wright, L.M., & Leahey, M. (Producers). (2010a). *Interviewing an Individual to Gain a Family Perspective With Chronic Illness: A Clinical Demonstration*. (DVD). Calgary, AB. Available at www.familynursingresources.com.

Wright, L.M., & Leahey, M. (Producers). (2010b). *Tips and Microskills for Interviewing Families of the Elderly*. (DVD). Calgary, AB. Available at www.familynursingresources.com.

Chapter **11**

How to Avoid the Three Most Common Errors in Family Nursing

Nurses working with families want to be helpful and to soften or alleviate emotional, physical, or spiritual suffering whenever possible (Wright, 2005). However, despite nurses' best efforts, sometimes errors, mistakes, and/or misjudgments occur. Whether nurses are beginners or experienced clinicians in family nursing, they can benefit from knowing the most common errors and how they might avoid or sidestep them. We have identified three errors that we believe occur most frequently in relational family nursing practice. They are:

1. Failing to create a context for change
2. Taking sides
3. Giving too much advice prematurely

Although we are experienced family nurses, we have committed, experienced, or witnessed these errors in our own practice and in the supervision of our students. But the most important aspect is to learn from these errors and to correct them immediately, if at all possible.

For each error, we will explain in what way we believe it is a mistake and how it can negatively impact the family. We also suggest practical ways for avoiding these errors and offer a clinical vignette for each error. It is our hope that by sidestepping the most prevalent mistakes, nurses can sustain and improve their nursing care of families. We have also produced an educational DVD entitled *Common Errors in Family Interviewing: How to Avoid & Correct* (Wright & Leahey, 2010) that demonstrates skills in actual clinical vignettes to avoid mistakes or errors.

Nurses will have more confidence and competence in their nursing practice if they can offer a context for clinical work that is more likely to be helpful and healing.

ERROR 1: FAILING TO CREATE A CONTEXT FOR CHANGE

Every nurse in every encounter and experience with a family, whether for 5 minutes or over 5 years, has the responsibility to create a context for healing and learning. Creating a context for change is the central and enduring foundation of the therapeutic process. It is key to the relationship between the clinician and family. It is not just a necessary prerequisite to the process of therapeutic change; it *is* therapeutic change in and of itself (Wright & Bell, 2009). In creating this context for change, both the nurse and family undergo change. From the first meeting, the nurse and family co-evolve together, with both the family and the nurse changing in response to the other and according to their own individual biopsychosocial-spiritual structures, which have been influenced by their history of interactions and their genetic makeup (Maturana & Varela, 1992).

What must happen in order to create a healing context for change? Empathy, mindfulness, and empathic responding are all necessary ingredients for creating a healing context (Block-Lerner, et al, 2007). Wright and Bell (2009) suggest that before a context for change can be created, all obstacles to change must be removed. Such obstacles can include a family member who does not want to be present or attends the session under duress, a family member who is dissatisfied with the progress of the clinical sessions, a family that has had previous negative experiences with health-care professionals, or a situation in which there are unclear expectations for the meetings.

At the Family Nursing Unit, University of Calgary, a hermeneutic research study conducted by Drs. Bell and Wright explored the process of therapeutic change (Bell, 1999). The focus of this study was to analyze the clinical work with three families who reported negative responses. These families suffered from serious illness and were seen in an outpatient clinic by a clinical nursing team of faculty and graduate nursing students.

Preliminary results of this study provided helpful feedback that can be used to improve family interviews. The most informative learning was that creating a context for change was either ignored or neglected among families that were dissatisfied with the nursing team's clinical work. Curiosity was absent on the part of the nurse interviewer. For example, the nurse interviewer did not seek clarification of the presenting problem or concern. Also, the nurse interviewer paid no attention to how the intervention "fit" the family's functioning. The nurse interviewer did not ascertain from the family if the intervention ideas offered were useful.

Another example of not creating a context for change was the error of commission of the clinical nursing team becoming too "married" to a particular way of conceptualizing the family's problems or dynamics that was not in harmony with the family's conceptualization.

These findings draw attention to the importance of the "common factors" Hubble, Duncan, and Miller (1999) discovered were associated with positive clinical outcomes. These included:

- Extratherapeutic factors, including client beliefs about change, strengths, resiliencies, and chance-occurring positive events in clients' lives (40%). Such events could include obtaining a new job, moving to a new city, and so on
- The client-therapist relationship experienced as empathic, collaborative, and affirmative in focusing on goals, methods, and pace of treatment (30%)
- Hope and expectancy about the possibility of change (15%)
- Structure and focus of a model or approach organizing the treatment (15%)

Blow, Sprenkle, and Davis (2007) argue that the clinician is a key change ingredient in most successful therapy and that it is the "fit" between the model and the clients' worldviews that is important. According to Miller, Hubble, and Duncan (2007, p. 28), "who provides the therapy is a much more important determinant of success than what treatment approach is provided." We believe that this same thought can be adapted to nurses providing care to families—that is, *who* provides the nursing care is a much more important determinant of healing than the particular nursing interventions that are offered.

The process of developing and maintaining a respectful and collaborative relationship between clinician and the family is one of the best predictors of success and therapeutic change (Garfield, 2004; Hubble, Duncan, & Miller, 1999; Martin, Garske, & Davis, 2000).

How to Avoid Failing to Create a Context for Change

1. **Show interest, concern, and respect for each family member.** The most useful way to do this is to invite to a family meeting anyone who is involved with or concerned about the problem or illness or who is suffering as a result of it. After introducing oneself and meeting each family member, the nurse should express his or her desire to learn from the family how this problem or illness has affected their lives and relationships. This articulation can convey to the family that the nurse is interested and willing to learn about them and their most pressing concerns. A nurse will find this task easier to accomplish if he or she embraces the belief that all families have strengths that are often unrealized or unappreciated (Wright & Bell, 2009).

2. **Obtain a clear understanding of the most pressing concern or greatest suffering.** Seek each family member's perspective on the problem/illness

and how it affects the family and their relationships. Even if the perspectives vary, each perspective offers the nurse the best understanding of the family's challenges and sufferings.

3. **Validate and acknowledge each member's experience.** Remember that no one view is the correct, right view or the truth about the family's functioning but is each family member's unique and genuine experience. Be open to all perspectives about the family's concerns. To bring understanding to the nurse and family, not only must each member's perspective be elicited, but each member's perspective must also be valued, acknowledged, and considered important.

4. **Acknowledge suffering and the sufferer.** Health providers' acknowledgment of clients' suffering can be a powerful starting point to begin understanding the family's situation and for healing to occur (Wright, 2005; Wright & Bell, 2009). Through these efforts to understand, the nurse–family relationship is enhanced and strengthened. When nurses acknowledge their clients' suffering and are compassionate and nonjudgmental, families are often more willing to disclose fears and worries. As a result, the potential for healing, growth, and change increases.

Clinical Example

Creating a context for change is often begun in the same manner as meeting a stranger for the first time. However, in the example that follows, the nurse excludes an introduction that is usually part of the greeting ritual with strangers. She also neglects to determine the goals for this meeting. Therefore, some of the important aspects of establishing a new relationship are omitted, and the therapeutic relationship starts down a slow, slippery slope to the point where the family is not interested in any further meetings.

The nurse first met the family at the patient's bedside on a busy medical unit in a large, urban hospital. Mr. Garcia had been admitted to the hospital because of his chronic obstructive pulmonary disease. A woman visited frequently and was usually crying during visits. On one occasion, the primary nurse asked the husband, "Do you know why your wife is crying?" Unfortunately, the nurse did not introduce herself to the woman who was visiting and made the assumption that it was the patient's wife. He responded, "No, this is not my wife. My wife and I are divorced; this is my sister." The nurse was somewhat embarrassed but responded, "Oh, I'm sorry. Well, do you know why your sister is crying? She cries on every visit." Mr. Garcia responded, "I'm not sure." At that point, his sister stopped crying and looked up but did not speak.

The nurse then made a premature conceptualization and offered her assessment by saying, "Well, I think she is crying because she is worried that you are not going to get better if you don't stop smoking. Isn't that right?" The sister shook her head to indicate no.

At this point, Mr. Garcia stated, "Well, it's too late even if I do stop smoking." The nurse then said she would like to come back at another time to discuss the issue with them more fully, at this point addressing the sister for the first time. However, the sister replied that she did not want to meet because this was her brother's problem. The nurse accepted this response and did not have any further discussions with this family.

This encounter illustrates many missed opportunities to create a context for change. First, the nurse should have introduced herself to the sister, clarifying the sister's relationship to the patient. By acknowledging the sister right at the start, the nurse may have encouraged the sister to be more forthcoming and more willing to have another meeting. In addition, the nurse could have asked Mr. Garcia and his sister if they had any questions about the patient's condition or if they had any worries or concerns. This would have given the nurse an opportunity to validate or acknowledge any concerns or sufferings they might have. The sister's weeping on each visit indicates that she may be suffering; however, the nature of her suffering and its cause is unclear. Finally, the nurse offers a quick conceptualization of the problem by assuming that the sister is worried about the brother's smoking habit and its relationship to his recovery. But the sister denies this conceptualization of her suffering, and, unfortunately, the nurse does not ask any therapeutic questions to ascertain the nature of the sister's distress.

The findings of the previously mentioned study by Bell and Wright (Bell, 1999) are clearly evident in this clinical example. There was no clear identification of the presenting concern or suffering, no acknowledgment of their suffering, and a conceptualization of suffering is offered too quickly without obtaining the perspective of each family member. Without these ingredients to create a context for change, there was no opportunity for healing to occur. Sadly, good manners were also missing.

ERROR 2: TAKING SIDES

One of the most common errors in family work is for the nurse to take sides or form an alliance with one family member or subgroup of the family. Although this is commonly done unintentionally, at times the nurse may do so deliberately, usually with a benevolent intent. However, aligning with one person or subgroup can often result in other family members feeling disrespected, disempowered, and noninfluential as the family pursues its goals with the nurse.

How to Avoid Taking Sides

1. **Maintain curiosity.** Be intensely interested in hearing each person's story about the health concern or problem. When each family member's perspective has been revealed, the nurse generally gains an understanding of the multiple forces interacting together to stimulate or trigger the problem. Families are always very complex, and the complexity is increased when an illness or problem emerges. Be open to experiencing an altered view of any family member and/or situation as more

information is revealed. This is particularly important when nurses work with the elderly, because there can be a temptation to take the side of the 55-year-old son (who is dressed in a suit) and not listen sufficiently to his 83-year-old mother lying passively in a bed in an extended care facility.

2. **Remember that the glass can be half full and half empty simultaneously.** There are multiple truths and therefore many ways to view a problem or illness. The more all-inclusive understanding from as many family members as possible, the more possible options for resolution. However, we wish to emphasize that we do not condone violence, and we do not fail to act in dangerous, illegal, or unethical situations.

3. **Ask questions that invite an exploration of both sides of a circular, interactional pattern.** Exploring each person's contribution to circular, interactional communication helps the nurse and family members understand that each person contributes to the problem rather than blaming one family member or taking one family member's side or position. (See Chapter 3 for more explanations about circular interactional patterns and the Calgary Family Assessment Model [CFAM].)

4. **Remember that all family members experience some suffering when there's a family problem or illness.** Invite family members to describe their suffering and the meaning they give to it. The nurse can also ask, "Who in the family is suffering the most?" Often it is surprising to find that the family member suffering the most is not the person with the illness diagnosis, but rather another family member (Wright, 2005).

5. **Give relatively equal "talk time" and interest to each family member.** This, of course, may vary with very young children or family members who are only able to minimally contribute verbally, such as those who are disabled or have dementia.

6. **Remember that information is, as Bateson (1972) described it, "news of a difference."** Treat all information as new discoveries; maintain a systems or interactional perspective regarding your understanding of the illness and family dynamics.

7. **Try not to answer phone calls or have "side conversations" involving one family member "telling on" another family member.** Instead, invite the person to bring the issue to the next family meeting. Alternatively, invite one parent to ask the other parent to join in the phone conversation. In this way, the conversation is transparent for all. Sometimes, e-mailing all parties participating in the family interviews also facilitates transparency.

Clinical Examples

A clinical example often encountered by community health nurses and nurse practitioners involves families and the eating habits of children. In our culture and worldwide, there is a tremendous concern about obesity and, in particular, childhood obesity. Given this situation, it is not uncommon for the nurse to believe wholeheartedly a mother's report about a school-age child's poor eating habits. In particular, the mother describes how the father is laid back about their son's eating habits. "It is like I have two children!" she says, referring to her husband's behavior as childlike. However, listening to the father's viewpoint, the nurse hears an entirely different story about how his son readily eats well in his presence. He describes how his wife becomes tense, screams, and gets "stressed out" by the boy's continuous eating of what she calls junk food.

The nurse then asks herself, "Who should I believe? Who is telling the truth?" If she sides with one parent, then she alienates the other. She misses opportunities to work with the entire family on helping them adjust to normal developmental child-care issues. This trap is especially easy to fall into if one parent negatively labels the other. For example, the husband may say, "You know my wife gets hysterical" or the wife may say, "My husband is so irresponsible; he struggles with depression. And furthermore, I think he may be addicted to watching porn. I can never get him away from the computer."

To address this situation, the nurse practitioner could (1) ask the mother, "When your husband shows you indifference, what do you find yourself doing?" (2) ask the father, "When your wife starts to scream at your son, what do you do?" and (3) invite both parents to a meeting together to talk about the challenges involved in raising a child to have healthy eating habits. Having obtained a circular view of the interaction, the nurse can look at them both and ask, "Which do you think would be harder: for your wife to give up screaming or for your husband to show more responsibility? Who, between the two of you, would find it easier to believe the other might change?"

Another clinical example concerns a family with a teenager dealing with anorexia. Sheena, age 16, is being seen by the unit nurse, Karin Johnson, age 51, to receive help developing more appropriate eating habits and to increase her socialization. Sheena has begun successfully to conquer the grip of anorexia and is very appreciative of Karin's assistance. She looks forward to individual meetings with Karin and compliments Karin frequently on wearing "fashionable clothes my mother never would wear." Karin believes she and Sheena have an "excellent" working relationship and is pleased that Sheena likes her taste in clothes.

Karin has agreed to alternate individual meetings with Sheena with family interviews that include both parents. During a family meeting in which Karin proudly described Sheena's recent accomplishments on the unit, Sheena's mom starts to downplay her daughter's successes. She tells Karin of the various "bad behaviors" Sheena engaged in during a recent pass home. Following this, Sheena bursts out to her mother, "How come you do not treat me as an adult like Karin does?"

By inadvertently aligning too much with Sheena (e.g., around clothes and a special relationship) and not sufficiently aligning with Sheena's parents (e.g., never seeing them as a couple alone to appreciate their challenges in raising a daughter who is in the grip of anorexia), Karin has sacrificed her ability and therapeutic leverage to be multipartial in the family meetings. Rather, the nurse is now perceived by the mother and daughter to be on the teen's side. This makes it difficult for the mother–daughter relationship to flourish and for Sheena's mother to acknowledge her daughter's changes. Rather, Sheena's mom may feel inadvertently competitive or usurped by the nurse. Indeed, nurses who take the side of one or more family members most often are not consciously trying to alienate, compete with, or usurp any particular family member. In fact, they are usually unaware of doing so, and thus it comes as a shock when other family members express dissatisfaction or begin to disengage or discontinue family meetings.

ERROR 3: GIVING TOO MUCH ADVICE PREMATURELY

Nurses have abundant knowledge to offer families and are in the socially sanctioned position of offering advice, information, and opinions about matters of health promotion, health problems, illness suffering, illness management, and relationship issues. We believe, similar to Couture and Sutherland (2006), that advice can have generative and healing potential when it is offered collaboratively. Families are often keen and receptive to nurses' expertise concerning health issues. However, each family is unique, as is each situation. Therefore, timing and judgment are critical for nurses to determine when and how to offer advice.

How to Avoid Giving Too Much Advice Prematurely

1. **Offer advice, opinions, or recommendations only after a thorough assessment has been done and a full understanding of the family's health concern or suffering has been gained and acknowledged.** Otherwise, advice and recommendations can appear too simplistic, patronizing, or lacking an in-depth understanding. Of course, in crisis situations or in a busy emergency or intensive care unit, a full family assessment may not be possible. When families are in shock, numb, or overwhelmed, they can benefit from clear, direct advice from a nurse, who, through professional experience and knowledge, can bring calm and structure in a time of crisis.

2. **Offer advice without believing that the nurse's ideas are the "best" or "better" ideas or opinions.** "Often there is a tendency and temptation among health-care providers to offer their own understandings, their own 'better' or 'best' meanings or beliefs for clients' suffering experiences with serious illness. One way to avoid this trap of prematurely offering explanations or advice to soften suffering is to remain insatiably curious about how clients and their families are managing in the midst of suffering" (Wright, 2005, p. 102). Specifically, nurses should ask themselves, "What do family members believe, and what meaning

do they give to their suffering?" (Wright & Bell, 2009). In working with the elderly, this is particularly important. Nurses should examine their own beliefs about whether they think seniors can change or whether they hold the belief that "the elderly are too old to change their ways." Health professionals who are insatiably curious put on the armor of prevention against blame, judgment, or the need to be "right."

3. **Ask more questions than offering advice during initial conversations with families.** Asking therapeutic or reflexive questions (Tomm, 1987; Wright & Bell, 2009) invites a person to explore and reflect on their own meanings of their health concerns or suffering, not the nurse's. Everyone, especially the elderly, has accumulated over the years a vast reservoir of personal local wisdom and knowledge about health and wellness. Hopefully, through reflections that happen in the therapeutic conversations we have with families, healing may be triggered as new thoughts, ideas, or solutions are brought forth about how a family can best live with illness (Wright, 2005).

4. **Obtain the family's response and reaction to the advice.** After offering advice, it is essential to obtain family members' reactions to the information. Specifically, does this information "fit" for the family with their own biopsychosocial-spiritual structures? We believe it is the manner in which advice is delivered, received, interpreted, and refined that is most critical in our clinical work. Relational practices and therapeutic conversations that include advice-giving are ongoing, collaborative, clarifying, and meaningful. There is a forward process to the conversation; advice-giving is not just a prescription of a particular course of action for the family to follow. (See Chapter 4 for an in-depth discussion about "fit," "meshing," and matching information offered to families with family functioning.)

Clinical Examples

Nurses commonly encounter families who are experiencing deep suffering and grief due to the anticipated or recent loss of a family member. One such family had recently experienced the loss of their 88-year-old father, William Li, who had lived with them for 10 years. Mr. Li had left Hong Kong after the death of his wife and moved to Canada to live with his son and son's family. Just 3 weeks after the death of the elderly father, his daughter-in-law, Ming-mei, presented with her husband, Shen, at a walk-in medical clinic with abdominal pain. Upon concluding a medical exam, a doctor determined that there were no physical reasons for her pain. A nurse was asked to meet with the husband and wife.

Shen told the story of the recent loss of his father, explaining that his wife had been the primary caregiver and had given up her employment to care for her father-in-law. He then offered his belief that his wife's pain was due to her extreme grief at the loss of her father-in-law. The nurse, upon hearing this story but without inquiring about the wife's extreme grief or the meaning of her loss and suffering, prematurely offered the following advice to the couple. To the husband she said, "You need to take your wife on a holiday. She is very tired after caring for your father." To Ming-mei, she said, "Your father-in-law was an elderly man and his time had come. And since he was not your father, but your husband's, you will get over his passing more quickly."

Understandably, the Li family did not find this advice helpful or comforting. If the nurse had asked a few assessment questions, even some structural assessment questions within the CFAM (see Chapter 3), she would have learned that Shen owns a small coffee shop and is unable to take holidays because he is the sole provider and works 7 days a week. Ming-mei also did not find the nurse's words healing, particularly because the nurse ignored the very close relationship she had had with her father-in-law.

By offering premature, albeit well-intentioned, advice, the nurse missed the opportunity to offer opinions and recommendations that would have been more healing. By not being more curious (through the asking of pertinent questions) and more interested in understanding the daughter-in-law's beliefs about the loss of her father-in-law, the nurse offered her own "best" ideas and advice, but the recommendations did not "fit" with this couple. Also, the nurse did not recognize the Chinese culture of the Li family and their sense of honoring and caring for their elderly family member. Sadly, this nurse missed a golden opportunity to commend the daughter-in-law for the care of her father-in-law. (See Chapter 4 for a more in-depth discussion of the intervention of commendations.)

CONCLUSIONS

Working with families in relational practice offers nurses many opportunities for helping them to live alongside and manage illness and increase their sense of wellness. Similar to other professionals, at times we make errors in our practice and are less helpful than we desire. It is our hope that by describing what we consider to be the three most common errors in relational family nursing practice, nurses will either avoid the errors, or if they do make a mistake, will find ways to rectify the situation and recoup with the family. The process of collaborating with families is rich with opportunities for creative healing despite the making of errors. By sidestepping the most frequent mistakes, nurses can offer a context for healing that is more likely to be helpful.

References

Bateson, G. (1972). *Steps to an Ecology of Mind: Collected Essays in Anthropology, Psychiatry, Evolution, and Epistemology.* New York: Ballantine Books.

Bell, J.M. (1999). Therapeutic failure: Exploring uncharted territory in family nursing. [Editorial]. *Journal of Family Nursing, 5*(4), 371–373.

Block-Lerner, J., et al. (2007). The case for mindfulness-based approaches in the cultivation of empathy: Does nonjudgmental, present-moment awareness increase capacity for perspective-taking and empathic concerns? *Journal of Marital and Family Therapy, 33*(4), 501–516.

Blow, A.J., Sprenkle, D.H., & Davis, S.D. (2007). Is who delivers the treatment more important than the treatment itself? The role of the therapist in common factors. *Journal of Marital and Family Therapy, 33*(3), 298–317.

Couture, S.J., & Sutherland, O. (2006). Giving advice on advice-giving: A conversation analysis of Karl Tomm's practice. *Journal of Marital and Family Therapy, 32*(3), 329–344.

Garfield, R. (2004). The therapeutic alliance in couples therapy: Clinical considerations. *Family Process, 43*(4), 457–465.

Hubble, M.A., Duncan, B.L., & Miller, S.D. (1999). Introduction. In M.A. Hubble, B.L. Duncan, & S.D. Miller (Eds.): *The Heart & Soul of Change: What Works in Therapy.* Washington, DC: American Psychological Association, pp. 1–19.

Martin, D.J., Garske, J.P., & Davis, K.M. (2000). Relation of the therapeutic alliance with outcome and other variables: A meta-analytic review. *Journal of Consulting and Clinical Psychology, 68*, 438–450.

Maturana, H.R., & Varela, F.G. (1992). *The Tree of Knowledge: The Biological Roots of Human Understanding* (rev. ed.). Boston: Shambhala.

Miller, S., Hubble, M., & Duncan, B. (2007). Supershrinks: Why do some therapists clearly stand out above the rest, consistently getting far better results than most of their colleagues? *Psychotherapy Networker, 31*(6), 26–35.

Tomm, K. (1987). Interventive interviewing—part ii. Reflexive questioning as a means to enable self-healing. *Family Process, 26*, 167–183.

Wright, L.M. (2005). *Spirituality, Suffering, and Illness: Ideas for Healing.* Philadelphia: F.A. Davis Co.

Wright, L.M., & Bell, J.M. (2009). *Belief and Illness: A Model to Invite Healing.* Calgary, AB: 4th Floor Press.

Wright, L.M., & Leahey, M. (Producers). (2010). *Common Errors in Family Interviewing: How to Avoid & Correct.* [DVD]. Calgary, Canada. Available at www.FamilyNursingResources.com.

Chapter **12**

How to Terminate With Families

Knowing how to successfully conclude or terminate clinical work with families is as important as knowing how to begin—perhaps even more so. When nurses part with families, they should do so in a manner that leaves the families with hope and confidence in their new and rediscovered strengths, resources, and abilities to manage their health and/or illness and relationships. If the family has been suffering with illness, loss, or disability, then at the conclusion of the clinical work, a highly desired outcome would be softened or alleviated suffering and increased healing.

To end professional relationships with families in a therapeutic fashion is one of the most challenging aspects of the family interviewing process for nurses. Reed and Tarko (2004) make the interesting observation that, in nursing, "the issue of termination has been often discussed in psychiatric nursing texts, making it seem as if no other nursing situations have issues surrounding termination" (p. 266). Termination continues to be the least examined of the treatment phases in clinical work with families.

Two important aspects of concluding with families is to end the nurse–family relationship therapeutically and to do so in a manner that will sustain the progress and foster hope for the future. Nurses commonly establish very intense and meaningful relationships with families and therefore may feel guilty or fearful about initiating termination. This is especially evident in nursing practice when the relationship has been a long-standing one, over months or even years, such as in nursing homes, extended-care facilities, and clients' homes.

In this chapter, we review the process of termination by examining the decision to terminate when it is initiated by the family or the nurse or as a result of the context in which the family members find themselves. In many cases, the nurse's decision to conclude with a family does not necessarily mean that the family will cease contact with all professionals. Therefore, we also discuss the process of referring families to other health professionals.

We provide specific suggestions for phasing out and concluding treatment and for evaluating the effects of the treatment process. We must emphasize that, just as other aspects of family interviewing are conducted in a collaborative manner, so, too, should the termination phase. Termination should occur with full participation and input from the family whenever possible.

DECISION TO TERMINATE

Nurse-Initiated Termination

It is important to emphasize that termination may occur before the presenting problem or illness is completely "cured" or resolved. However, it is the family's ability to master or live alongside problems or illness, although hopefully with softened emotional, physical, and spiritual suffering, that is the impetus for initiating termination. In most cases, it is unrealistic for nurses to attempt to completely eliminate the presenting concern or illness, and such a goal can frequently leave families feeling more discouraged and hopeless and nurses feeling inadequate or unhelpful. It is by softening suffering or increasing healing and awareness that enables a family to live with their problems or illness in a more peaceful and manageable way. If the family's presenting concern is related to health promotion, then greater knowledge or increased expertise by the family might be an indicator for termination.

The termination stage evolves easily if the beginning and middle phases of engagement and treatment have progressed successfully. However, the most difficult decision for any nurse to make in regard to termination relates to time. When is the right time for termination? This question is directly related to the new views, beliefs, ideas, and solutions that the family and nurse have generated to resolve current problems. If new solution options have been discovered and consequently the family functions differently, particularly with the presenting concern, it is time to terminate, because change has occurred. The skills necessary for nurse-initiated termination are given in the "Phasing Out and Concluding Treatment" section of this chapter and in Chapter 5.

In contexts where family meetings have occurred over time, then the nurse and family may collaboratively decide that additional meetings are not necessary. In these situations, the termination phase of treatment has begun. First and most importantly during this phase, we prefer to help families expand their perspectives to focus on strengths, positive behaviors, and changes in beliefs or feelings that have occurred or reemerged rather than focus exclusively on troublesome or problematic behaviors. We encourage families not to associate these new behaviors with our work but instead with their own efforts. For example, we would ask a family what positive changes they have noticed over the last 3 months rather than ask what positive changes they have noticed since working with a nurse.

White and Epston (1990) offer another useful clinical idea for nurses terminating with families; they recommend that the interviewer "expand the audience" to describe and acknowledge the family's unique outcomes and progress. For example, we commonly ask families to tell us what advice they would have for other families confronting similar health problems. Sometimes we have families write letters to other families to offer suggestions regarding what has or has not worked in coping with a particular illness. (It is essential that the family that receives the letter has given permission for the letter to be sent.) For example, one woman, who was experiencing multiple sclerosis (MS) but was successfully living with her illness, wrote a letter to a younger woman who was not yet as successful in managing her illness. The younger woman found that it gave her hope and encouragement. The older woman expressed that writing the letter was a very "cathartic" experience for her. She went on to say, "MS is still here, but it does not dominate our lives and occupies only a small space over in the corner. I did experience a minor flare-up after Christmas but it cleared quickly. I remain optimistic."

The nurse should highlight and become enthusiastic about the family's ideas and advice as a way of both reinforcing positive ideas for change and the family's new beliefs about themselves and generating useful information for other families. Thus, the family's competencies, resources, and strengths are overtly acknowledged.

When the nurse initiates termination of the therapeutic relationship, the emphasis throughout this process is to identify, affirm, amplify, and solidify the changes that have taken place within and between family members. Consequently, it is essential that change be distinguished to become a reality (Bell & Wright, 2011; Wright & Bell, 2009). One way to distinguish change is to obtain the perspective of family members. The nurse can accomplish this by asking questions such as, "What changes do you notice in your wife since she has adopted this new idea that 'illness is a family affair'?" or "What else would your family or friends notice that is different in you since your depression about experiencing cancer has dissipated?"

Initiating rituals at the time of termination can also emphasize change and give families courage to live their lives without the involvement of healthcare professionals. If the initial concern involves a child, we have had parties (balloons, cake, and all) to celebrate the child's mastery of the particular problem, whether it be enuresis, fighting fears, or putting chronic pain in its place. In addition, we have given children a certificate indicating that he or she has overcome the problem. This practice helps families to acknowledge change through celebration.

Some clinical settings send a closing letter at the end of the clinical work to each family highlighting what the clinical nursing team has learned from the family and what ideas the team offered the family (Bell, Moules, & Wright, 2010; Moules, 2002, 2003, 2009; Wright & Bell, 2009). These therapeutic letters serve as closing rituals. They provide the opportunity to highlight the family's strengths and document in a personal way the family and individual interventions that were offered. The letters also acknowledge that family nursing is not a one-way street with nurses assisting families. Rather, by stating what the nurse and clinical team have learned from the family, the nurse honors the reciprocal and relational influence between the family and the clinical nursing team. More information about closing letters is provided in Chapter 4.

Family-Initiated Termination

When a family takes the initiative to terminate, it is very important for the nurse to acknowledge their desire and then to gain more explicit information in a nonjudgmental fashion regarding their reasons for wanting to terminate. This information helps the nurse to understand the family's responses to the interviewing process. Has the family discovered new solutions to their problems or challenged their beliefs to soften their suffering? For example, have they found a way to have respite from caring for their ill child without feeling excessive guilt? Has the family challenged some of their constraining beliefs about the illness experience (Bell & Wright, 2011; Wright & Bell, 2009)? For example, have they now stopped blaming themselves for the husband suffering a coronary in part because of having to work two jobs? Are the family and nurse able to identify and agree on significant changes that have occurred in both individual and family functioning? Is the family also aware of how to sustain these changes? For example, if a son refuses to give his own insulin injections in the future, what will the family do differently?

If the family specifically states that they wish to terminate but the nurse believes this would be premature or even enhance their suffering, it is important for the nurse to take the initiative to review the family's decision. In so doing, the nurse reconceptualizes the progress the family has made and recognizes what problems remain and what goals and solutions might yet be achieved.

One way to do this is to have family members discuss with one another their desires to continue or discontinue sessions and explore who most disfavors termination. Also, the specifics of the decision may be helpful, such as when the family decided to terminate and what prompted the decision. After establishing who is most eager to continue, the nurse can invite that family member to share with the other family members the anticipated benefit of further sessions. It is helpful for families to be specific and emphasize the benefits that could be achieved if family interviewing were to continue. However, there are times when termination is inevitable. At such a point, it is reasonable and ethical to accept the family's initiative to terminate and to do so without applying undue pressure, even though the nurse may disagree with their decision.

We strongly urge nurses not to engage in linear blame of either families or themselves when they believe that families have prematurely or abruptly left treatment. Rather, we encourage nurses to hypothesize about the factors that may have contributed to the termination. These factors may include such nurse-related behaviors as being too aligned with children, too slow to intervene, or too "married" to a particular hypothesis about the family's functioning, or not attending to the family's main concern (see Chapter 11 for errors to avoid). Family-related behaviors such as concurrent involvement with other agencies should also be considered.

Nurses may also encounter cases in which a family states that they want to continue treatment but initiate termination indirectly. Indications include late arrivals for meetings, missed appointments, and the absence from sessions of certain family members who were asked to attend. Another indicator that families are perhaps considering termination is their expression of dissatisfaction with the course of treatment or complaints about the logistical difficulties of attending or the loss of time from work. In these situations, we suggest that the same steps be taken as when the family initiates termination directly.

The challenge of family-initiated termination is to determine whether it is premature. It could be, as Slive and Bobele (2011) suggest, that the family has received all the assistance they needed and choose not to return for meetings. In the nursing literature, there is a dearth of research to provide insights into reasons for premature termination. Therefore, nurses must rely on their own clinical judgment to ascertain if termination is premature. Future research studies should address this area in nursing practice with families who are seen on an outpatient basis.

In our clinical experience, we have found that families who miss the first meeting are at high risk for dropping out over the course of treatment. The implication of missed appointments refers back to the importance of the engagement stage and even to the initial contact with families on the telephone. We have also found that the referral source has a direct correlation with the family's continuing treatment. Families who are referred by institutions (such as a school or court) are more likely to discontinue treatment before achieving treatment goals than families who were individually referred (such as by physicians or mental health professionals). Families who are self-referred tend to complete the treatment process.

It is critically important to help families understand the nature of the treatment contract. Many families' understandings of what takes place in family interviewing are markedly different than the understandings held by nurses. Therefore, these families may relate to nurses as they do to physicians, imams, or clergy, whereby they use the services as they wish and discontinue when they desire. For this reason, we find it particularly useful when seeing families on an outpatient basis to contract for a certain number of sessions and then reevaluate as progress occurs. This approach may help to prevent premature or abrupt termination. It also keeps the focus on time-effective, change-oriented conversation.

Context-Initiated Termination

In some settings, such as hospitals (particularly those in managed health-care systems), it is not the nurse or the family who initiates termination but the health-care system or insurance company. In these situations, it is very important for the nurse to assess whether the family needs further treatment on an outpatient basis or can continue to resolve problems and discover solutions on their own. If the family needs to be referred, the nurse requires some specific skills in this area. The referral process will be discussed in a later section of this chapter.

PHASING OUT AND CONCLUDING TREATMENT

In Chapter 5, we highlighted some of the specific skills required for therapeutic termination in the form of learning objectives. We will now expand on these particular skills.

Review Contracts

For families seen on an outpatient basis, we strongly encourage periodic review of the present status of the family's problems and changes. The use of a contract for a specific number of sessions provides a built-in way to set a time limit to the meetings and to ensure periodic review. In one outpatient clinic, all families contracted for four sessions and then evaluated change (Wright & Bell, 2009). In some cases, four sessions were not necessary; families could save unused sessions to be used at a later time if desired. If the family required additional sessions at the conclusion of the four-session contract, then another contract was made between the family and the nurse, and reevaluation occurred again at the end of those sessions. Interestingly, families who contracted for more sessions rarely wanted another 5 or 10 sessions but usually requested just 1 or 2 more sessions. This finding is consistent with the literature that posits change occurs early in treatment and improvement declines as the number of therapy sessions increase (Bloom, 2001).

Contracts help nurse interviewers to be mindful of the progress and direction of their work with families rather than seeing families endlessly and without purpose beyond the vague good intention of "helping." We prefer a designated number of sessions to open-ended sessions. However, nurses need to be flexible about the frequency and duration of sessions. Normally, the frequency decreases as problems improve, suffering has softened, and confidence and hopefulness has increased. Periodic reviews allow family members the opportunity to express their pleasure or displeasure with the progress that is being made.

Decrease Frequency of Sessions

When adequate progress has been made, as evidenced by reduced suffering, the time is ideal to begin to decrease the frequency of sessions. In our experience, we have found that families are able to work toward termination more readily and with more confidence when they recognize the improvement in their own ability to solve problems. However, many families find it difficult to acknowledge changes. In these circumstances, we suggest the use of a question such as, "What would each of you have to do to bring the problem back?" to elicit a more explicit understanding or statement from family members regarding the changes that have been made.

Another significant time to decrease the frequency of sessions is when the nurse has inadvertently fostered undue dependency. We have had many family situations presented to us in which nursing students or professional nurses provide "paid friendship" with mothers. These nurses have become the mother's major support system because they have failed to mobilize other supports, such as husbands, friends, or relatives. In situations in which this dependency has occurred and is recognized, we strongly suggest that the nurse help foster other supports for the family and decrease the frequency of sessions. Regular consultation with colleagues or a supervisor will assist the nurse to ascertain if a dependent relationship has occurred between the nurse and the family.

If a nurse encounters hesitancy or reluctance to decrease the frequency of sessions or to terminate completely, the nurse should encourage a discussion of the fears related to termination and solicit support from other family members. It has been our experience that family members commonly fear that if sessions are decreased or discontinued, they will not be able to cope with their problems or their problems will become worse. Thus, asking a question such as, "What are you most concerned would happen if we discontinued our meetings now?" can get to the core of the matter very quickly. By clarifying family members' fears openly, other family members (who may be less fearful) have an opportunity to provide support.

Give Credit for Change

Nurses often choose the nursing profession because they have a strong desire to help individuals and families obtain optimal health and soften their suffering. Their efforts are usually helpful, and they are commonly given all or much of the credit for the changes and improvements. However, it has been our experience in family work that it is vitally important that the family receive the credit for change. There are several reasons for this:

1. Families experience the tension, conflict, suffering, and anxiety of working through problems related to their health or illness and relationships; therefore, they deserve the credit for improvement.

2. If the identified patient is a child and the nurse accepts credit for change, the nurse can be seen to be in a competitive relationship with the parents.

3. Perhaps the most important reason for giving the family credit for change is that doing so increases the chance that the positive effects of treatment will last. Otherwise, the nurse may inadvertently convey the message that the family cannot manage without him or her, and they will become indebted or too dependent. Termination provides an opportune time to comment on the positive changes that have already happened during the course of treatment.

4. Praising the family for their accomplishments in having helped or corrected the original presenting problem provides them with confidence to handle future problems. Statements such as "You did the work" or

"You people are being far too modest" can reinforce to family members the idea that their efforts were essential in making the change.

It is never possible to know for certain what precipitated, perturbed, or initiated the change that occurs within families. In many cases, nurses create a context for change by helping family members explore solution options to their difficulties or suffering. Wright and Bell (2009) suggest that creating a context for change constitutes the central and enduring foundation of the therapeutic process. They further propose that it is not just a necessary prerequisite to the process of therapeutic change; it is therapeutic change in and of itself. Sometimes the very effort of bringing a family together in a room to discuss important family issues and their suffering can be the most significant intervention (Robinson & Wright, 1995).

If families present themselves at termination with concerns about progress, nurses must express their appreciation for the family's positive efforts to solve problems constructively, even when no significant improvement has occurred. In such cases, we strongly recommend that nurses discuss with their clinical supervisors some hypotheses about why the interview sessions did not seem to be effective. Perhaps the goals of the family or the nurse were too high or demanding. If a family does not progress, it is usually the result of our inability to discover an intervention that "fits" or "meshes" with the family. Too often, nurses excuse themselves from making further efforts to intervene by labeling families as noncompliant, unmotivated, or resistant (Wright & Levac, 1992). But it is very important that nurses believe that families have worked hard despite minimal progress, and it is important to praise them for having done so.

However, we do not mean to imply that because we are encouraging nurses to give families the credit for change that the nurse cannot enjoy the change. Family work can be very rewarding, and certainly the nurse is part of the change process.

Evaluate Family Interviews

It is important to provide a formal closure to the end of the treatment process with a face-to-face discussion, whenever possible. Madsen (2007) refers to this part of the termination process as a *consolidation interview*. In a consolidation or termination interview, the nurse asks particular questions to review the process of the work that the family and clinician have done together and then discusses the work the family seeks to accomplish on its own in the future. This kind of interview is a way to reduce feelings of anxiety, fear, or loss on the part of the clinician, family, or both.

During this final session, it is very valuable to evaluate the effectiveness of the treatment process and the effect of changes on various family members. We recommend evaluating the impact not only on the whole-family system but also on various subsystems, such as the marital subsystem and individual family member functions. Questions such as "What have you learned about yourself and ALS?" or "What have you come to appreciate about your marriage?" or "What have you come to understand is the most effective way you can live with your grief?" invite reflections from the family about its changes.

We also believe in sharing the family's wisdom and will frequently ask, "When you meet with other families with chronic illness, from what you know now, what would you advise them or offer them?"

An even more dramatic evaluation can occur by having each family member and the nurse write about their reflections on the family meetings, emphasizing what they learned, what has changed, and what new ideas or beliefs they have about their problems or illness. One such family clinical nursing team wrote poignant descriptions about dealing with their grief (Levac, et al, 1998).

We also suggest asking family members the following questions: "What things did you find most and least helpful during our work together?" and "What things did you wish or were hoping would happen during our work together that did not?" or "Based on what you've accomplished and learned, what suggestions do you have for me or other nurses in trying to help other families suffering with similar issues?" This behavior demonstrates that the nurse is also open and receptive to feedback. It is important at this time that the nurse not become defensive to any of the feedback. Rather, he or she can express appreciation to the family and inform them that this feedback will assist and educate him or her to be even more helpful in work with future families. Participatory evaluation research turns the traditional evaluation process on its head. Outsiders are no longer the "experts" but instead empower families to become leaders in evaluation and change throughout the interviewing process (Duhamel & Talbot, 2004).

Extend an Invitation for Follow-Up

Nurses often place themselves or are placed in situations of "follow-up." However, follow-up is frequently a negative experience for both the nurse and the family. For example, community health nurses (CHNs) have reported that they are often requested to "check" on family members to assess their functioning. However, those who request the visit (be they physicians or Departments of Child Welfare) often make no clear statement to the family about the purpose of the visit. Follow-up in this manner can give a very unfortunate and unpleasant message to the family that further problems are anticipated. Therefore, the nurse is in a very awkward position. We strongly discourage nurses from placing themselves in these kinds of situations unless there has been clear, direct communication with the family by the requesting party. It is better to make clear to the family that progress has been made and that the sessions are finished. However, if they would like input again in the future, indicate that you would be willing to see them. Families usually appreciate knowing that backup support by professionals is available to them in times of stress.

For nurses employed in hospitals, a follow-up session is usually not possible, but referral can be made to a CHN, emergency room outreach worker, or home-care nurse if deemed appropriate. Our experience has been that families do appreciate knowing whether they will have future contact with the nurse who has worked intimately with them.

Closing Letters

Another way to punctuate the end of treatment positively is to send the family a letter giving a summary of the family sessions. This letter provides the opportunity to highlight the family strengths, reinforce the changes made, offer the family a review of their efforts and what they have accomplished, and list the ideas (interventions) that were offered to them (Bell, Moules, & Wright, 2009; Hougher Limacher & Wright, 2006; Moules, 2002, 2003, 2009; Wright, 2005; Wright & Bell, 2009). Many families have commented about how much they appreciate the letters and how they frequently refer to them. Additional information about closing letters is provided in Chapter 4.

The following example illustrates a typical closing letter:

Dear Family Barbosa:

Greetings from the Family Nursing Unit. We had the opportunity to meet with various members of your family on eight occasions. I have also had several phone conversations with both Venicio and Fatima in recent months.

What Our Team Offered Your Family. Throughout our work together, our clinical nursing team has been very impressed with your family. Although a great many challenges have been presented to all of you over the past years, your family was able to overcome many obstacles and search for ways of helping each other through these difficult times.

1. We offered you the idea that most families find it very difficult to talk openly about an impending loss or death of a family member but that talking can be very healing. You have shown us that this was the case in your family.

2. We offered you a few books to read about other families who have experienced a similar tragedy as yours.

3. We offered you the idea that resolving issues in a relationship that has been conflictual can bring great peace and comfort, particularly following the death of a loved one.

What Our Team Learned From Your Family. Our experience with your family has taught our clinical nursing team a great deal. The following is a synthesis:

1. Families that have a member dealing with a life-shortening illness have the strength to deal with unresolved issues of

blame, guilt, and shame. Even though there has been a great deal of pain and hurt in a family, they can heal their relationships and move on.

2. Although it can be a common response for family members to distance themselves from the possibility of death with a life-shortening illness and to be afraid of dying, it is possible for them to make peace with each other and find peace in themselves, giving them the courage to go on.

3. Although a mother and son may reside in different places and may not see each other often, they can still play a significant part in each other's lives. No matter how old a child and parent are, the knowledge that they love and accept each other for who they are can make a significant difference in their lives.

4. The uncertainty involved with a life-shortening illness can be the most difficult thing for families to handle. Family members can help each other with the uncertainty by discussing the situation openly among themselves.

5. Grandparents and grandsons have very special relationships that are different from those of parents and sons.

As you all continue to face the many challenges that are ahead, we trust that you will draw on your own special strengths as well as on more open communication to help you meet these challenges. It was truly a privilege to work with you. We wish you continued strength for the future.

Should you desire further consultation at any time, you can arrange this by contacting the Family Nursing Unit's secretary. A research assistant will be in contact with you in approximately 6 months to ask you to participate in our outcome study to ascertain your satisfaction with the Family Nursing Unit.

Sincerely,

Jane Nagy, RN   Lorraine M. Wright, RN, PhD
Masters Student   Director, Family Nursing Unit
Professor, Faculty of Nursing

Therapeutic letters, whether sent during clinical work with families or at the end of treatment, have proved a very useful and often potent intervention to invite families to reflect on ideas offered within the session and on changes they have made over the course of sessions (Bell, Moules, & Wright 2009; Hougher Limacher & Wright, 2006; Levac, et al, 1998; Moules, 2002, 2003; Watson & Lee, 1993; White & Epston, 1990; Wright, 2005; Wright & Bell, 2009; Wright & Nagy, 1993; Wright & Watson, 1988).

REFERRAL TO OTHER PROFESSIONALS

Referral to other professionals may be advisable for various reasons. We will list some specific tasks that are required to make a smooth transition for the family from one professional to another. First, however, we will discuss some of the more common reasons for nurses to refer families to other professionals.

With the expanding specialty areas within nursing, it is becoming impossible and totally unrealistic to expect nurses to be experts in all areas. Therefore, when problems are quite complex, it may be appropriate for nurses to seek the input of additional professional resources. A nurse may refer families or specific family members for consultation or ongoing treatment. For example, if a senior within a family is experiencing temporal headaches, it is very important that any organic or biological origin of this problem be ruled out. Therefore, a nurse might refer the family for consultation with a neurologist and may suspend treatment until the consultation is complete. Similarly, the nurse may discover that a particular child has a learning disability that is out of the realm of the nurse's expertise. The nurse may suggest referring the child to an education center where personnel have greater expertise in dealing with children with learning difficulties. Nurses need to be open to referring individuals or entire families for consultation without perceiving this as an inadequacy in their repertoire of skills. To refer wisely, nurses need an extensive knowledge of professional resources within the community.

Although not as common, other situations nurses may encounter that require them to refer families to other professionals include when the family moves, is transferred to another setting, or is discharged before treatment is over. It is very important that the nurse, especially in hospital settings, maximize opportunities to do family work. A beautiful illustration of this was given by one of our graduate nursing students. After some university seminars on the importance of family involvement, this student, who was working part-time in a rural hospital, invited the parents of an asthmatic child to a family interview. The student obtained much valuable information regarding the interrelationship of the child's asthmatic problem with other family dynamics. Shortly thereafter, the child was discharged. The nursing student ascertained that the family was interested in changing the recurring problem of frequent admissions for this young child. The student made an appropriate referral to the mental health services within the community. This highlights the point that with only one family interview, an assessment can be made and a significant intervention completed through referral for a recurring problem. Some of the specific skills required in making appropriate referrals are described in the following paragraphs.

Prepare Families

Nurses must adequately prepare families so that they understand the nature of the referral to a new professional. Useful referrals can be done by explaining to families the reason for the referral and why the nurse feels that the family would benefit from it. Another method that can be useful for ensuring openness and clarity about the nature of the referral is for the nurse to write a summary and then to review this summary with the family. This summary can then be sent to the new professional and a copy made available to the family. In this way, the family is not left wondering what information will be shared with the new professional. Also, an important implicit message is given that this information is confidential and private about them, so they have a right to know what is shared.

Selecting a new professional can sometimes pose a challenge. If a nurse is known in the community, it is wise to solicit the help of colleagues for ideas and advice on which agencies or professionals are best for the type of treatment needed or to seek information from community information directories, booklets, and online resources.

Meet the New Professional

It has been our experience that the transition to the new professional is much more effective and efficient if the nurse can be present with the family at the first meeting. In this way, a more personal referral is made. It often reduces the fears and anxieties that families may have about starting "fresh" with someone new. Before the referral, opportunities should be given to the family to express concerns or ask questions about the referral. At the first meeting, the family may wish to clarify with the new professional their expectations and understanding of the reason for the referral, and any misconceptions can be dealt with at that time. A conjoint meeting with the family, nurse, and new professional can also serve as a "marker" for the end of the nurse's relationship with the family.

Keep Appropriate Boundaries

Despite increased interdisciplinary collaboration in health care, it is still very important that when a family has been referred, boundaries of responsibility are clear. Otherwise, there is a potential for the nurse to inadvertently become triangulated between the family and the new professional. For example, a home-care nurse regularly visited an elderly patient who lived with her adult daughter. The purpose of the visits by the home-care nurse was to assist with colostomy care. The nurse observed and assessed a severe and long-standing conflict between the elderly parent and the adult daughter. This conflict was having a negative effect, deterring the elderly patient from assuming more responsibility for her physical care. Because of her family assessment skills, the nurse was able to make an important referral to a family therapy program where more in-depth work on the intergenerational conflict began. However, in future visits, the elderly patient expressed to the nurse complaints about the adult daughter that the patient was not discussing in the family meetings. Also, the family therapist called the nurse and asked the nurse to apply pressure on the elderly parent to be more cooperative in attending sessions. Thus, very quickly the nurse had become "caught in the middle" between the family and the therapist. The nurse dealt with the situation by requesting to join in a meeting with the family and the therapist to clarify expectations of all parties. In this one session, the nurse was able to "detriangulate" herself from any alliance by clarifying her present role with the family and the new professional. See Chapter 3 for more discussion about alliances and coalitions.

Transfers

In our more than 35 years of clinical experience, we have not found the practice of transferring families from one clinician to another to be very successful. We view the process of transfers as very different from referrals. A referral is usually made to another health-care professional with different expertise. A transfer, on the other hand, is usually made to another colleague of similar expertise and competence. We recommend, if possible, that nurses conclude treatment with the families they are working with rather than transfer them to another colleague. In our experience, families frequently disengage with the new nurse in various ways (e.g., by missing appointments, not showing up, or not stating any particular concern). It is understandable that families do not wish to "start over" with another nurse. We hypothesize that transfers are frequently made to assuage the nurse's feelings about leaving versus the family's desires about continuing treatment.

If, however, a transfer is necessary, we recommend that the "old" nurse use language indicating an ending of her relationship with the family. For example, she can say, "Now that my work with you is coming to an end, what would you like to work on with Sanjeshna, the new nurse?" In addition, we encourage the new nurse to directly ask the family about their relationship with previous nurses. Such questions as "What do you anticipate will be different in our work together versus your work with Li?" are useful. This type of conversation punctuates a change rather than a continuance of the same work. It fosters engagement and is important for the new nurse and the family in establishing a collaborative relationship.

Another way to increase engagement is for the current nurse to ask the family to take a break before the family initiates setting up an appointment with the new nurse. This again emphasizes the change in the working relationship and encourages the family to be self-directive in initiating the new contact rather than simply responding to the professionals.

Success of Treatment in Family Work

Although interventions may obtain positive and possibly dramatic results during treatment, the real success of family work is the positive changes that are maintained or continue to evolve weeks and months after nurses have terminated treatment with particular families. We strongly encourage professional nurses and nursing students to make it a pattern of practice to obtain data from the family regarding outcomes in order to determine best practices. When nurses focus on outcomes, they orient their work toward change, focus on problems that can be changed, and think about how families will cope without them in the future. We also suggest that nurses explain to families that follow-up is a normal pattern of practice (e.g., by saying, "We normally contact families with whom we have worked within 6 months to gain information on how things are evolving"). It is also important to use this follow-up contact and have specific goals in mind. A very useful reason for follow-up can be for research purposes. In our experience, beginning family nurse interviewers tend to be more focused on what is going on in the family, whereas more experienced nurses focus on more specific goals for treatment.

To facilitate evaluation, we suggest formalizing follow-up of families, particularly those seen on an outpatient basis, by live interview, questionnaire, telephone, e-mail, or online survey. At present, we favor the use of a face-to-face discussion and questionnaire that is answered by all available family members.

One outcome study at an outpatient education and research clinic, namely the Family Nursing Unit, University of Calgary (Bell, 2008; Wright & Bell, 2009), was designed to evaluate the services provided to families. The variables examined by this study were the family's satisfaction with the services provided, satisfaction with the nurse interviewer, and change in the presenting problem and family relationships. A semistructured questionnaire designed for this study asked for each family member's perspective on each of the variables. Questions were asked in relation to two periods: at the conclusion of the family sessions and at the time of the survey. Results from the survey indicated that the most helpful aspects of family sessions were the opportunity to ventilate family concerns, thereby increasing communication among family members, and to obtain support from the clinical nursing team. Families ranked the interview process and the suggestions from the clinical nursing team as the second most helpful aspects.

Family members reported satisfaction with nurse interviewers, who were either master's or doctoral students or faculty members specializing in family systems nursing. They indicated that the friendly, professional, and non-threatening manner of the graduate nursing students made them comfortable. More than 75% of the family members reported that the presenting problem was better at the time of the survey. Regardless of the presenting problem, positive changes in the marital relationship, such as increased communication, improved relationships, and decreased tension, were also reported, suggesting support for the systems-theory tenet that change in one part of the system affects change in other parts.

This type of outcome study suggests that change should be evaluated at the individual, parent–child, marital, and family system levels. We believe that a higher level of positive change has occurred when improvement is evidenced in systemic (total family) or relationship (dyadic) interactions than when it is evidenced in individuals alone—that is, individual change does not

336 Nurses and Families: A Guide to Family Assessment and Intervention

logically require system change, but stable system change does require individual change and relationship change, and relationship change requires individual changes.

Nurses can contribute significantly to family outcome research by focusing on follow-up with families in which particular family members experience a health problem. This area of family work is just beginning to be researched and lends itself beautifully to the active involvement of nurses in its evolution.

CONCLUSIONS

Concluding treatment in a therapeutic and constructive way is a challenge for any nurse working with families. Unfortunately, much more has been written in the literature about how to begin with and treat families than how to effectively and therapeutically terminate with them. However, we want to emphasize the extreme importance of terminating contact with families in a manner that will increase the likelihood that diminished suffering will be sustained and that changes and hopefulness in family relationships will be maintained, celebrated, and expanded.

References

Bell, J.M. (2008). The Family Nursing Unit, University of Calgary: Reflections on 25 Years of Clinical Scholarship (1982–2007) and Closure Announcement. *Journal of Family Nursing, 14*(3), 275–288.

Bell, J.M., Moules, N.J., & Wright, L.M. (2009). Therapeutic letters and the Family Nursing Unit: A legacy of advanced nursing practice. *Journal of Family Nursing, 15*(1), 6–30.

Bell, J.M., & Wright, L.M. (2011). Creating practice knowledge for families experiencing illness suffering: The Illness Beliefs Model. In E. Svavarsdottir & H. Jonsdottir (Eds.): *Family Nursing in Action.* Reykjavik, Iceland: University of Iceland Press.

Bloom, B.L. (2001). Focused single-session psychotherapy: A review of the clinical and research literature. *Brief Treatment and Crisis Intervention, 1,* 75–86.

Duhamel, F., & Talbot, L. (2004). A constructivist evaluation of family interventions in cardiovascular nursing practice. *Journal of Family Nursing, 10*(1), 12–32.

Hougher Limacher, L.H., & Wright, L.M. (2006). Exploring the therapeutic family intervention of commendations: Insights from research. *Journal of Family Nursing, 12,* 307–331.

Levac, A.M., et al. (1998). A "Reader's Theater" intervention to managing grief: Posttherapy reflections by a family and a clinical team. *Journal of Marital and Family Therapy, 24*(1), 81–93.

Madsen, W. (2007). Working within traditional structures to support a collaborative clinical practice. *International Journal of Narrative Therapy and Community Work, 2,* 51–61.

Moules, N.J. (2002). Nursing on paper: Therapeutic letters in nursing practice. *Nursing Inquiry, 9*(2), 104–113.

Moules, N.J. (2003). Therapy on paper: Therapeutic letters and the tone of the relationship. *Journal of Systemic Therapies, 22*(1), 33–49.

Moules, N.J. (2009). Therapeutic letters in nursing: Examining the character and influence of the written word in clinical work with families experiencing illness. *Journal of Family Nursing, 15*(1), 31–49.

Reed, K., & Tarko, M.A. (2004). Using the nursing process with families. In P.J. Bomar (Ed.): *Promoting Health in Families: Applying Family Research and Theory to Nursing Practice* (3rd ed.). Philadelphia: Saunders.

Robinson, C.A., & Wright, L.M. (1995). Family nursing interventions: What families say makes a difference. *Journal of Family Nursing, 1*(2), 327–345.

Slive, A., & Bobele, M. (Eds.). (2011). *When One Hour Is All You Have: Effective Therapy for Walk-in Clients.* Phoenix, AZ: Zeig, Tucker & Theisen.

Watson, W.L., & Lee, D. (1993). Is there life after suicide? The systemic belief approach for "survivors" of suicide. *Archives of Psychiatric Nursing, 7*(1), 37–43.

White, M., & Epston, D. (1990). *Narrative Means to Therapeutic Ends.* New York: Norton.

Wright, L.M. (2005). *Spirituality, Suffering, and Illness: Ideas for Healing.* Philadelphia: F.A. Davis.

Wright, L.M., & Bell, J.M. (2009). *Beliefs and Illness: A Model for Healing.* Calgary, AB: 4th Floor Press.

Wright, L.M., & Levac, A.M. (1992). The non-existence of non-compliant families: The influence of Humberto Maturana. *Journal of Advanced Nursing, 17*(8), 913–917.

Wright, L.M., & Nagy, J. (1993). Death: The most troublesome family secret of all. In E. Imber-Black (Ed.): *Secrets in Families and Family Therapy.* New York: W.W. Norton & Co., pp. 121–137.

Wright, L.M., & Watson, W.L. (1988). Systemic family therapy and family development. In C.J. Falicov (Ed.): *Family Transitions: Continuity and Change Over the Life Cycle.* New York: Guilford Press, pp. 407–430.

INDEX

Transfers, 334
difference from referrals, 334
Transgendered family life cycle, 121–123
*Tree of Knowledge, The: The Biological
Roots of Human Understanding,* 46
Triangles, 141
Twin-spirited family life cycle, 121–123
Two-spirited, definition of, 59

V

Validating emotional responses, 161–162
Verbal communication, 127
questions to ask the family, 127

W

Whole greater than the sum of its parts,
28–29
"Why" questions, 43
World Health Organization (WHO) Family
Health Nurse Multinational Study, 3

Y

Young adult, launching, 95, 98–99, 99f
attachments, 99, 99f
questions to ask the family, 99
tasks, 98–99

The "How to" Family Nursing DVD Series

www.familynursingresources.com
Available in DVD and/or .mov files, streaming video format
Developed and demonstrated by:
Lorraine M. Wright, RN, PhD, and Maureen Leahey, RN, PhD
Produced by FamilyNursingResources.com

This series presents live clinical scenarios that demonstrate how to practice family nursing. Interviews are with a family with young children, middle-aged families, and later-life families. The health problems and health-care settings are varied as are the ethnic and racial groups. Intended for practicing nurses, educators, undergraduate students, and graduate nursing students, these educational programs will increase nurses' skills in assisting families experiencing illness.

These actual family nursing interviews are a perfect accompaniment to Wright and Leahey's highly acclaimed, award-winning text, **Nurses and Families: A Guide to Family Assessment and Intervention.**

#1: How to Do a 15-Minute (or Less) Family Interview (length 23:18)

Featuring real-life clinical scenarios, Wright and Leahey demonstrate key family nursing skills such as how to use manners to engage families in a short period, how to start therapeutic conversations with families, and how to routinely ask key therapeutic questions of families.

#2: Calgary Family Assessment Model: How to Apply in Clinical Practice (length 26:47)

Wright and Leahey, co-developers of the Calgary Family Assessment Model (CFAM), demonstrate the model in clinical practice. Highlighting the structural, developmental, and functional categories of CFAM in clinical interviews, they present examples of specific questions the nurse can ask the family, illustrate the helpfulness of the genogram and ecomap, and demonstrate how to construct circular interactional diagrams in clinical settings.

#3: Family Nursing Interviewing Skills: How to Engage, Assess, Intervene, and Terminate With Families (length 22:32)

Observe the four stages of a family nursing interview, from engagement through termination. Wright and Leahey define and demonstrate key perceptual, conceptual, and executive skills; show how to apply these skills in family nursing clinical practice; offer sample questions for nurses to explore family concerns/solutions; and show key interventions to help families change.

#4: How to Intervene With Families With Health Concerns (length 27:54)

Focus on intervention and change! Wright and Leahey demonstrate interventions in new clinical interviews: encouraging the telling of illness narratives, validating affect, drawing forth family strengths/support, encouraging respite, offering commendations, and offering information/opinions. These interventions focus on strengthening, promoting and/or sustaining effective family functioning in cognitive, emotional, and behavioral domains.

#5: How to Use Questions in Family Interviewing (length 26:45)

Increase your interviewing skills by using questions that are effective and time-efficient! Wright and Leahey demonstrate how to use questions that engage all family members and focus the meeting, assess the impact of the illness/problem on the family, elicit family coping strategies/strengths, intervene and invite change, and request family feedback.

#6: Common Errors in Family Interviewing: How to Avoid and Correct (length 27:04)

How to avoid and correct errors in family interviewing is essential for relational practice and for healing to occur. Interviewing skills are demonstrated in new actual clinical vignettes. Specifically shown is how to create a context for change and work collaboratively with all family members in the room without taking sides. Both physical and mental health issues are explored.

#7: Tips and Microskills for Interviewing Families of the Elderly (length 27:22)

An interview with a clinician and two senior children at the time of their mother's transition to a care facility demonstrates the microskills for assisting families of the elderly with a potentially difficult life transition. Tips for how to engage with family members quickly, obtain a brief relevant history, and discuss caregiver impact and burden are provided. Interviewing skills for how to collaborate with senior children and respond to suggestions about their mother's care are also demonstrated in new clinical vignettes.

#8: Interviewing an Individual to Gain a Family Perspective With Chronic Illness: A Clinical Demonstration (length 28:15)

A brief clinical interview honors the notion that illness is a family affair and demonstrates skills for how to assess the impact of chronic illness on one's life and relationships (work, family, marriage, and children). Interventions of commendations and rituals are also illustrated.

PURCHASE INFORMATION

Products are available in DVD format. For information about licensing agreements, .mov files, and streaming video, see www.familynursingresources.com. These DVDs have been translated into Japanese and are available at www.igakueizou.co.jp

$329 per DVD includes shipping and handling. Additional charge if courier delivery is requested.

Canadian residents pay in Canadian funds and add GST/HST.

United States and international residents pay in U.S. funds.

Payment can be made by: check, money order, or bank wire transfer. Institutional purchase orders are accepted.

Make check payable to: efamilynursing.com

To order by phone: North America 902-243-3454 or 403-830-3445 (12 noon to 3 p.m. Monday–Friday)

To order by email: mleahey@bellaliant.net or lmwright@ucalgary.ca

To order by Internet: www.FamilyNursingResources.com

To order by mail: efamilynursing.com, 291 Pugwash Point Road, Pugwash, Nova Scotia, Canada, B0K 1L0

Name:_____Dept./Title:_____

Organization:_____

Address:_____

City:_____Province/State:_____Code/Zip:_____Country_____

Telephone: ()_____Purchase Order#_____Signature:_____

E-mail:_____

PROGRAM NAME	QUANTITY	UNIT PRICE	GST/HST	TOTAL
1. 15 Minute				
2. CFAM				
3. Family Nursing Skills				
4. Interventions				
5. Questions				
6. Common Errors				
7. Tips and Microskills— Elderly				
8. Interviewing Individual				
Total				

(Revised 11/1/12; price subject to change without notice)

www.familynursingresources.com

daybook, *n.* a book in which the events of the day are recorded; *specif.* a journal or diary

DAYBOOK
of Critical Reading and Writing

FRAN CLAGGETT

LOUANN REID

RUTH VINZ

Great Source Education Group
a Houghton Mifflin Company
Wilmington, Massachusetts

www.greatsource.com

W9-CAM-714

The Authors

Fran Claggett, currently an educational consultant for schools throughout the country and teacher at Sonoma State University, taught high school English for more than thirty years. She is author of several books, including *Drawing Your Own Conclusions: Graphic Strategies for Reading, Writing, and Thinking* (1992) and *A Measure of Success* (1996).

Louann Reid taught junior and senior high school English, speech, and drama for nineteen years and currently teaches courses for future English teachers at Colorado State University. Author of numerous articles and chapters, her first books were *Learning the Landscape* and *Recasting the Text* with Fran Claggett and Ruth Vinz (1996).

Ruth Vinz, currently a professor and director of English education at Teachers College, Columbia University, taught in secondary schools for twenty-three years. She is author of several books and numerous articles that discuss teaching and learning in the English classroom as well as a frequent presenter, consultant, and co-teacher in schools throughout the country.

Printed in the United States of America

International Standard Book Number: 0-669-46431-7

9 10 11 12 13 14 - VHG - 09 08 07 06 05

Focus/Strategy	Lesson	Author/Literature

TABLE OF CONTENTS

3

5

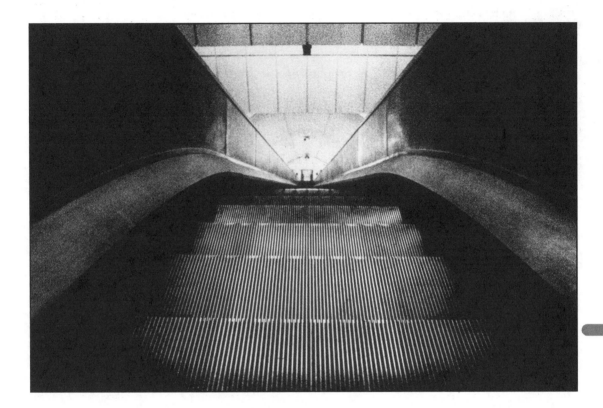

Angles of Literacy

Literacy means being able to understand what you read. It also means being able to communicate your ideas clearly to other people. In many ways, a written text is like a conversation: you must listen to what it has to say and respond to what you have understood.

Throughout the *Daybook* you will be asked to read and respond to a wide variety of literature. To help you, the *Daybook*

is organized into five "angles of literacy." Each angle is a different way of looking at what you read and what you write.

In this first unit you will read poems by the American poet Li-Young Lee. You will also practice five approaches we refer to as angles of literacy:

- interacting with a text by marking and high-lighting
- making connections to the story

- shifting the perspective to examine point of view
- studying the language and craft
- considering how the life and works of a writer enter into a text.

One Interactions with the Text

As you read, it is important to interact with a text, personalizing it by marking your questions and reactions. Some readers think of it as having a dialogue or conversation with the words on the page. Things you should consider doing include:

- circling any vocabulary words that you do not know
- underlining key phrases
- keeping track of the story or idea as it unfolds
- noting word patterns and repetitions or anything that strikes you as confusing or important
- writing down questions in the margins

As you read "Early in the Morning" by Li-Young Lee notice how one active reader has marked up the poem.

Response notes

Does "long grain" mean rice?

I. Description

Who: mother
father
child = poet
When: an adult looking back to childhood

Who's the speaker?

II. Commentary

Early in the Morning
Li-Young Lee

While the long grain is softening
in the water, gurgling
over a low stove flame, before
the salted Winter Vegetable is sliced
for breakfast, before the birds,
my mother glides an ivory comb
through her hair, heavy
and black as calligrapher's ink.

She sits at the foot of the bed.
My father watches, listens for
the music of the comb
against hair.

My mother combs,
pulls her hair back
tight, rolls it
around two fingers, pins it
in a bun to the back of her head.
For half a hundred years she has done this.
My father likes to see it like this.
He says it is kempt.

But I know
it is because of the way
my mother's hair falls
when he pulls the pins out.
Easily, like the curtains
when they untie them in the evening.

Now read "The Gift." Use the interactive reading strategies, such as marking vocabulary and underlining key phrases, as you read. Write your reactions to the poem in the response notes.

Response notes

The Gift
Li-Young Lee

To pull the metal splinter from my palm
my father recited a story in a low voice.
I watched his lovely face and not the blade.
Before the story ended, he'd removed
the iron sliver I thought I'd die from.

I can't remember the tale,
but hear his voice still, a well
of dark water, a prayer.
And I recall his hands,
two measures of tenderness
he laid against my face,
the flames of discipline
he raised above my head.

Had you entered that afternoon
you would have thought you saw a man
planting something in a boy's palm,
a silver tear, a tiny flame.
Had you followed that boy
you would have arrived here,
where I bend over my wife's right hand.

Look how I shave her thumbnail down
so carefully she feels no pain.
Watch as I lift the splinter out.
I was seven when my father
took my hand like this,
and I did not hold that shard
between my fingers and think,
Metal that will bury me,
christen it Little Assassin,
Ore Going Deep for My Heart.
And I did not lift up my wound and cry,
Death visited here!
I did what a child does
when he's given something to keep.
I kissed my father.

11

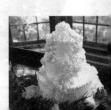

➤ Write a summary of "The Gift" as you understand it. What is it about? What do you know about the speaker and the situation? Who is the speaker addressing when he says "you"? Include your own reactions to the poem. Do not be afraid to give an honest opinion, but be sure to have reasons for any statement you make. Using examples from the text is important to good writing.

Active readers interact with what they read, responding to the work's ideas.

Two
Story Connections

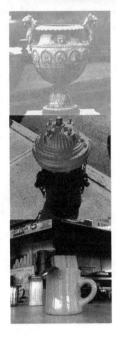

Another important part of reading and understanding literature is making connections to the stories. Not everything you read will be a story with a beginning, middle, and end. But writers generally recall stories from their lives or imagine events that could have occurred. You can find real and imaginary experiences in what you read. Three important strategies for making story connections are:

- analyzing the stories being told
- speculating on the significance or meaning of incidents
- connecting stories to your own experience

In "Early in the Morning," the speaker of the poem recalls an event that has happened so often ("half a hundred years") that it is more like a ritual. While breakfast is cooking, the mother sits on the edge of the bed and combs her hair. Then, she rolls it around her fingers and "pins it in a bun to the back of her head." That is the central incident in this poem. But the incident means much more than the mere actions suggest. When the speaker tells about the father's reaction to this ritualized event in the last two lines of the third **stanza**, we can almost see how much the parents love each other.

Now make a story chart for "The Gift." Discuss this poem with a partner. What are the important incidents? What is the significance or meaning of each one? What personal connections can you make with similar incidents from your own experience or from experiences you have heard or read about?

13

Incident in "The Gift"	Meaning of Incident	Similar Incident I know of

> Analyze the story or stories each writer is trying to tell. It helps you understand what you've read.

Shifting Perspectives

Shifting **perspectives** means looking at what you read and write from many **points of view**. First, try to get a basic understanding of the poem. Ask yourself questions. Who is the speaker? What is the subject? What is happening? What ideas or images do I get as I read? Answering these questions becomes automatic for active readers. In "Early in the Morning," Lee expects you to understand that the narrator is looking back on an event that happened repeatedly rather than just once.

After you get the basic meaning, think about the text in other ways. You will find that trying different perspectives gives you a clearer, deeper understanding of the poem. You can get a different perspective by:

- exploring various versions of an event
- comparing texts
- forming interpretations
- changing **point of view**

Response notes

14

Eating Together
Li-Young Lee

In the steamer is the trout
seasoned with slivers of ginger,
two sprigs of green onion, and sesame oil.
We shall eat it with rice for lunch,
brothers, sister, my mother who will
taste the sweetest meat of the head,
holding it between her fingers
deftly, the way my father did
weeks ago. Then he lay down
to sleep like a snow-covered road
winding through the pines older than him,
without any travelers, and lonely for no one.

Did you mark up the poem as you read? In the response notes, write down your initial impressions of the poem. Who is speaking? What are the circumstances? Reflect on the subject and your feelings after reading the poem.

With a partner, discuss how you might read this poem differently if:

- you believed the speaker of the poem is female
- you believed that the speaker hated the father
- the feelings of every person in the family were described
- you have yourself experienced the loss of a parent

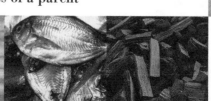

●❖ Write an interpretation of "Eating Together." Consider your initial impressions, the basic meaning of the poem, and the perspectives you have explored. Tell what you think the poem is about and explain why you think so.

15

Look at a piece of literature from several angles. Think about "what if" situations that might change how you perceive a text.

Four

Language and Craft

It is important to pay attention to the words an author uses and the ways they are arranged. There are many strategies you can use to understand the words and structure of what you read. Some of them are:

- looking at the way the author uses words
- understanding figurative language
- comparing the style with other writers'
- studying various kinds of literature

Look at how Lee uses words. Make a vocabulary chart to help you understand words that you do not know. Go back to the poems you have read so far. Put the vocabulary words you circled in the first column of the chart below. To fill in the "meaning" column, you should make an educated guess about the meaning of the word by looking at the other words around it. Then use a dictionary to look up the word. The example words are from "Early in the Morning."

vocabulary	meaning	what is implied
"long grain"	guess--rice is the only grain I know of that is "long" and it is probably the most common kind of grain that people would eat for breakfast	rice for breakfast
"kempt"	dictionary--neat and tidy.	that the father likes order

16

Another way to study how an author uses words is to look at key words and phrases. As you read "Mnemonic," pay attention to Lee's choice of words and how he arranges these words to present his ideas. Circle any words that catch your attention.

Mnemonic
Li-Young Lee

I was tired. So I lay down.
My lids grew heavy. So I slept.
Slender memory, stay with me.

I was cold once. So my father took off his blue sweater.
He wrapped me in it, and I never gave it back.
It is the sweater he wore to America,
this one, which I've grown into, whose sleeves are too long,
whose elbows have thinned, who outlives its rightful owner.
Flamboyant blue in daylight, poor blue by daylight,
it is black in the folds.

A serious man who devised complex systems of numbers
    and rhymes
to aid him in remembering, a man who forgot nothing, my
    father
would be ashamed of me.
Not because I'm forgetful,
but because there is no order
to my memory, a heap
of details, uncatalogued, illogical.

For instance:
God was lonely. So he made me.
My father loved me. So he spanked me.
It hurt him to do so. He did it daily.

The earth is flat. Those who fall off don't return.
The earth is round. All things reveal themselves to men
    only gradually.

I won't last. Memory is sweet.
Even when it's painful, memory is sweet.

Once, I was cold. So my father took off his blue sweater.

17

⬥ Use a double-entry log to help you understand the language of this poem.

Words or phrases from the poem that catch my attention, puzzle, or interest me	Why I chose the word or phrase

•◆ Now, write about how the title organizes the poem. Why does Li-Young Lee title this poem "Mnemonic"? What is a mnemonic device? What item in the poem serves as one? Could the poem itself be a mnemonic device for the speaker? What if the poem were called "My Father's Sweater" instead? Write a paragraph that begins "The best title for this poem is _____ because." Explain your ideas.

18

Five

Focus on the Writer

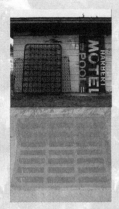

You can often gain insights into a work of literature by knowing about the writer's life. Not all works are autobiographical, but many authors do draw on their experiences. Using biographical insights is another angle for understanding a text. The following strategies will help you do that:

- making inferences about the connections between the author's life and work
- analyzing the author's style
- noticing the author's subject matter and sources of inspiration
- paying attention to repeated themes and topics
- reading what an author says about his or her own work and what critics say

MEET THE WRITER

Li-Young Lee

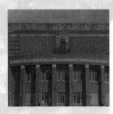

LI-YOUNG LEE was born in 1957 in Jakarta, Indonesia. He now lives in Chicago with his wife and two sons. His father was the personal physician to the Chinese leader Mao Tse-tung in the 1950s. He was later a political prisoner of Indonesia's President Sukarno and escaped to Hong Kong where he became a preacher. Lee writes, "When my father preached between 1963 and 1964, on the island of Hong Kong, he drew crowds in such numbers that rows of folding chairs had to be set up in the very lobbies of the theaters where his revival meetings took place, while loudspeakers were set up outside, where throngs of sweating believers stood for hours in the sun, listening to him speak and pray." When Lee was six years old, the family moved to Pennsylvania, where his father became a Presbyterian minister.

Li-Young Lee tells his family history in *The Winged Seed: A Remembrance*. But he also suggests it in his two collections of poems (*Rose* and *The City In Which I Love You*) where the speakers detail family rituals, express passion and grief, and explore the tensions between past and present and between silence and speech.

Two people are especially prominent in Lee's work—his father and his wife, Donna. Jonathan Spence wrote in his review of *The Winged Seed* that "Lee creates an all-enveloping portrait of his father as man-of-God, political prisoner, tyrant, toucher of souls, and weaver of spells." Lee himself says that Donna is "everything that's not melancholy [in my work]."

19

Read this excerpt from *The Winged Seed*. As you read, mark the text, circling or highlighting phrases that strike you. For example, you might focus on Lee's descriptions or a phrase that reminds you of something from one of his poems.

from ***The Winged Seed*** by Li-Young Lee

←Response notes→

Our first Christmas Eve in America, our parents took us to the Sears & Roebuck in East Liberty where we were each given a quarter to spend at the gum ball and novelty vending machines that stood arrayed at the department store's entrance. We had little money; my father, at the age of forty, was starting a new life as a student at the Pittsburgh Theological Seminary; my mother had already pawned a jade carving of a hare to see us through the months of November and December. At home, a leafless branch my father broke off a tree served as our Tannenbaum, which he and my mother decorated with white paper birds they made, no two alike, and each bearing inside it a birthday candle.

It was my sister's idea that the children should exchange gifts by allowing each to ask of his siblings one thing each desired from among the other's belongings. So it was, she laid out her keepsakes on the kitchen table, from which I chose two walnuts, reddish-brown from her constant fondling in her coat pocket, and my brothers each chose a fountain pen and a comic book. Then each of us laid out our own treasures, and I gave up a new pencil, a lock without a key, and a magnet. At midnight, our mother brought out a bowl of oranges, and we all sat in our parents' bedroom telling stories and eating the fruit our mother peeled with such skill we tasted no skin or rind.

20

●◆ Readers naturally make inferences about the connections between an author's life and work. You may not have found a direct connection between Lee's life and his poems, but you can still make good inferences—guesses based on evidence. Using evidence from *The Winged Seed* and "Meet the Writer," make two good inferences about the connections between Lee's life and any of the poems you have read. The example is from "Early in the Morning."

EVIDENCE FROM THE AUTHOR'S LIFE	INFERENCE	COMPARISON TO THE POEMS
"...we all sat in our parent's bedroom telling stories...."	It is not unusual for the family to gather in the parents' bedroom	The narrator watches his mother as "She sits at the foot of the bed" combing her hair.

Knowing about a writer's life can help you better understand his or her work.

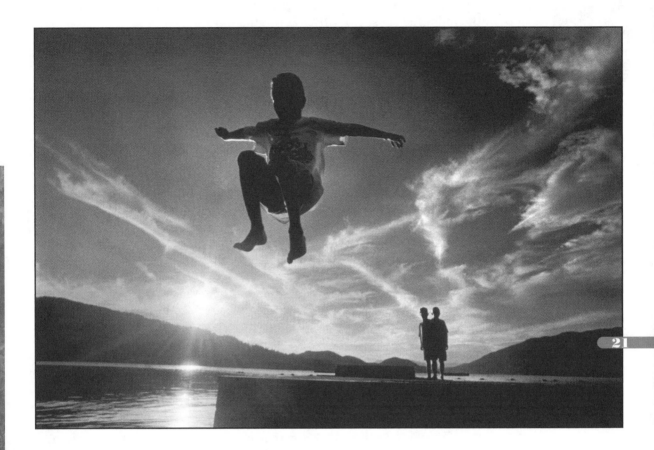

Connecting With Stories

Where the Wild Things Are is a picture book that tells the story of Max's adventures when he sails to the island of the Wild Things (Monsters) after his mother sends him to bed without his supper. The author, Maurice Sendak, was asked why he did not describe the mother, who is a central character in the story. Sendak responded, "you should only imagine what she looks like. . . . I leave the mother to the imagination. But you feel her there. By her absence she is more available." His comment is a reminder that the author and reader work together. Each expects something from the other. For example, Sendak went on to say that the reader could imagine the mother as scarier than he could create her in words.

You expect the author to communicate ideas important to the meaning of the story, provide details and images that help you visualize what is taking place, and highlight events that are important to the development of the story. The author expects you to understand the connections between the subject of the story, the plot, characters, or other important devices the author uses to tell the story.

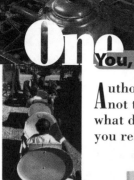

One

Authors invite you, as reader, to enter the world they create in stories. Whether or not the story can hold you in its world depends on both you and the writer. Just what does it mean to "get into" a story? Keep track of where your mind travels as you read the following short story by Bel Kaufman.

"Sunday in the Park" by Bel Kaufman

←— *Response notes* —→

It was still warm in the late-afternoon sun, and the city noises came muffled through the trees in the park. She put her book down on the bench, removed her sunglasses, and sighed contentedly. Morton was reading the *Times Magazine* section, one arm flung around her shoulder; their three-year-old son, Larry, was playing in the sandbox: a faint breeze fanned her hair softly against her cheek. It was five-thirty of a Sunday afternoon, and the small playground, tucked away in a corner of the park, was all but deserted. The swings and seesaws stood motionless and abandoned, the slides were empty, and only in the sandbox two little boys squatted diligently side by side. *How good this is*, she thought, and almost smiled at her sense of well-being. They must go out in the sun more often; Morton was so city-pale, cooped up all week inside the gray factorylike university. She squeezed his arm affectionately and glanced at Larry, delighting in the pointed little face frowning in concentration over the tunnel he was digging. The other boy suddenly stood up and with a quick, deliberate swing of his chubby arm threw a spadeful of sand at Larry. It just missed his head. Larry continued digging; the boy remained standing, shovel raised, stolid and impassive.

"No, no, little boy." She shook her finger at him, her eyes searching for the child's mother or nurse. "We mustn't throw sand. It may get in someone's eyes and hurt. We must play nicely in the nice sandbox." The boy looked at her in unblinking expectancy. He was about Larry's age but perhaps ten pounds heavier, a husky little boy with none of Larry's quickness and sensitivity in his face. Where was his mother? The only other people left in the playground were two women and a little girl on roller skates leaving now through the gate, and a man on a bench a few feet away. He was a big man, and he seemed to be taking up the whole bench as he held the Sunday comics close to his face. She supposed he was the child's father. He did not look up from his comics, but spat once deftly out of the corner of his mouth. She turned her eyes away.

At that moment, as swiftly as before, the fat little boy threw another spadeful of sand at Larry. This time some of it landed on his hair and forehead. Larry looked up at his mother, his mouth tentative; her expression would tell him whether to cry or not.

Her first instinct was to rush to her son, brush the sand out of his hair, and punish the other child, but she controlled it. She always said that she wanted Larry to learn to fight his own battles.

"Sunday in the Park" by Bel Kaufman

← Response notes →

"Don't *do* that, little boy," she said sharply, leaning forward on the bench. "You mustn't throw sand!"

The man on the bench moved his mouth as if to spit again, but instead he spoke. He did not look at her, but at the boy only.

"You go right ahead, Joe," he said loudly. "Throw all you want. This here is a *public* sandbox."

She felt a sudden weakness in her knees as she glanced at Morton. He had become aware of what was happening. He put his *Times* down carefully on his lap and turned his fine, lean face toward the man, smiling the shy, apologetic smile he might have offered a student in pointing out an error in his thinking. When he spoke to the man, it was with his usual reasonableness.

"You're quite right," he said pleasantly, "but just because this is a public place. . . ."

The man lowered his funnies and looked at Morton. He looked at him from head to foot, slowly and deliberately. "Yeah?" His insolent voice was edged with menace. "My kid's got just as good right here as yours, and if he feels like throwing sand, he'll throw it, and if you don't like it, you can take your kid the hell out of here."

The children were listening, their eyes and mouths wide open, their spades forgotten in small fists. She noticed the muscle in Morton's jaw tighten. He was rarely angry; he seldom lost his temper. She was suffused with a tenderness for her husband and an impotent rage against the man for involving him in a situation so alien and so distasteful to him.

"Now, just a minute," Morton said courteously, "you must realize. . . ."

"Aw, shut up," said the man.

Her heart began to pound. Morton half rose; the *Times* slid to the ground. Slowly the other man stood up. He took a couple of steps toward Morton, then stopped. He flexed his great arms, waiting. She pressed her trembling knees together. Would there be violence, fighting? How dreadful, how incredible. . . . She must do something, stop them, call for help. She wanted to put her hand on her husband's sleeve, to pull him down, but for some reason she didn't.

Morton adjusted his glasses. He was very pale. "This is ridiculous," he said unevenly. "I must ask you. . . ."

"Oh, yeah?" said the man. He stood with his legs spread apart, rocking a little, looking at Morton with utter scorn. "You and who else?"

For a moment the two men looked at each other nakedly. Then Morton turned his back on the man and said quietly, "Come on, let's get out of here." He walked awkwardly, almost limping with self-consciousness, to the sandbox. He stooped and lifted Larry and his shovel out.

At once Larry came to life; his face lost its rapt expression and he began to kick and cry. "I don't *want* to go home, I want to play better, I don't *want* any supper, I don't *like* supper. . . ." It became a chant as they walked, pulling their child between them, his feet dragging on

23

the ground. In order to get to the exit gate they had to pass the bench where the man sat sprawling again. She was careful not to look at him. With all the dignity she could summon, she pulled Larry's sandy, perspiring little hand, while Morton pulled the other. Slowly and with head high she walked with her husband and child out of the playground.

Her first feeling was one of relief that a fight had been avoided, that no one was hurt. Yet beneath it there was a layer of something else, something heavy and inescapable. She sensed that it was more than just an unpleasant incident, more than defeat of reason by force. She felt dimly it had something to do with her and Morton, something acutely personal, familiar, and important.

Suddenly Morton spoke. "It wouldn't have proved anything."

"What?" she asked.

"A fight. It wouldn't have proved anything beyond the fact that he's bigger than I am."

"Of course," she said.

"The only possible outcome," he continued reasonably, "would have been—what? My glasses broken, perhaps a tooth or two replaced, a couple of days' work missed—and for what? For justice? For truth?"

"Of course," she repeated. She quickened her step. She wanted only to get home and to busy herself with her familiar tasks; perhaps then the feeling, glued like heavy plaster on her heart, would be gone. *Of all the stupid, despicable bullies*, she thought, pulling harder on Larry's hand. The child was still crying. Always before she had felt a tender pity for his defenseless little body, the frail arms, the narrow shoulders with sharp, winglike shoulder blades, the thin and unsure legs, but now her mouth tightened in resentment.

"Stop crying," she said sharply. "I'm ashamed of you!" She felt as if all three of them were tracking mud along the street. The child cried louder.

If there had been an issue involved, she thought, *if there had been something to fight for. . . . But what else could he possibly have done? Allow himself to be beaten? Attempt to educate the man? Call a policeman? "Officer, there's a man in the park who won't stop his child from throwing sand on mine. . . ."* The whole thing was as silly as that, and not worth thinking about.

"Can't you keep him quiet, for Pete's sake?" Morton asked irritably.

"What do you suppose I've been trying to do?" she said.

Larry pulled back, dragging his feet.

"If you can't discipline this child, I will," Morton snapped, making a move toward the boy.

But her voice stopped him. She was shocked to hear it, thin and cold and penetrating with contempt. "Indeed?" she heard herself say. "You and who else?"

24

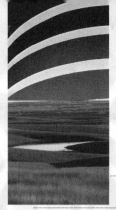

Jot comments in your response notes to indicate what you were focusing on at particular moments in the story. Then, write a response to the question: where were you, mentally and physically, while you were reading this story? Be as detailed and honest as possible. Describe what you remember seeing, thinking, and feeling as you read. Where were you most involved or detached from what was happening? Other reactions?

....

....

....

....

....

....

....

25

Compare what you wrote with that of a classmate. Discuss similarities and differences in how each of you involved yourselves in the story. Work together to write statements of advice for other readers about how to "get into" a story.

....

....

....

....

....

....

....

....

....

Readers enter the imaginative world created by authors and locate themselves in the story.

Two

Reading Experiences

Your memories and experiences influence the way you read a story. For example, a character, a scene, or a single phrase in a story may cause you to react in a certain way because of an experience you've had.

● Write about a personal experience that connects in some way to the incident or characters in "Sunday in the Park."

● "What really knocks me out is a book that, when you're all done reading it, you wish the author that wrote it was a terrific friend of yours and you could call him up on the phone whenever you felt like it." This statement from J. D. Salinger's novel *The Catcher in the Rye* reminds us that readers are not passive. Think of a time when you had a particularly strong reaction to something you read. Write a paragraph about what in your own life experiences may have influenced how you responded. What did you connect to most in the story? What did you carry away from the reading?

Your memories and experiences influence the way you read. Because of that, a story can sometimes have a different meaning for each reader.

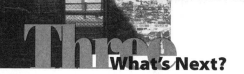

Three

What's Next?

The story unfolds as you read it. For example, here's a story start: "One rainy day I'm walking through a narrow alleyway, and as I turn the corner around a pile of battered garbage cans. . . ." What goes through your mind when you reach the word "cans"?

As your experience with the previous sentence might suggest, predicting is one of the ways that readers keep actively involved in a story. As you read the following story by the late Salvadoran writer and painter Salazar Arrué, notice what clues he gives that help you anticipate what might happen next.

"We Bad" by Salazar Arrué

Goyo Cuestas and his youngster pulled up stakes and lit out for Honduras with the phonograph. The old man carried the works over his shoulder, the kid the bag of records and the beveled trumpet element, tooled like a monstrous tin-plated bellflower that gave off the fragrance of music.

"They say there's money in Honduras."

"Yeah, Dad, and they say they've never heard of phonos there."

"Get a move on, boy—you've been dogging it since we left Mepatán."

"It's just that this saddle's about worn my crotch raw!"

"That's enough—watch your tongue!"

They laid up for a nap under the whistling and aromatic pines. Over an ocote-wood fire they warmed up coffee. Rabbits huddled in an uneasy quiet in the *sapote* grove, browsing. Goyo and the boy were approaching the wild Chamelecón. Twice they saw traces of the *carretía* snake, thin as the track of a belt. When they stopped to rest, they put on a fox trot and ate tortillas with Santa Rosa cheese. For three days they made their way through mud up to their knees. The boy broke down crying; the old man cursed and laughed at him.

The priest in Santa Rosa had cautioned Goyo not to sleep in the shelters, because gangs of thieves constantly patrolled for travelers. So at nightfall Goyo and the boy went deep into the underbrush; they cleared a little spot at the foot of a tree and there they spent the night, listening to the singing of cicadas and the buzzing of blue-tailed mosquitoes as big as spiders, not daring to breathe hard, trembling with cold and fear.

"Dad, you seen *tamagases* snakes?"

"No, boy, I checked the trunk when we turned in, and there weren't any hollows."

"If you smoke, pull down your hat, Dad. If they see the embers they'll find us."

"OK, take it easy, man. Go to sleep."

"It's just I can't sleep all bunched up."

"Stretch out, then."

"I can't, Dad, it's freezing."

"The devil with you! Curl up against me then!"

And Goyo Cuestas, who had never in his life hugged his son, took

← *Response notes* →

27

him against his foul skin, hard as a rail, and, circling his arms around him, warmed him until he was sleeping on top of him, while he, his face twisted in resignation, waited for daybreak to be signaled by some far-off rooster.

The first daylight found them there, half frozen, aching, worn out with fatigue, with ugly mouths open and driveling, half folded up in their ragged blankets, dirty, and striped like zebras.

But Honduras is deep in the Chamelecón. Honduras is deep in the silence of its rough, cruel mountains; Honduras is deep in the mystery of its terrible snakes, wildcats, insects, men. Human law does not reach to the Chamelecón; justice does not extend that far. In that region, as in primitive times, it is up to men to be good- or bad-hearted, to be cruel or magnanimous, to kill or to spare according to their own free will. Clearly the right belongs to the strong.

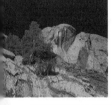

●◆ Reread the opening section and note places that hint at what might happen. Then, write your predictions below.

28

The four bandits entered through the fence and then settled in the little square of their camp, that camp stranded like a shipwreck in the wild cane plantation. They put the phonograph works between them and tried to connect the trumpet element. The full moon made flashes of silver appear on the apparatus. From a beam of their lean-to hung a piece of stinking venison.

"I tell you it's a phonograph."

"You seen how it works?"

"Yeah! In the banana plantations I seen it."

"Youdunnit!"

The trumpet worked. The highwaymen cranked it up and then opened the bag of records and lifted them to the moonlight like so many other black moons.

The bandits laughed, like children from an alien planet. Their peasant clothes were stained with something that looked like mud and that was blood.

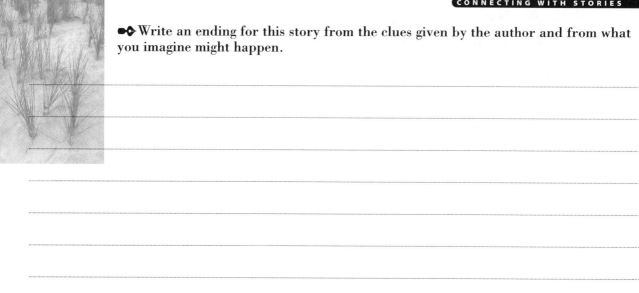

●◆ Write an ending for this story from the clues given by the author and from what you imagine might happen.

_____

_____

_____

_____

_____

_____

_____

_____

"We Bad" by Salazar Arrué

29

←—Response notes —→

In the nearby gully, Goyo and his youngster fled bit by bit in the beaks of vultures; armadillos had multiplied their wounds. Within a mass of sand, blood, clothing, and silence, their illusions, dragged there from far away, remained only as fertilizer, perhaps for a willow, perhaps for a pine.

The needle touched down, and the song flew forth on the tepid breeze like something enchanted. The coconut groves stilled their palm trees and listened in the distance. The large morning star seemed to swell and shrink, as if, suspended from a line, it was moistening itself by dipping into the still waters of the night.

A man played the guitar and sang a sorrowful song in a clear voice. It had a tearful accent, a longing for love and glory. The lower strings moaned, sighed with desire, while the lead strings hopelessly lamented an injustice.

When the phonograph stopped, the four cutthroats looked at one another. They sighed.

One of them took off, sobbing into his poncho. Another bit his lip. The oldest looked down at the barren ground, where his shadow served as his seat, and, after thinking hard, he said:

"We bad."

And the thieves of things and of lives cried, like children from an alien planet.

Stop to predict what might happen next. Take time to think about what characters will say and do or what events might take place.

Discuss with a partner or small group your reactions to the end of the story. Is it generally what you would have anticipated? How different is it from your prediction? Describe what clues were given that would help you anticipate or be surprised by the ending.

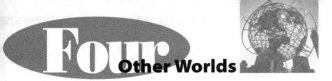

Four
Other Worlds

Stories about bullies, kids fighting in the park, and the tension between parents are not a far stretch from everyday events. You have probably read accounts of highway robbers or bandits taking advantage of people who have very little. But how do you, as reader, make sense of a story that isn't based on events that might happen in the real world?

➥ Write about your expectations for a story titled "Why Tortoise's Shell Is Not Smooth." What kind of story might this be? Does the title remind you of anything you have read before?

"Why Tortoise's Shell Is Not Smooth" by Chinua Achebe

←—Response notes—→

Low voices, broken now and again by singing, reached Okonkwo from his wives' huts as each woman and her children told folk stories. Ekwefi and her daughter, Ezinma, sat on a mat on the floor. It was Ekwefi's turn to tell a story.

"Once upon a time," she began, "all the birds were invited to a feast in the sky. They were very happy and began to prepare themselves for the great day. They painted their bodies with red cam wood and drew beautiful patterns on them with *uli*."

"Tortoise saw all these preparations and soon discovered what it all meant. Nothing that happened in the world of the animals ever escaped his notice; he was full of cunning. As soon as he heard of the great feast in the sky his throat began to itch at the very thought. There was a famine in those days and Tortoise had not eaten a good meal for two moons. His body rattled like a piece of dry stick in his empty shell. So he began to plan how he would go to the sky."

"But he had no wings," said Ezinma.

"Be patient," replied her mother. "That is the story. Tortoise had no wings, but he went to the birds and asked to be allowed to go with them."

" 'We know you too well,' said the birds when they had heard them. 'You are full of cunning and you are ungrateful. If we allow

"Why Tortoise's Shell Is Not Smooth" by Chinua Achebe

←—Response notes—→

you to come with us you will soon begin your mischief.' "

" 'You do not know me,' said Tortoise. 'I am a changed man. I have learned that a man who makes trouble for others is also making it for himself.' "

"Tortoise had a sweet tongue, and within a short time all the birds agreed that he was a changed man, and they each gave him a feather, with which he made two wings."

"At last the great day came and Tortoise was the first to arrive at the meeting place. When all the birds had gathered together, they set off in a body. Tortoise was very happy and voluble as he flew among the birds, and he was soon chosen as the man to speak for the party because he was a great orator."

" 'There is one important thing which we must not forget,' he said as they flew on their way, 'when people are invited to a great feast like this, they take new names for the occasion. Our hosts in the sky will expect us to honor this age-old custom.' "

"None of the birds had heard of this custom but they knew that Tortoise, in spite of his failings in other directions, was a widely-traveled man who knew the customs of different peoples. And so they each took a new name. When they had all taken one, Tortoise also took one. He was to be called *All of you*."

"At last the party arrived in the sky and their hosts were very happy to see them. Tortoise stood up in his many-colored plumage and thanked them for their invitation. His speech was so eloquent that all the birds were glad they had brought him, and nodded their heads in approval of all he said. Their hosts took him as the king of the birds, especially as he looked somewhat different from the others."

"After kola nuts had been presented and eaten, the people of the sky set before their guests the most delectable dishes Tortoise had even seen or dreamed of. The soup was brought out hot from the fire and in the very pot in which it had been cooked. It was full of meat and fish. Tortoise began to sniff aloud. There was pounded yam and also yam pottage cooked with palm-oil and fresh fish. There were also pots of palm-wine. When everything had been set before the guests, one of the people of the sky came forward and tasted a little from each pot. He then invited the birds to eat. But Tortoise jumped to his feet and asked: 'For whom have you prepared this feast?' "

" 'For all of you,' replied the man."

"Tortoise turned to the birds and said: 'You remember that my name is *All of you*. The custom here is to serve the spokesman first and the others later. They will serve you when I have eaten.' "

"He began to eat and the birds grumbled angrily. The people of the sky thought it must be their custom to leave all the food for their king. And so Tortoise ate the best part of the food and then drank two pots of palm-wine, so that he was full of food and drink and his body filled out in his shell."

"The birds gathered round to eat what was left and to peck at the bones he had thrown all about the floor. Some of them were too angry to eat. They chose to fly home on an empty stomach. But before they left, each took back the feather he had lent to Tortoise. And there he

31

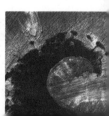

←—Response notes —→

stood in his hard shell full of food and wine but without any wings to fly home. He asked the birds to take a message for his wife, but they all refused. In the end Parrot, who had felt more angry than the others, suddenly changed his mind and agreed to take the message."

" 'Tell my wife,' said Tortoise, 'to bring out all the soft things in my house and cover the compound with them so that I can jump down from the sky without very great danger.'"

"Parrot promised to deliver the message, and then flew away. But when he reached Tortoise's house he told his wife to bring out all the hard things in the house. And so she brought out her husband's hoes, machetes, spears, guns and even his cannon. Tortoise looked down from the sky and saw his wife bringing things out, but it was too far to see what they were. When all seemed ready he let himself go. He fell and fell and fell until he began to fear that he would never stop falling. And then like the sound of his cannon he crashed on the compound."

"Did he die?" asked Ezinma.

"No," replied Ekwefi. "His shell broke into pieces. But there was a great medicine man in the neighborhood. Tortoise's wife sent for him and he gathered all the bits of shell and stuck them together. That is why Tortoise's shell is not smooth."

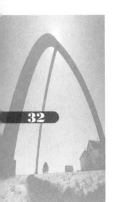

32

Writers who invite you into other worlds—through galaxies and magical forests or where turtles fly—have to help you believe.

What details in the story helped you live in this world temporarily? List some of the things that Achebe asks you to believe in the left column of the chart below. In the right column, explain how he helps you to believe. For example, the turtle flies because the birds lend him feathers.

Elements of Fantasy in Story	What Makes Them Believable
a flying turtle	the birds lend him feathers

> Sometimes writers stretch our minds as readers by taking us to far off, magical worlds built in their imaginations.

Five

Beginnings, Beginnings

Authors have to hook you and keep you interested in their stories. Usually this responsibility starts with the beginning. What can the opening of a story accomplish? Reread the opening paragraph of "Sunday in the Park," "We Bad," and "Why Tortoise's Shell Is Not Smooth." Look closely at what each author introduces and how the story starts. What do you think each author accomplishes in the opening paragraphs? What is the effect of each on you as a reader? Record what is introduced and its effect in the chart below.

	How the Story Starts	Effects on You
Sunday in the Park	sunny and peaceful	pleasant day
We Bad		
Tortoise's Shell		

33

As a reader, beginnings may help locate you, hook you, or give you necessary background. An opening not only sets the stage for what is to come but also provokes you into imagining other stories—that is, predicting from this beginning moment what might happen and how it might happen. In one way or another, a writer needs to get a reader immediately interested.

Here are some ways of beginning.

The Hook: "I knew when I decided to walk through that door that I'd be sorry for the rest of my life."

Introducing Character: "If Charlene Roberts hadn't been a flaming redhead with buck teeth and glasses thick as bottle caps, she never would have found herself in Casper, Wyoming."

Scene Setting: "The smog settled in like a thick blanket."

A Telling Detail: "The door had been left ajar. . ."

Dialogue: "Nobody said life's fair. Who sent you here to torment me?"

Read the following openings and describe in the response notes the type of story you expect will follow.

Response notes

> My father had a small romance with danger. He followed sirens, for one. Even if we were eating dinner, he'd get in his car and pursue a police car or fire engine. And he was a gambler, though he wasn't at the racetrack or the poker table when he lost everything.
>
> Stephen Dunn, from
> "Gambling: Remembrances and Assertions"

> Years later, when Lalla was almost a grandmother, she was standing in the rain at the Pettah market on her way to a party. Money was not so easily available and she did not own a car. When the bus arrived she herded herself in with the rest and, after ten minutes of standing in the aisle, found a seat where three could sit side by side. Eventually the man next to her put his arm behind her shoulder to give them all more room.
>
> Michael Ondaatje, from
> "The War Between Men and Women"

> The children were bored. It was a stifling, hot, and dusty Sunday afternoon. The children's bare feet sank ankle-deep into the dust of the great courtyard enclosed by the flour mill to the left and the house on the right. Their eyebrows were grey with dust, and when they spat, dust grated in their teeth.
> "What should we play now?" asked Manci. She was sitting on the porch steps staring at the dust in front of her. The other children hung lazily around her, standing first on one leg and then on the other; they were silent. Kalman, the watchmaker's son, wiped dust off his glases with a large walnut leaf.
>
> Tibor Déry, from "The Circus"

Authors try to hook readers with the beginnings of their stories. Strong beginnings create interest and get readers involved with a story.

Compare your charts and response notes with others. Discuss characteristics that you believe make an effective beginning for a story. Explain how looking carefully at beginnings may help you as a reader.

34

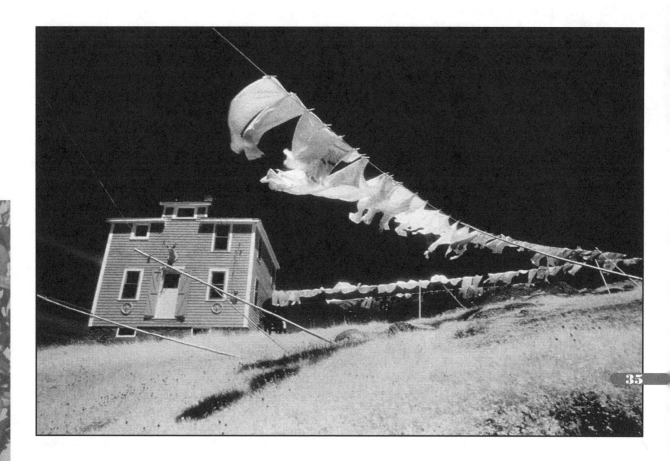

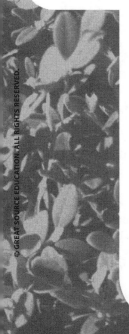

The Stories We Tell

My writing expects, demands partici- patory reading, and that I think is what lit- erature is supposed to do. It's not just about telling the story; it's about in- volving the reader. The reader supplies the emo- tions. The reader supplies even some of the color, some of the sound. My language has to have holes and spaces so the reader can come into it. He or she can feel some- thing visceral, see some- thing striking. Then we [you, the reader, and I, the author] come together to make this book, to feel this experience

The Nobel Prize-win- ning author Toni Morrison wrote this expressing her idea of the reader and the writer. Telling a good story is a challenge: How in a small amount of time or space can the writer create a memorable and persua- sive experience for the reader or listener? This is the challenge for every writer, but as Morrison points out, the reader must also work hard.

Writing stories your- self is an important part of learning about how to tell them. One of the most com- mon pieces of advice to young writers is to "write what you know." In this exploration of story, you'll read and write stories of the self, the personal nar- ratives that stick close to what's familiar.

One

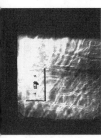

When the Subject Is "I"

Personal narratives are stories that tap into an individual's life experiences. In such stories, writers recapture memorable moments—trips, accidents, first loves, family stories. Whatever the subject matter, personal narratives have one thing in common—the story is told with "I," the first-person point of view. Why would anyone write about events they have already lived? How do these stories of self get told in effective ways? To begin, read the following excerpt from Isabel Allende's autobiographical work, *Paula*.

---

from *Paula* by Isabel Allende

← Response notes →

I place one hand over my heart, close my eyes, and concentrate. There is something dark inside. At first it is like the night air, transparent shadow, but soon it is transformed into impenetrable lead. I try to lie calmly and accept the blackness that fills my inner being as I am assaulted by images from the past. I see myself before a large mirror. I take one step backward, another, and with each step decades are erased and I grow smaller, until the glass returns the reflection of a seven-year-old girl. Me.

It has been raining for several days; I am leaping over puddles, my leather bag bouncing against my back. I am wearing a blue coat that is too large for me and a felt hat pulled down to my ears; my shoes are sodden. The huge wooden entry door, swollen by rain, is stuck; it takes all my weight to pull it open. In the garden of my grandfather's house is a gigantic poplar with roots growing above the ground, a scrawny sentinel standing guard over property that appears abandoned—shutters hanging from their hinges, paint peeling from walls. Outdoors it is just getting dark, but inside it is already deepest night. All the lights are off except in the kitchen. I walk through the garage toward the light. The walls of the cavernous kitchen are spotted with grease, and large blackened saucepans and spoons hang from iron hooks. One or two fly-specked lightbulbs cast a dull light on the scene. Something is bubbling in a pot and the kettle is whistling; the room smells of onion, and an enormous refrigerator purrs in a corner. Margara, a large woman, with strong Indian features and a thin braid wound around her head, is listening to a serial on the radio. My brothers are sitting at the table with cups of hot cocoa and buttered bread. Margara does not look up. "Go see your mother, she's in bed again," she scolds. I take off my coat and hat. "Don't strew your things about; I'm not your slave, I don't have to pick up after you." She turns up the volume on the radio. I leave the kitchen and confront the darkness in the rest of the house. I feel for the light switch and a pale glow barely fills the hall with its several doors. A claw-footed table holds the marble bust of a pensive girl; there is a mirror with a heavy wood frame, but I don't look because the Devil might be reflected in it. I shiver as I climb the stairs; currents of air swirl through an incomprehensible hole in the strange architecture. Clinging to the handrail, I reach the second floor. The climb seems interminable. I am aware of silence and shadows. I walk to the closed

from *Paula* by Isabel Allende

door at the end of the hall and tiptoe in without knocking. A stove furnishes the only illumination; the ceilings are covered with the accumulation of years of paraffin soot. There are two beds, a bunk, a sofa, tables and chairs—it is all I can do to make my way through the furniture. My mother, with Pelvina López-Pun asleep at her feet, is lying beneath a mountain of covers, her face half-hidden on the pillow: straight nose, high cheekbones, pallid skin, finely drawn eyebrows above closed eyes. "Is it you?" A small, cold hand reaches out for mine.

"Does it hurt a lot, Mama?"

"My head is bursting."

"I'll go get you a glass of warm milk and tell my brothers not to make any noise."

"Don't leave. Stay here with me. Put your hand on my forehead, that helps."

I sit on the bed and do as she asks, trembling with sympathy, not knowing how to free her from that crushing pain. Blessed Mary, Mother of God, pray for us sinners now and at the hour of our death, Amen. If she dies, my brothers and I are lost; they will send us to my father. The mere idea terrifies me. Margara is always telling me that if I don't behave I will have to go live with him. Could it be true? I have to find out, but I don't dare ask my mother, it would make her headache worse. I mustn't add to her worries or the pain will grow until her head explodes. I can't mention it to Tata, either, no one may speak my father's name in his presence. "Papa" is a forbidden word, and anyone who says it stirs up a hornet's nest. I'm hungry, I want to go down to the kitchen and drink my cocoa, but I must not leave my mother, and besides, I don't have the courage to face Margara. My shoes are wet and my feet feel like ice. I stroke my mother's poor head and concentrate: everything depends on me now. If I don't move, and pray hard, I can make the pain go away.

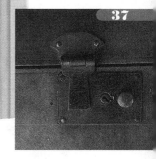

●◆ Begin with a word that accurately describes the strongest impression, image, or reaction that you had while reading this incident. Then, write about how that word helps explain what you find most interesting and effective in Allende's story.

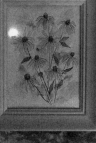

Share what you have written with others. Then, discuss what you think Allende is trying to say about herself in this scene. Explain what you think Allende might get out of writing this particular story.

Reading Allende's personal narrative may have got you thinking about some of your own experiences that would be worth writing. As she said: "I take one step backward, another, and with each step decades are erased and I grow smaller, until the glass returns the reflection of a seven-year-old girl."

As a way for you to "step backward" in time, create a memory catalog of your experiences. The catalog will include important events from your life that you think might be interesting as subjects for your writing.

List topics under each of the category headings provided below. Include words, phrases, or names that will remind you of specific experiences that you might write about. Space is provided for you to create headings of your own.

MEMORY CATALOG

Accidents	Trips	Firsts	Secrets

Special Places	Family Stories	_____	_____

Memories— and telling about them in rich detail—are what make personal narratives interesting and powerful. A memory catalog can help you find subjects to write your own personal stories.

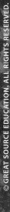

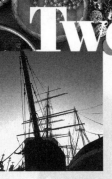

Two Story Descriptions

Your catalog probably represents the swirl of memories in your head. All of the events, people, places, possessions, and experiences that you listed have the potential to be written into personal narratives. Much of the art of writing and reading narratives is knowing how descriptions contribute to the mood or meaning of the story. It is important to understand how descriptive details create the overall effect of stories.

●◆ Reread the excerpt from Allende's *Paula* and circle three or four phrases of description that you think are particularly strong. Write about how each helps you to see, feel, or understand this incident.

....

....

....

....

....

....

39

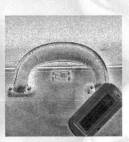

Descriptions that activate the senses are referred to as sensory descriptions. They serve to emphasize a mood or certain qualities in objects, places, or people. Sensory details evoke colors, textures, sounds, odors, visual images, and other sensations. For example, look at Allende's first paragraph description: "At first it is like the night air, transparent shadow, but soon it is transformed into impenetrable lead." There is the heaviness of feeling associated with the description of "impenetrable lead." What senses come into play with an image such as "night air, transparent shadow"? How does the description help you understand Allende's mood?

Select one sense (sight, sound, taste, smell, or touch) and trace it through the Allende excerpt, underlining every example you can find that relies on that particular sense. Then, complete the following sensory description chart.

Descriptive Details	Effect on Meaning
"impenetrable lead"	overcome by heavy feelings

[continued on next page]

SENSORY DESCRIPTION CHART

Descriptive Details	Effect on Meaning

40

●◆ Compare your sensory description chart with that of a partner's. Collaborate on writing at least two statements that explain how sensory descriptions can help intensify meaning for the reader.

Sensory descriptions not only help readers locate themselves in the story but also intensify the meaning of the story.

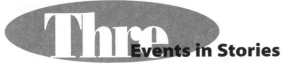

Three
Events in Stories

Stories rely on events that are interesting enough to keep the reader curious about what will happen next. As the events unfold and get resolved, various forms of suspense, tension, or conflict keep the story going. The story's plot, or how the author moves the action forward, is usually based on a three-part structure: conflict (the problem), complications (attempts to solve), and a resolution. A story plot, then, is a series of events that complicates as well as attempts to resolve the conflict.

As you read the following story, an excerpt from the novel *Annie John* by Jamaica Kincaid, notice how the relationship between events creates tension that will involve the reader in attempts to predict and participate in the steps toward resolution.

---

from ***Annie John*** by Jamaica Kincaid

← Response notes →

One afternoon, after making some outlandish claim of devotion to my work at school, I told my mother that I was going off to observe or collect —it was all the same to me—one ridiculous thing or other. I was off to see the Red Girl, of course, and I was especially happy to be going on that day because my gift was an unusually beautiful marble—a marble of blue porcelain. I had never seen a marble like it before, and from the time I first saw it I wanted very much to possess it. I had played against the girl to whom it belonged for three days in a row until finally I won all her marbles—thirty-three—except for that one. Then I had to play her and win six games in a row to get the prize—the marble made of blue porcelain. Using the usual slamming-the-gate-and-quietly-creeping-back technique, I dived under the house to retrieve the marble from the special place where I had hidden it. As I came out from under the house, what should I see before me but my mother's two enormous, canvas-clad feet. From the look on my face, she guessed immediately that I was up to something; from the look on her face, I guessed immediately that everything was over. "What do you have in your hand?" she asked, and I had no choice but to open my hand, revealing the hard-earned prize to her angrier and angrier eyes.

My mother said, "Marbles? I had heard you played marbles, but I just couldn't believe it. You were not off to look for plants at all, you were off to play marbles."

"Oh, no," I said. "Oh, no."

"Where are your other marbles?" said my mother. "If you have one, you have many."

"Oh, no," I said. "Oh, no. I don't have marbles, because I don't play marbles."

"You keep them under the house," said my mother, completely ignoring everything I said.

"Oh, no."

"I am going to find them and throw them into the deep sea," she said.

My mother now crawled under the house and began a furious and incredible search for my marbles. If she and I had been taking a walk in the Amazon forest, two of my steps equaling one of her strides, and after a while she noticed that I was no longer at her side, her search for me then would have equaled her search for my marbles now. On and on went her search—behind some planks my father had stored

41

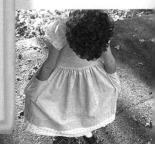

years ago for some long-forgotten use; behind some hatboxes that held old Christmas and birthday cards and old letters from my mother's family; tearing apart my neat pile of books, which, if she had opened any one of them, would have revealed to her, stamped on the title page, these words: "Public Library, Antigua." Of course, that would have been a whole other story, and I can't say which would have been worse, the stolen books or playing marbles. On it went. "Where are the marbles?" she asked. "I don't have any marbles," I would reply. "Only this one I found one day as I was crossing the street to school."

Of course I thought, at any minute I am going to die. For there were the marbles staring right at me, staring right at her. Sometimes her hand was actually resting on them. I had stored them in old cans, though my most valued ones were in an old red leather handbag of hers. There they were at her feet, as she rested for a moment, her heel actually digging into the handbag. My heart could have stopped.

My father came home. My mother postponed the rest of the search. Over supper, which, in spite of everything, I was allowed to eat with them, she told him about the marbles, adding a list of things that seemed as long as two chapters from the Old Testament. I could hardly recognise myself from this list—how horrible I was—though all of it was true. But still. They talked about me as if I weren't there sitting in front of them, as if I had boarded a boat for South America without so much as a goodbye. I couldn't remember my mother's being so angry with me ever before; in the meantime all thoughts of the Red Girl vanished from my mind. Trying then to swallow a piece of bread that I had first softened in gravy, I thought, Well, that's the end of that; if tomorrow I saw that girl on the street, I would just act as if we had never met before, as if her very presence at any time was only an annoyance. As my mother went on to my father in her angry vein, I rearranged my life: Thank God I hadn't abandoned Gwen completely, thank God I was so good at rounders that the girls would be glad to have me head a side again, thank God my breasts hadn't grown and I still needed some tips about them.

Days went by. My mother kept up the search for the marbles. How she would torment me! When I left for school, she saw me out the gate, then watched me until I was a pin on the horizon. When I came home, there she was, waiting for me. Of course, there was no longer any question of going off in the late afternoon for observations and gatherings. Not that I wanted to anyway—all that was finished. But on it would go. She would ask me for the marbles, and in my sweetest voice I would say I didn't have any. Each of us must have secretly vowed to herself not to give in to the other. But then she tried this new tack. She told me this: When she was a girl, it was her duty to accompany her father up to ground on Saturdays. When they got there, her father would check on the plantain and banana trees, the grapefruit and lime and lemon trees, and check the mongoose traps. Before returning they would harvest some food for the family to eat in the coming week: plantains, green figs, grapefruit, limes, lemons, coffee beans, cocoa beans, almonds, nutmegs, cloves, dasheen, cassavas, all

from *Annie John* by Jamaica Kincaid

depending on what was ripe to be harvested. On one particular day, after they had loaded up the donkeys with the provisions, there was an extra bunch of green figs, and my mother was to carry it on her head. She and her father started off for their home, and as they walked my mother noticed that the bunch of figs grew heavier and heavier—much heavier than any bunch of figs she had ever carried before. She ached, from the top of her neck to the base of her spine. The weight of the green figs caused her to walk slowly, and sometimes she lost sight of her father. She was alone on the road, and she heard all sorts of sounds that she had never heard before and sounds that she could not account for. Full of fright and in pain, she walked into her yard, very glad to get rid of the green figs. She no sooner had taken the load from her head when out of it crawled a very long black snake. She didn't have time to shout, it crawled away so quickly into the bushes. Perhaps from fright, perhaps from the weight of the load she had just gotten rid of, she collapsed.

When my mother came to the end of this story, I thought my heart would break. Here was my mother, a girl then, certainly no older than I, travelling up that road from the ground to her house with a snake on her head. I had seen pictures of her at that age. What a beautiful girl she was! So tall and thin. Long, thick black hair, which she wore in two plaits that hung down past her shoulders. Her back was already curved from not ever standing up straight, even though she got repeated warnings. She was so shy that she never smiled enough for you to see her teeth, and if she ever burst out laughing she would instantly cover her mouth with her hands. She always obeyed her mother, and her sister worshipped her. She, in turn, worshipped her brother, John, and when he died of something the doctor knew nothing about, of something the obeah woman knew everything about, my mother refused food for a week. Oh, to think of a dangerous, horrible black snake on top of that beautiful head; to think of those beautifully arched, pink-soled feet (the feet of which mine were an exact replica, as hers were an exact replica of her mother's) stumbling on the stony, uneven road, the weight of snake and green figs too much for that small back. If only I had been there, I would not have hesitated for even a part of a second to take her place. How I would have loved my mother if I had known her then. To have been the same age as someone so beautiful, someone who even then loved books, someone who threw stones at monkeys in the forest! What I wouldn't have done for her. Nothing would ever be too much. And so, feeling such love and such pity for this girl standing in front of me, I was on the verge of giving to my mother my entire collection of marbles. She wanted them so badly. What could some marbles matter? A snake had sat on her head for miles as she walked home. The words, "The marbles are in the corner over there" were on the very tip of my tongue, when I heard my mother, her voice warm and soft and treacherous, say to me, "Well, Little Miss, where are your marbles?" Summoning my own warm, soft, and newly acquired treacherous voice, I said, "I don't have any marbles. I have never played marbles, you know."

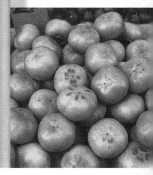

43

If this story reminds you of particular incidents in your own life worth writing about, list those in your memory catalog for future reference.

It is important to emphasize that a story needs more than a sequence of events. It needs a plot—a structure that links events to a pattern of problem, complication, and resolution. Describe the plot of Kincaid's story in the chart below.

- List four key events on the numbered lines below.
- On the lettered lines, list the two complications or conflicts that cause the tension.

1. _____

      A. _____

      B. _____

2. _____

      A. _____

      B. _____

3. _____

      A. _____

      B. _____

4. _____

      A. _____

      B. _____

●◆ Using your chart as a guide, explain the plot in three sentences.

_____
_____
_____
_____
_____
_____
_____
_____

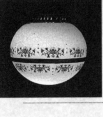

●◆ At what point in the story is the tension greatest? Describe the moment and explain how Kincaid dramatizes the tension.

_____

_____

_____

_____

_____

_____

_____

●◆ Choose one experience from your memory catalog that had some tension associated with it. In a short paragraph dramatize the situation. Try to recreate the feeling of tension.

_____

_____

_____

_____

_____

_____

_____

_____

_____

_____

_____

Plots in stories generally follow a three-part structure. The beginning introduces a conflict or problem. The middle describes a series of complications in the attempt to solve a problem. The end generally provides a resolution.

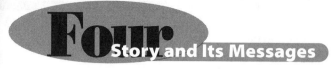
Four

When reading personal narratives, you have the opportunity to examine other people's heritage and experiences. This can, in turn, lead you to compare their experiences with yours. Personal narratives can help you understand others and the worlds in which they live. The following story, "I Get Born," is from Zora Neale Hurston's autobiography *Dust Tracks on the Road*.

from **"I Get Born"** by Zora Neale Hurston

←—Response notes—→

This is all hear-say. Maybe, some of the details of my birth as told me might be a little inaccurate, but it is pretty well established that I really did get born.

The saying goes like this. My mother's time had come and my father was not there. Being a carpenter, successful enough to have other helpers on some jobs, he was away often on building business, as well as preaching. It seems that my father was away from home for months this time. I have never been told why. But I did hear that he threatened to cut his throat when he got the news. It seems that one daughter was all that he figured he could stand. My sister, Sarah, was his favorite child, but that one girl was enough. Plenty more sons, but no more girl babies to wear out shoes and bring in nothing. I don't think he ever got over the trick he felt that I played on him by getting born a girl, and while he was off from home at that. A little of my sugar used to sweeten his coffee right now. That is a Negro way of saying his patience was short with me. Let me change a few words with him—and I am of the word-changing kind—and he was ready to change ends. Still and all, I looked more like him than any child in the house.

Of course, by the time I got born, it was too late to make any suggestions, so the old man had to put up with me. He was nice about it in a way. He didn't tie me in a sack and drop me in the lake, as he probably felt like doing.

People were digging sweet potatoes, and then it was hog-killing time. Not at our house, but it was going on in general over the country, like, being January and a bit cool. Most people were either butchering for themselves, or off helping other folks do their butchering, which was almost just as good. It is a gay time. A big pot of hasslits cooking with plenty of seasoning, lean slabs of fresh-killed pork frying for the helpers to refresh themselves after the work is done. Over and above being neighborly and giving aid, there is the food, the drinks and the fun of getting together.

So there was no grown folks close around when Mama's water broke. She sent one of the smaller children to fetch Aunt Judy, the mid-wife, but she was gone to Woodbridge, a mile and a half away, to eat at a hog-killing. The child was told to go over there and tell Aunt Judy to come. But nature, being indifferent to human arrangements, was impatient. My mother had to make it alone. She was too weak after I rushed out to do anything for herself, so she just was lying

46

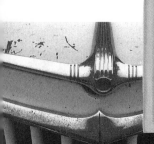

from **"I Get Born"** by Zora Neale Hurston

there, sick in the body, and worried in mind, wondering what would become of her, as well as me. She was so weak, she couldn't even reach down to where I was. She had one consolation. She knew I wasn't dead, because I was crying strong.

Help came from where she never would have thought to look for it. A white man of many acres and things, who knew the family well, had butchered the day before. Knowing that Papa was not at home, and that consequently there would be no fresh meat in our house, he decided to drive the five miles and bring a half of a shoat, sweet potatoes, and other garden stuff along. He was there a few minutes after I was born. Seeing the front door standing open, he came on in, and hollered, "Hello, there! Call your dogs!" That is the regular way to call in the country because nearly everybody who has anything to watch, has biting dogs.

Nobody answered, but he claimed later that he heard me spreading my lungs all over Orange County, so he shoved the door open and bolted on into the house.

He followed the noise and then he saw how things were, and being the kind of a man he was, he took out his Barlow Knife and cut the navel cord, then he did the best he could about other things. When the mid-wife, locally known as a granny, arrived about an hour later, there was a fire in the stove and plenty of hot water on. I had been sponged off in some sort of a way, and Mama was holding me in her arms.

As soon as the old woman got there, the white man unloaded what he had brought, and drove off cussing about some blankety-blank people never being where you could put your hands on them when they were needed.

He got no thanks from Aunt Judy. She grumbled for years about it. She complained that the cord had not been cut just right, and the belly-band had not been put on tight enough. She was mighty scared I was going to have a weak back, and that I would have trouble holding my water until I reached puberty. I did.

The next day or so a Mrs. Neale, a friend of Mama's, came in and reminded her that she had promised to let her name the baby in case it was a girl. She had picked up a name somewhere which she thought was very pretty. Perhaps, she had read it somewhere, or somebody back in those woods was smoking Turkish cigarettes. So I became Zora Neale Hurston.

There is nothing to make you like other human beings so much as doing things for them. Therefore, the man who grannied me was back next day to see how I was coming along. Maybe it was pride in his own handiwork, and his resourcefulness in a pinch, that made him want to see it through.

47

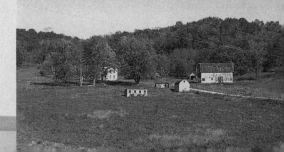

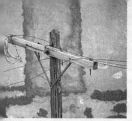

Does Hurston's story remind you of stories related to your birth, how your name was chosen, or other related incidents? Add any remembrances to your memory catalog.

As a way of summing up the message of the story, write a short reflective piece in which you explain:

• the message of the story

• what details from the story support the message

• what you learned about yourself and others from this piece

Five
On With the Story

ere's a little piece of advice from the writer Natalie Goldberg:

If I had a topic to begin with, it was easier to get started. Almost any topic was okay, because once you began, you entered your own mind and your mind had its own paths to travel. You just needed to step out of the way, but a topic was a first footstep or the twist of a doorknob into the entry of yourself. I began to look for topics, made a list of them in the back of my notebook: apples in August, shoes, my grandmother's feet, stairs I climbed. . . . When I sat down to write I could grab one of these topics off the list and begin.

from *Long, Quiet Highway*

You have a rich list of topics in your memory catalog. Choose one of the topics and write a topic sentence describing what the topic means to you. Then outline a short story on the topic.

TOPIC SENTENCE

OUTLINE

49

●◆ Write a draft with as much detail as you can remember. Use the three-part plot structure to order your story. If it is helpful, study how Allende, Kincaid, and Hurston constructed their stories to encourage the reader's participation. Use any of their techniques to help you get started or to shape and craft the story you tell.

Choosing a topic is the first step in writing a story. But how that story gets told is what creates a memorable and participatory experience for the reader.

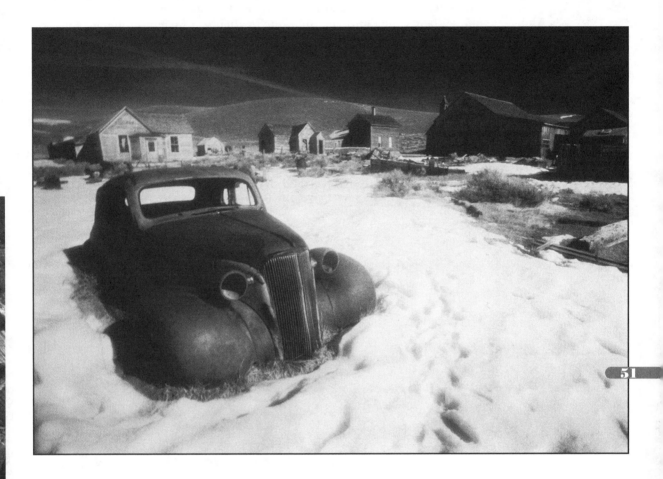

Framing and Focusing

Imagining the sensory details of the text, or doing what some readers call "making movies in the mind," is an important strategy for critical reading. We make sense of what we read by creating mental images of the people, places, and action. Often we even include sound in our mental movies.

Writers help us form mental images by the details they select. They arrange details in the most effective ways to convey their ideas. This is similar to what a photographer or filmmaker does as he or she "frames" and "focuses" a scene.

Framing and focusing are ways of shifting perspectives in reading. Active readers constantly shift from the big picture to the details and back again. Our initial impressions become more complete as we closely observe the details in the text.

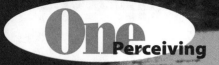

One
Perceiving

Understanding details in reading and using them in writing requires close observation. When seeing and reading, our brains first form an immediate impression about what is in front of our eyes. The image or picture of what we see gradually becomes more and more specific the longer we look. This is true with images stored in our brains, too.

Doodling as you read or listen to a poem is a way to tap into your visual images. Read or listen to someone read "The Last Wolf." In the response notes, draw pictures or symbols that come to you. Let this be subconscious, rather than conscious. The pictures and symbols you draw may not look like anything in the poem, or you may end up representing key images. If you need to, you can use some words, too, but try to rely more on pictures. You may have to read or hear the poem several times before you are finished doodling.

Response notes

52

The Last Wolf
Mary TallMountain

the last wolf hurried toward me
through the ruined city
and I heard his baying echoes
down the steep smashed warrens
of Montgomery Street and past
the few ruby-crowned highrises
left standing
their lighted elevators useless

passing the flicking red and green
of traffic signals
baying his way eastward
in the mystery of his wild loping gait
closer the sounds in the deadly night
through clutter and rubble of quiet blocks

I heard his voice ascending the hill
and at last his low whine as he came
floor by empty floor to the room
where I sat
in my narrow bed looking west, waiting
I heard him snuffle at the door and
I watched
he trotted across the floor

he laid his long gray muzzle
on the spare white spread
and his eyes burned yellow
his small dotted eyebrows quivered

Yes, I said.
I know what they have done.

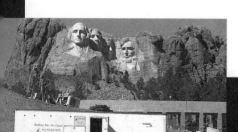

●◆ Look back at your doodling. Describe how your impression of the poem changed as you drew the figures. Then describe your impression of either the subject of the poem or the feeling the poem gives you.

53

Think about the first impression a piece of writing makes. Then shape or fine-tune your impression later as you reread.

We, as readers, want enough detail that we can actually see a scene as we read the text. We want the author to use the most significant details and organize them effectively. This framing by the author helps us visualize the text.

Note the details that Ernie Pyle has included in this excerpt about the Allied landing in Normandy during World War II. Circle the details that strike you.

---

from *Brave Men* by Ernie Pyle

←—Response notes—→

I took a walk along the historic coast of Normandy in the country of France. It was a lovely day for strolling along the seashore. Men were sleeping on the sand, some of them sleeping forever. Men were floating in the water, but they didn't know they were in the water, for they were dead.

The water was full of squishy little jellyfish about the size of a man's hand. Millions of them. In the center of each of them was a green design exactly like a four-leafed clover. The good-luck emblem. Sure. Hell, yes.

I walked for a mile and a half along the water's edge of our many-miled invasion beach. I walked slowly, for the detail on that beach was infinite.

The wreckage was vast and startling. The awful waste and destruction of war, even aside from the loss of human life, has always been one of its outstanding features to those who are in it. Anything and everything is expendable. And we did expend on our beachhead in Normandy during those first few hours.

For a mile out from the beach there were scores of tanks and trucks and boats that were not visible, for they were at the bottom of the water swamped by overloading, or hit by shells, or sunk by mines. Most of their crews were lost.

There were trucks tipped half over and swamped, partly sunken barges, and the angled-up corners of jeeps, and small landing craft half submerged. And at low tide you could still see those vicious six-pronged iron snares that helped snag and wreck them.

On the beach itself, high and dry, were all kinds of wrecked vehicles. There were tanks that had only just made the beach before being knocked out. There were jeeps that had burned to a dull gray. There were big derricks on caterpillar treads that didn't quite make it. There were halftracks carrying office equipment that had been made into a shambles by a single shell hit, their interiors still holding the useless equipage of smashed typewriters, telephones, office files.

There were LCTs turned completely upside down, and lying on their backs, and how they got that way I don't know. There were boats stacked on top of each other, their sides caved in, their suspension doors knocked off.

In this shore-line museum of carnage there were abandoned rolls of barbed wire and smashed bulldozers and big stacks of thrown-away life belts and piles of shells still waiting to be moved. In the water floated empty life rafts and soldiers' packs and ration boxes, and mysterious oranges. On the beach lay snarled rolls of telephone wire and big rolls of steel matting and stacks of broken, rusting rifles.

54

from *Brave Men* by Ernie Pyle

←—Response notes—→

On the beach lay, expended, sufficient men and mechanism for a small war. They were gone forever now. And yet we could afford it.

We could afford it because we were on, we had our toehold, and behind us there were such enormous replacements for this wreckage on the beach that you could hardly conceive of the sum total. Men and equipment were flowing from England in such a gigantic stream that it made the waste on the beachhead seem like nothing at all, really nothing at all.

But there was another and more human litter. It extended in a thin little line, just like a high-water mark, for miles along the beach. This was the strewn personal gear, gear that would never be needed again by those who fought and died to give us our entrance into Europe.

There in a jumbled row for mile on mile were soldiers' packs. There were socks and shoe polish, sewing kits, diaries, Bibles, hand grenades. There were the latest letters from home, with the address on each one neatly razored out one of the security precautions enforced before the boys embarked.

There were toothbrushes and razors, and snapshots of families back home staring up at you from the sand. There were pocketbooks, metal mirrors, extra trousers, and bloody, abandoned shoes. There were broken-handled shovels, and portable radios smashed almost beyond recognition, and mine detectors twisted and ruined.

There were torn pistol belts and canvas water buckets, first-aid kits, and jumbled heaps of life belts. I picked up a pocket Bible with a soldier's name in it, and put it in my jacket. I carried it half a mile or so and then put it back down on the beach. I don't know why I picked it up, or why I put it down again.

Soldiers carry strange things ashore with them. In every invasion there is at least one soldier hitting the beach at H-hour with a banjo slung over his shoulder. The most ironic piece of equipment marking our beach—this beach first of despair, then of victory—was a tennis racket that some soldier had brought along. It lay lonesomely on the sand, clamped in its press, not a string broken.

Two of the most dominant items in the beach refuse were cigarettes and writing paper. Each soldier was issued a carton of cigarettes just before he started. That day those cartons by the thousand, water-soaked and spilled out, marked the line of our first savage blow.

Writing paper and air-mail envelopes came second. The boys had intended to do a lot of writing in France. The letters now forever incapable of being written that might have filled those blank abandoned pages!

Always there are dogs in every invasion. There was a dog still on the beach, still pitifully looking for his masters.

He stayed at the water's edge, near a boat that lay twisted and half sunk at the waterline. He barked appealingly to every soldier who approached, trotted eagerly along with him for a few feet, and then, sensing himself unwanted in all the haste, he would run back to wait in vain for his own people at his own empty boat....

55

●✦ Use a double-entry log to examine the impression you get from this text. In the left column, list the details you circled. In the right column, tell how they made you feel.

Details	Impressions, Feelings

56

Noticing detail is essential to getting an impression of a scene.

Three
Framing the Scene

Read the excerpt from *Brave Men* again. This time, study how Pyle has organized or arranged the details. Then, discuss this excerpt with a partner. What is your reaction to it? What details did you both mark as striking? If you were a filmmaker, reading this scene as a series of shots, how would you describe Pyle's use of wide-angle shots, close-ups, and long shots? Do you think Pyle frames and focuses this scene effectively or would you suggest other ways that he might present the same details?

Pyle has created a "verbal snapshot," a written description of a place or moment in time. It is framed like a photograph to reveal some aspects of the scene but not all of them. Now, do your own framing of Pyle's text. Select one part of the scene. It might be a wide-angle shot or a close-up. Draw what you see. Your artistic ability does not matter here; the emphasis is on your perceptions.

57

Visualize the pictures writers create through the arrangements of details in descriptions.

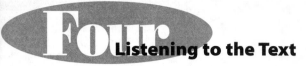

Four
Listening to the Text

Another part of visualizing a text is hearing it. Gone are the days of silent movies; we expect dialogue and soundtracks to accompany the action of today's films. Read the following excerpt from *Woodsong*, an autobiography by Gary Paulsen. Then work with the text to help you hear it better.

1. Imagine that you are going to film just a part of this scene. Select 20–25 lines of the text and add the dialogue. Dialogue could be "voice over," that is, the narrator or someone else telling the story as you see it happen. Or, you could have the main character talking to himself or the dogs.

2. Add sound effects, as suggested by the text or as you feel are necessary. They can include music or specific sounds, such as cracking branches.

Mark the text and write out the dialogue and sound effects in the margins.

from *Woodsong* by Gary Paulsen

←—Response notes—→

There was a point where an old logging trail went through a small, sharp-sided gully—a tiny canyon. The trail came down one wall of the gully—a drop of fifty or so feet—then scooted across a frozen stream and up the other side. It might have been a game trail that was slightly widened or an old foot trail that had not caved in. Whatever it was, I came onto it in the middle of January. The dogs were very excited. New trails always get them tuned up and they were fairly smoking as we came to the edge of the gully.

I did not know it was there and had been letting them run, not riding the sled brake to slow them, and we virtually shot off the edge.

The dogs stayed on the trail, but I immediately lost all control and went flying out into space with the sled. As I did, I kicked sideways, caught my knee on a sharp snag, and felt the wood enter under the kneecap and tear it loose.

I may have screamed then.

The dogs ran out on the ice of the stream but I fell onto it. As these things often seem to happen, the disaster snowballed.

The trail crossed the stream directly at the top of a small frozen waterfall with about a twenty-foot drop. Later I saw the beauty of it, the falling lobes of blue ice that had grown as the water froze and refroze, layering on itself. . . .

But at the time I saw nothing. I hit the ice of the stream bed like dropped meat, bounced once, then slithered over the edge of the waterfall and dropped another twenty feet onto the frozen pond below, landing on the torn and separated kneecap.

I have been injured several times running dogs—cracked ribs, a broken left leg, a broken left wrist, various parts frozen or cut or bitten while trying to stop fights—but nothing ever felt like landing on that knee.

I don't think I passed out so much as my brain simply exploded.

Again, I'm relatively certain I must have screamed or grunted, and then I wasn't aware of much for two, perhaps three minutes as I squirmed around trying to regain some part of my mind.

When things settled down to something I could control, I opened my eyes and saw that my snow pants and the jeans beneath were ripped in a jagged line for about a foot. Blood was welling out of the tear,

58

from **Woodsong** by Gary Paulsen

←—Response notes—→

soaking the cloth and the ice underneath the wound.

Shock and pain came in waves and I had to close my eyes several times. All of this was in minutes that seemed like hours, and I realized that I was in serious trouble. Contrary to popular belief, dog teams generally do not stop and wait for a musher who falls off. They keep going, often for many miles.

Lying there on the ice, I knew I could not walk. I didn't think I could stand without some kind of crutch, but I knew I couldn't walk. I was a good twenty miles from home, at least eight or nine miles from any kind of farm or dwelling.

It may as well have been ten thousand miles.

There was some self-pity creeping in, and not a little chagrin at being stupid enough to just let them run when I didn't know the country. I was trying to skootch myself up to the bank of the gully to get into a more comfortable position when I heard a sound over my head.

I looked up, and there was Obeah looking over the top of the waterfall, down at me.

I couldn't at first believe it.

He whined a couple of times, moved back and forth as if he might be going to drag the team over the edge, then disappeared from view. I heard some more whining and growling, then a scrabbling sound, and was amazed to see that he had taken the team back up the side of the gully and dragged them past the waterfall to get on the gully wall just over me.

They were in a horrible tangle, but he dragged them along the top until he was well below the waterfall, where he scrambled down the bank with the team almost literally falling on him. They dragged the sled up the frozen stream bed to where I was lying.

On the scramble down the bank Obeah had taken them through a thick stand of cockleburs. Great clumps of burrs wadded between their ears and down their backs.

He pulled them up to me, concern in his eyes and making a soft whine, and I reached into his ruff and pulled his head down and hugged him and was never so happy to see anybody probably in my life. Then I felt something and looked down to see one of the other dogs—named Duberry—licking the wound in my leg.

She was licking not with the excitement that prey blood would cause but with the gentle licking that she would use when cleaning a pup, a wound lick.

I brushed her head away, fearing infection, but she persisted. After a moment I lay back and let her clean it, still holding on to Obeah's ruff, holding on to a friend.

And later I dragged myself around and untangled them and unloaded part of the sled and crawled in and tied my leg down. We made it home that way, with me sitting in the sled; and later, when my leg was sewed up and healing and I was sitting in my cabin with the leg propped up on pillows by the wood stove; later, when all the pain was gone and I had all the time I needed to think of it . . . later I thought of the dogs.

How they came back to help me, perhaps to save me. I knew that somewhere in the dogs, in their humor and the way they thought, they had great, old knowledge; they had something we had lost.

And the dogs could teach me.

59

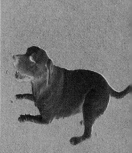

●◆ Now add the visual element. Make a story board for your 20-25 lines of *Woodsong*. Put together drawings, dialogue, and sound effects to show an action sequence. Don't worry about your artistic ability. Feel free to draw stick figures.

1.

2.

3.

4.

5.

6.

Adding sound effects and dialogue as you read helps you visualize the scene.

Five
Making Mental Movies

Sound is an essential element in understanding poetry. To read "A Poem for 'Magic,'" you need not know all of the technical terms for the sounds of poetry, such as **alliteration** or **assonance**, but you do need to "listen" carefully with both your eyes and your ears to get the full meaning of the text. Quincy Troupe provides both sound and visual images in this poem.

Read the poem silently once or twice. In the margins, write your initial impressions.

Response notes

A Poem for "Magic"
for Earvin "Magic" Johnson, Donnell Reid, and Richard Franklin
Quincy Troupe

take it to the hoop, "magic" johnson
take the ball dazzling down the open lane
herk & jerk & raise your six foot nine inch
frame into air sweating screams of your neon name
"magic" johnson, nicknamed "windex" way back in high
    school
'cause you wiped glass backboards so clean
where you first juked & shook
& wiled your way to glory
a new styled fusion of shake & bake energy
using everything possible you created your own space
to fly through any moment now we expect your wings
to spread feathers for that spooky take-off of yours
then shake & glide till you hammer home
a clotheslining deuce off glass
now, come back down with a reverse hoodoo gem
off the spin, & stick it in sweet popping nets
clean from twenty feet right side

put the ball on the floor, "magic"
slide the dribble behind your back, ease it deftly
between your bony stork legs, head bobbin everywhichaway
up & down, you see everything on the court, off the high
yoyo patter, stop & go dribble, you shoot
a threading needle rope pass sweet home to kareem
cutting through the lane, his skyhook pops the cords
now lead the fastbreak, hit worthy on the fly
now blindside a behind the back pinpointpass, for two more
off the fake, looking the other way
you raise off balance into tense space sweating chants of your
    name, turn 360 degrees

61

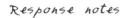
A Poem for "Magic" (continued)

on the move your legs scissoring space like a swimmer's
yoyoing motion in deep water, stretching out now
towards free flight, you double pump through human trees
hang in place, slip the ball into your left hand
then deal it like a las vegas card dealer off squared glass
into nets living up to your singular nickname, so "bad"
you cartwheel the crowd towards frenzy
wearing now your electric smile, neon as your name

in victory we suddenly sense your glorious uplift
your urgent need to be champion
& so we cheer, rejoicing with you for this quicksilver,
      quicksilver, quicksilver
moment of fame, so put the ball on the floor again, "magic"
juke & dazzle, shaking & baking down the lane
take the sucker to the hoop, "magic" johnson
recreate reverse hoodoo gems off the spin
deal alley-oop-dunk-a-thon-magician passes, now
double-pump, scissor, vamp through space, hang in place
& put it all in the sucker's face, "magic" johnson
& deal the roundball like the juju man that you am
like the sno-nuff shaman man that you am
"magic," like the shonuff spaceman you am

62

Listen to someone else read the poem. Circle all the words that describe sound, such as "cheer."

Look at the poem again. Troupe has created sound in it with his selection and arrangement of words. He has paid special attention to the **rhythm** of his subject. For example, what is the effect if you say aloud "quicksilver, quicksilver, quicksilver"? How else might Troupe have suggested a player dribbling a basketball? To understand his technique, use the chart on the next page to make lists of the ways Troupe has employed sound and visual images in this verbal snapshot of a remarkable basketball player.

SOUND WORDS	WORDS SELECTED AND ARRANGED TO SUGGEST A SPECIFIC SOUND
cheer	quicksilver, quicksilver, quicksilver

WORDS SELECTED AND ARRANGED TO SUGGEST A CHANGE IN MOVEMENT

'cause you wiped glass backboards so clean
where you first juked & shook
& wiled your way to glory

63

WORDS THAT PAINT PICTURES

double-pump, scissor, vamp through space, hang in place

Create a word bank to describe a performer. Select a basketball player, actor, actress, golfer, gymnast, musician, or someone similar. List details of sound and sight that capture the performer in action.

Performer: ....

Sound	Sight

●◆ Write a poem about the person using your sight and sound words.

Notice the ways writers play with words and images to convey both sight and sound.

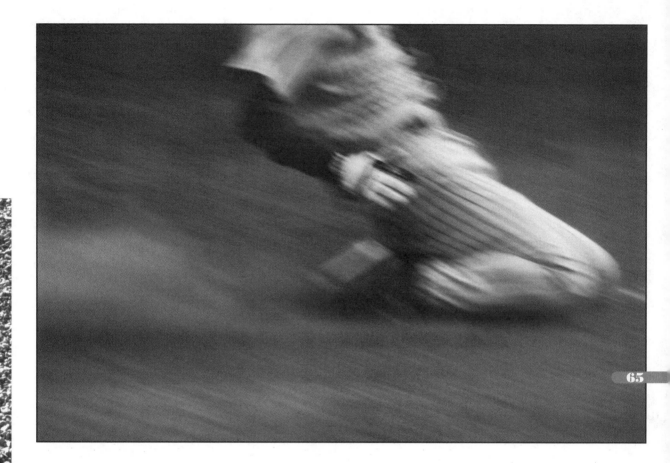

Perspectives on a Subject: Baseball

Exploring a single topic from several perspectives enriches our understanding of it. Not surprisingly, it also enriches each additional book or article we read on that topic. Actively reading each text, we compare what the writer says to our own experience and to the comments of other writers. We shape, re-shape, and express our own ideas.

Writers usually select a topic from a larger subject area. The essay, story, or poem is carefully shaped to appeal to the audience and to meet the writer's purpose. You can see how a topic is selected and shaped by focusing on one subject. In this case, the subject is baseball.

Baseball, and every-thing related to it, occu-pies a central place in the culture of the United States. For some, there is nothing more American than baseball, even when the sport isn't their personal favorite as a pastime.

One

Finding a Topic

A subject can be explored from many perspectives. Writers often think about a subject by clustering all the aspects of it they can think of. Then they narrow their focus to one topic, rather than trying to write about all of the perspectives at once. Start thinking about baseball by making a subject cluster.

As you can see below, the word "players" on the line is one perspective of the center subject "baseball." The name in the corner circle is more specific than "players," and the phrase in the smaller circle is an even more specific topic. With a partner, write words and phrases on the lines. Fill in the circles connected to those lines.

Jackie Robinson

Players

First black player in the Major Leagues

Baseball

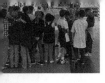

After you read the paragraph by Shirley Jackson, create a miniature subject cluster for the topic in the response notes.

from **_Raising Demons_** by Shirley Jackson

Before the children were able to start counting days till school was out, and before Laurie had learned to play more than a simple scale on the trumpet, and even before my husband's portable radio had gone in for its annual check-up so it could broadcast the Brooklyn games all summer, we found ourselves deeply involved in the Little League. The Little League was new in our town that year. One day all the kids were playing baseball in vacant lots and without any noticeable good sportsmanship, and the next day, almost, we were standing around the grocery and the post office wondering what kind of manager young Johnny Cole was going to make, and whether the Weaver boy—the one with the long arm—was going to be twelve this August, or only eleven as his mother said, and Bill Cummings had donated his bulldozer to level off the top of Sugar Hill, where the kids used to go sledding, and we were all sporting stickers on our cars reading "We have contributed" and the fundraising campaign was over the top in forty-eight hours. There are a thousand people in our town, and it turned out, astonishingly, that about sixty of them were boys of Little League age. Laurie thought he'd try out for pitcher and his friend Billy went out for catcher. Dinnertime all over town got shifted to eight-thirty in the evening, when nightly baseball practice was over. By the time our family had become accustomed to the fact that no single problem in our house could be allowed to interfere in any way with the tempering of Laurie's right arm, the uniforms had been ordered, and four teams had been chosen and named, and Laurie and Billy were together on the Little League Braves. My friend Dot, Billy's mother, was learning to keep a box score. I announced in family assembly that there would be no more oiling of baseball gloves in the kitchen sink.

$\longleftarrow$ Response notes $\longrightarrow$

67

●◆ Write a two- or three-sentence summary of Jackson's perspective on baseball. How did this story affect your perspective on the subject? Explain.

....

....

....

....

....

....

....

....

Understanding how writers focus on topics can help readers understand the structure and details of a story, poem, or essay.

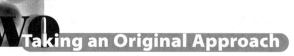

Two

Taking an Original Approach

How writers approach topics depends primarily on two factors—**audience** and **purpose**. They ask themselves questions: Who am I writing for? What is the **main idea** that I want to communicate? What reaction do I want? How can I select and shape the **details** about my topic to suit the particular audience?

Readers want to read something new and fresh, but there are only so many topics available. So writers often need to find a fresh approach to a familiar topic. Little League is a fairly common subject. Shirley Jackson approached it from the point of view of a parent, describing how family life revolved around the new team. Annie Dillard takes a different approach.

from *An American Childhood* by Annie Dillard

← Response notes →

On Tuesday summer evenings I rode my bike a mile down Braddock Avenue to a park where I watched Little League teams play ball. Little League teams did not accept girls, a ruling I looked into for several years in succession. I parked my bike and hung outside the chainlink fence and watched and rooted and got mad and hollered, "Idiot, catch the ball!" "Play's at first!" Maybe some coach would say, "Okay, sweetheart, if you know it all, you go in there." I thought of disguising myself. None of this was funny. I simply wanted to play the game earnestly, on a diamond, until it was over, with eighteen players who knew what they were doing, and an umpire. My parents were sympathetic, if amused, and not eager to make an issue of it.

At school we played softball. No bunting, no stealing. I had settled on second base, a spot Bill Mazeroski would later sanctify: lots of action, lots of talk, and especially a chance to turn the double play. Dumb softball: so much better than no ball at all, I reluctantly grew to love it. As I got older, and the prospect of having anything to do with young Ricky up the street became out of the question, I had to remind myself, with all loyalty and nostalgia, how a baseball, a real baseball, felt.

A baseball weighted your hand just so, and fit it. Its red stitches, its good leather and hardness like skin over bone, seemed to call forth a skill both easy and precise. On the catch—the grounder, the fly, the line drive—you could snag a baseball in your mitt, where it stayed, snap, like a mouse locked in its trap, not like some pumpkin of a softball you merely halted, with a terrible sound like a splat. You could curl your fingers around a baseball, and throw it in a straight line. When you hit it with a bat it cracked and your heart cracked, too, at the sound. It took a grass stain nicely, stayed round, smelled good, and lived lashed in your mitt all winter, hibernating.

There was no call for overhand pitches in softball; all my training was useless. I was playing with twenty-five girls, some of whom did not, on the face of it, care overly about the game at hand. I waited out by second and hoped for a play to the plate.

68

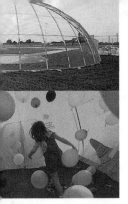

●◆Imagine you are Annie Dillard and answer the questions as she might have in the space below.

1. Who am I writing for?

2. What is the main idea that I want to communicate?

3. What reaction do I want?

4. How can I select and shape the details to suit the audience?

   Consider the commentary she includes, like "None of this was funny."

69

Topics do not have to be original, but writers need to find a fresh approach or angle on the

Developing a Topic Through a Portrait

Another approach to developing a topic is through portraits or character studies. Reading about a person related to the subject is a good way to learn about the subject. Baseball is full of potential character studies. You could learn about character, talent, and drama by reading about Hank Aaron, Pete Rose, Ty Cobb, Babe Ruth, Cal Ripken, and countless others. One major-league player stands out not only for his talent but also for his place in American history.

Jackie Robinson entered the Baseball Hall of Fame in 1962, five years after retiring from baseball. Sam Lacy of the *Baltimore Afro-American* was there to cover the induction ceremony.

"Hall of Famer Still on Cloud 9" by Sam Lacy

←— Response notes —→

Baseball ushered Jackie Robinson into immortality Monday morning, and by so doing added a touch of realism to its Hall of Fame.

The former star of the Brooklyn Dodgers was inducted along with ex-Cleveland pitcher Bob Feller, former manager Bill McKechnie, and oldtime outfielder Edd Roush, bringing to 90 the total number of onetime stars accorded the national pastime's highest honor.

Because they are done in bronze, the busts of none of the other 89 immortals enshrined here can be as lifelike as that of the first colored man to win a pedestal in the famed museum.

Not since 1936, when Ty Cobb, Babe Ruth, Honus Wagner, Christy Mathewson, and Walter Johnson became the Hall's initial honorees has the induction ceremony attracted such wide attention.

This tiny hamlet, situated between Albany and Rochester and pinpointed only on the most detailed maps of New York State, is accessible to neither train nor plane. And only two bus arrivals daily invade the quiet life of its inhabitants.

Yet thousands of persons converged on Cooperstown Sunday night, taxing its limited housing facilities to the utmost, so as to be on hand for the 10:30 a.m. ceremony.

The family of George Brown, a retired letter carrier, slept in the car in which father, mother and three children drove down from Boston Sunday evening.

"I was at Braves Field when Jackie played his first game there in 1947," Brown told the *Afro*. "I was there when Larry Doby and Satchel Paige came in for the 1948 World Series with Cleveland. And Alice [Mrs. Brown] and I used to go to Nashua [New Hampshire] and Pawtucket [Rhode Island] on weekends to watch [Roy] Campanella and [Don] Newcombe play before they were brought up.

"Wheelchair and crutches couldn't have stopped this old mailman from being here today," he beamed.

Of greater importance to Jackie, however, was the fact that the

70

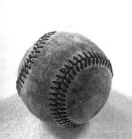

"Hall of Famer Still on Cloud 9" by Sam Lacy

←—Response notes—→

huge audience included the three persons he said "did the most in helping me attain this honor."

Watching ceremonies commemorating the event were Jackie's mother, Mrs. Mallie Robinson; his wife, Rachel; and Branch Rickey, the man who, as general manager of the Dodgers, broke baseball's color line by signing him in 1945.

In the 70-odd years of Branch Rickey there have been many thrills—too many to sift through to find his biggest.

But the induction of Jackie Robinson into baseball's Hall of Fame here Monday morning gave the kindly old man his "Greatest satisfaction."

"Robinson himself gave me many thrills," said Rickey upon renewing an old friendship. "But the term 'thrill' is too much of a generalization.

"In my time I've been thrilled by a youngster throwing a ball or stealing a base; by a minister's sermon; by a well-written book.

"This ritual today is of another category. Witnessing this final acknowledgment of the success of a wonderful experiment is highly satisfying.

"Even the six pennants for which some have said I was responsible [St. Louis in 1946, Brooklyn in 1947–49–52–53, and Pittsburgh in 1960] failed to arouse the satisfaction I get from this experience here.

"Jackie's enshrinement is perhaps the greatest satisfaction I shall derive from a life time of baseball. . . . ."

"This could not have happened," Robinson told the hushed crowd, "without the guidance and advice of Mr. Rickey, my mother and my wife."

Continuing in a voice that betrayed an inward battle to hold back the tears, Robinson declared: "I have been on 'Cloud Nine' since learning of the election last winter, and I don't think I'll ever come down."

Smiling broadly as the crowd applauded was 15-year-old Jackie Jr. On either side were the Robinsons' other two children, Sharon, aged 13, and David 10.

So it was here Monday as the ivy-covered shrine witnessed a baseball drama as ironic as it was touching.

One of the more vocal figures at the time Robinson was signed by Rickey was Feller, the ace of a formidable Cleveland pitching staff.

He unhesitatingly predicted that Jackie would be unable to make the major leagues because of "too many batting flaws."

According to the Tribe right-hander, Robinson couldn't even make the league, not to mention Hall of Fame.

On Monday, they mounted the museum's four steps to immortality together.

71

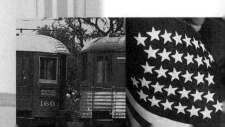

Because Sam Lacy was writing a feature story for his newspaper, he used very short paragraphs. That is common newspaper style. He also used techniques of characterization that writers of both fiction and nonfiction employ. To understand how a subject is developed through a character, go back through the feature story and mark the text with the appropriate characterization code.

Code

CS Character is revealed through what the character says to or about other people.

OS Character is revealed through what others say about him.

OD Character is revealed through what others do.

CD Character is revealed through what the character does.

DD Character is revealed through direct description by the author.

➥ Now describe someone you know. Develop your portrait by using some of the techniques explained above.

Reading about a person related to a subject provides a personal perspective on it and helps hold interest in your subject.

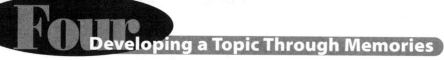

Subjects can be infused with personal feelings and memories. Reading what the writer remembers can trigger our own memories. Read Ann Hood's memoir, marking anything that connects to any of your own memories.

"Memoir" by Ann Hood

←——Response notes ——→

Baseball is in my blood. Like the light hair and eyes I inherited from my father, and the hot Italian temper I got from my mother, a love of baseball runs through my veins. Until recently, I was not sure where my passion for the sport came from. Sometimes I thought it began long ago, on summer trips to Fenway Park, when my family would drive in our oversized Chevy to Boston, park in a garage near Government Center, and take the T out to the ballpark.

As I grew older and more accustomed to our routine, my father's neatly arranged exact subway fare used to annoy me. In his pocket, I knew, he carried small bills to pay for hot dogs and beer and a souvenir program. In his wallet he had the exact amount needed to retrieve the car at day's end. What about the unknown? I used to think. But for us, that lay in the game itself. The great catch by Carlton Fisk. The Yaz home run. The pitching of Luis Tiant and Bill Lee.

It was around that same time, when my father's proclivity for careful planning bothered me, that I fell in love with the Red Sox third baseman. He was blond and blue-eyed, Number 8. I used to watch, awestruck, as he ran for balls. Once I saw him race into the dugout and emerge, arm raised high, fist clutching the baseball for an out. On our way home from games, as my father drove exactly 55, I lounged in the back seat and recalled Butch Hobson at bat, or running the bases.

In college, I dragged friends to shopping malls when he made appearances. There I would stand, in a crowd of ten-year-old boys, at Lincoln Mall, waiting for a closer look at Butch and an 8 by 10 signed photo. That photo still sits in my parent's garage, pressed into a scrapbook, surrounded by movie ticket stubs and matchbook covers and dried corsages from boys now forgotten. Sometimes I even gave Butch Hobson credit for my love of baseball.

I moved to New York City on an early summer day in 1983. It was, I remember, a perfect day for baseball. I like to think I went right then out to a ballpark, but I know this is not true. My first trip was a few days later, out to Yankee Stadium, where I was yelled at for rooting against the home team. But how could a girl from Rhode Island, a loyal Red Sox fan, become a Yankees fan? Impossible.

Like my need for a good book beside my bed, and coffee in the morning, I need baseball. So the next time the need to see a game struck me that first summer here, I boarded the number 7 train for Shea Stadium, where a young Mets team was just being formed. Butch Hobson had long ago left Boston; my heart was free. I developed a crush on the Mets' catcher, Gary Carter. I had a new apartment in a new city, a boyfriend who, in a certain light, even resembled Carter,

"Memoir" by Ann Hood

and a baseball stadium just a subway ride away. I had found my home away from home.

←—Response notes—→

Last year I won a bet. A man at a wedding I attended bet me I couldn't name the entire 1976 Red Sox team. It was a foolish bet. I had already won three margaritas from him on Mets stats.

"I know baseball," I warned him.

"Sure," he said. "Sure, you do. *Anybody* can know about the Mets. All you have to do is read the paper. But the Red Sox? 1976? Forget it."

I took a breath and began. "Yaz played first that year," I told him. He narrowed his eyes.

I continued. The names sounded almost magical. As I recited them, I remembered those trips to Fenway Park, when a ride on the T from Government Center seemed brave and exciting. "Dwight Evans," I said, like a special incantation. "Jim Rice. Fred Lynn."

The man cleared his throat. He looked at his friend. "I've never seen a girl who knows baseball like this," he said. Then he looked at me. "Third base," he said.

I smiled. "Third base," I repeated, and imagined a long ago summer when my heart soared as I watched Number 8 leap into the dugout and emerge victorious. "Third base was Butch Hobson," I said, and collected my win.

"How did you get to be such a baseball fan?" the man said, shaking his head.

Even then I did not know that it was genetic, inherited from a woman I never got to know. That day I just shrugged and said, "I love the game. That's all."

Last year I found Butch Hobson again. My father called and told me he was managing the Pawtucket Red Sox. "Remember what a crush you had on him?" He sent me clippings from the sports pages of the *Journal*, inky arrows pointing to Butch.

When he was named the new manager of the Red Sox, my father called to tell me. "Maybe you'll come back where you belong," he said. "A Red Sox fan again."

That's when I asked him, Did he remember when my love of baseball began?

He didn't. Instead, he told me this: "My mother," he said, "loved the Cincinnati Reds. Listened to every game on the radio. The saddest day in our house was when the catcher blew the World Series, went back to his hotel room, and killed himself. I'll never forget that. I was just a kid. It was the early thirties and my mother cried when she heard the news."

I never knew my father's mother. In old faded photographs she looks back at me like a stranger. Now I know she isn't. It is because of her that baseball is in my blood. Like most things, it was passed on to me, the way these days, when I leave my apartment to catch the number 7 train to Shea Stadium, I have in my pocket exactly enough change for two subway tokens, one to get me to the game, and the other to take me back home.

75

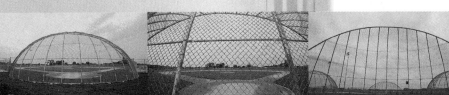

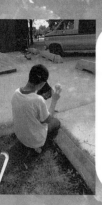

A memoir is autobiographical, but it does not have to describe the entire life of the writer. Instead, it is more of a snapshot, a significant or vivid moment or collection of moments arranged around one idea. Note how Hood organizes her memoir around a search for an answer: "Until recently, I was not sure where my passion for the sport came from." Two times in the memoir she approaches the answer, once with a hint and the second time with the conclusion. Find those places in the text and put a star by them.

◖◗Ann Hood is writing about more than baseball. Write about what stories or connections this memoir triggers for you, which may not be about baseball at all.

Some writers approach a subject through memories and personal feelings, using their experiences to reflect on an idea.

Five

Exploring the Significance of a Subject

The language of baseball can be found throughout our everyday speech. We talk about "striking out," "throwing a curve," or "heading home." These phrases represent an additional layer of meaning or significance. Circle or highlight the places in Roger Angell's essay that show the significance of certain baseball terms.

from "Celebration" by Roger Angell

← Response notes →

We were driving through East Harlem, heading for a ballgame. "Where does 'bullpen' come from?" my companion said, "I heard Ralph Kiner talking about it the other night, and he said it was from those Bull Durham tobacco billboards on the outfield fences, back in the old days. The pitchers warmed up out there, so the name carried over. That sounds logical, but it's almost too neat, don't you think? Now I suppose it's all going to get mixed up with this movie *Bull Durham*. But it would be good to know. And where does 'home plate' come from? That's a better question. I keep coming back to it, because it says so much about baseball and about other things. About ourselves. Home—'Safe at home,' 'Home is the sailor, home from sea,' and the rest of it. I make a lot of that *nostos*. But who gave it the name 'home' in baseball? It's never called 'fourth base,' you know. It must go way back to the beginnings of the game."

The light changed, and we crossed Second Avenue and swung up onto the Triborough ramp. We were on our way to Shea, and the Mets against the Reds.

"Well, there's 'Home' in Parcheesi, isn't there?" I said, digging out change for the toll. "Isn't it printed out there in the middle of the board, in that funny lettering? That's an old game, too."

"I guess so," he said.

"And what about that eighteenth-century nursery quatrain they keep reprinting in all the baseball anthologies?" I said. "You know— 'The ball once struck, off speeds the boy' . . . something, something . . . 'then home with joy'?"

"Yes, I know it," he said. "That must have been about rounders, or some other children's game. So the usage was there before there was any baseball. Sometimes I think baseball was invented just to remind us of things. It's a living memory, and it has an epic quality—you can't get away from it. Think of the man at the plate and what he wants to do up there—travel that long way around, and all just to get back where he started from, back home. He's a pioneer. He has to wander and explore, but it's dangerous out there, and he remembers the other need as well—the need to get back home. You can die at second base."

"Base runners die at third, too," I said. "Look at the Yankees lately."

"Yes, but mostly you die at second, don't you?" he went on. "I don't know why, except that it's the farthest place from home. And if you forget the home place you're lost."

"You're out," I said.

"You've got it," he said. We laughed.

"But then you have to do it again and again, and then again, no matter how hard it is," he said, not quite as an afterthought. "It's the eternal return. It's that repetition and impediment that are so much a part of the game and the legend."

"Even talking about it, it's O.K. to repeat ourselves," I said.

"Absolutely," he said, with satisfaction. "We participate in the epic by talking about it while it's in progress. It's a celebration."

●◆ With a partner, brainstorm as many baseball terms as you can. Then, pick one to explore. Write a paragraph about the significance of that term beyond baseball.

78

Searching for the significance of a subject can enlarge our understanding of it.

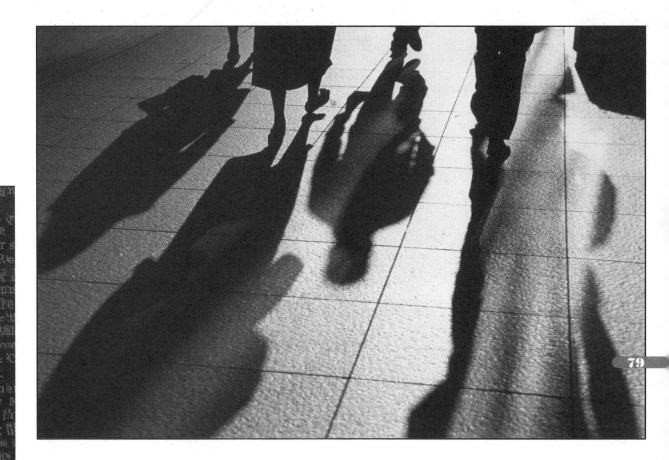

The Universe of Language

We define our world with words. They stand for all the things we know and recognize. We think with words. We talk with words. We write with words. In our reading, when we come across words that we do not know, we often skip over them. We hardly even notice them. If the same unfamiliar words occur often enough or in contexts that are important to us, we slow down, think about them, and try to understand what they mean. We then add these words to our way of perceiving the world. Our personal universe expands.

Some writers are easy for you to read. Others are more difficult. Why? One reason is that writers easy for you to read share many words that are in your universe of language. This is more than just a question of vocabulary. The words that writers select show how they view the world. Instead of seeing the world in terms of primary colors (red, yellow, blue), some writers will see the in-between colors (green, orange, purple). If you can see what a writer sees, hear what a writer hears, you will be drawn into that writer's world. Expanding your personal universe of language will let you enter new worlds and explore new ideas.

Computer experts can feed into the computer all the words used by any writer and make a wordmap of that author. It is unlike the wordmap of any other person. Read Eve Merriam's poem as an introduction to the idea of creating your own wordmap. As you read, make notes about any words that strike you as unusual, words that are a special part of Eve Merriam's wordmap. Make a note about any words that you especially like or that you think might become part of your own wordmap.

Response notes

Thumbprint
Eve Merriam

In the heel of my thumb
are whorls, whirls, wheels
in a unique design:
mine alone.
What a treasure to own!
My own flesh, my own feelings.
No other, however grand or base,
can ever contain the same.
My signature,
thumbing the pages of my time.
My universe key,
my singularity.
Impress, implant,
I am myself,
of all my atom parts I am the sum.
And out of my blood and my brain
I make my own interior weather,
my own sun and rain.
Imprint my mark upon the world,
whatever I shall become.

Words reveal an individual's way of looking at the world. How do you see the world? Find out by creating your own wordmap in the chart on the next page.

- First, make a list of 16 words for each of the five senses. Select words that are important to you. Most people tend to think first about things they can see. By selecting the same number of words for each of the senses, you pay attention to sound, smell, taste, and touch as well as sight. In choosing these words, search for the exact word to convey your meaning. For example, you might write *tomato*, not *red*, for a favorite color; *apple*, not *fruit*, for taste; *cat fur*, not *smooth*, for touch; or *horn*, not *music*, for sound.

- Next, select 10 words showing action. You may choose words that end in *-ing*, like *running*, *stretching*, *dancing*, or the simple form of a verb like, *run*, *stretch*, or *dance*.

- Now select nine "free" words: words that are important to you and don't fit anywhere else. You can include words just for the sound of them or for how they make you feel.

- Last, choose one abstraction or concept word. An abstraction represents an idea that you cannot know through your senses. For example, you cannot touch or see the concept *happiness*, but two children playing with a puppy gives you the idea of happiness. Before deciding on your abstraction, write down all of the ideas you value, such as *love*, *peace*, or *independence*. Circle one. Then create a word cluster for the word you chose as your abstraction.

81

Ideas You Value

Universe of Language Word Chart

	Sight Words	Sound Words	Taste Words	Touch Words	Smell Words	Action Words	Free Words
1							
2							
3							
4							
5							
6							
7							
8							
9							
10							
11							Abstract Word
12							
13							
14							
15							
16							

Words are sensory and authors choose them carefully to reflect the way we perceive the world with our five senses.

TWO Mapping Your Universe

Construct a wordmap or drawing of your universe of language. Include all 100 of your words in a design that reflects the way you perceive your world. You might want to use colored markers or pencils to help organize your map. Here are several ideas for drawing your world:

- Choose one word, perhaps the concept word, to provide a central picture for your map. For example, think of a way that you can make your concept word concrete. Charles Schulz, the creator of Charlie Brown and Snoopy, made the concept word *happiness* concrete when he wrote "happiness is a warm puppy." You can see and touch a warm puppy. This image expresses the feeling of the abstract idea.

- Draw an outline of the neighborhood, city, state, or country that represents your universe. You could even draw a map of an imaginary world.

- Pick any word on your sensory list that is really important to you. Use it as the outline of your world. For instance, you could draw your world inside the shape of a kitten or a convertible.

Use all of your words to make the map of your universe. Use words to make the outline of your map. Make some big, some little. Give them funny shapes or shapes of the things that they represent. Use colors, shapes, and drawings however you like, just so the map reflects how you perceive the world.

83

Thinking visually with words can help us understand how we perceive the world and what words mean to us.

It's not just the individual words in your universe that are important, it's also how you put them together to communicate your world to others that counts. Construct a poem using the words from your word chart. Your poem should show the connections between your concept word and the other words on your list. Begin by using concrete words to describe the concept. For example, if the concept word is friendship, you could start to fill in the chart like this:

Friendship is like:

Sight Words	Sound Words	Taste Words	Touch Words	Smell Words	Action Words	Free Words
a dove	guitar	honey	velvet	popcorn	a quick hug	summer vacation
the lake in a storm	a tennis ball hitting my racket	french fries with ketchup	freshly washed hair	chocolate cookies in the oven	running	old shoes

Now try it with words from your list.

_____ is like:

Sight Words	Sound Words	Taste Words	Touch Words	Smell Words	Action Words	Free Words

●◆Now, use your chart to make up a poem. Following the example below, create your poem.

The Model	Example
1. _____ is like (taste word).	Friendship is like the taste of honey.
2. _____ is like (sound word).	Friendship is like the sound of a guitar.
3. _____ is like (smell word).	Friendship is like the smell of popcorn.
4. _____ is like (touch word).	Friendship is like the feel of velvet.
5. _____ is like (free word).	Friendship is like summer vacation.
6. _____ is like (action word).	Friendship is like a quick hug.

Title: _____

85

_____
_____
_____
_____
_____
_____
_____
_____
_____
_____
_____

Working with words helps you understand how they can be used to express your thoughts, feelings, and sensations.

Every author has his or her personal wordmap. Explore one writer's universe of language by reading "The Flowers" by Alice Walker. Use the margin to write your ideas, ask questions, and note interesting words or expressions as they come up.

Response notes

The Flowers
Alice Walker

It seemed to Myop as she skipped lightly from hen house to pigpen to smokehouse that the days had never been as beautiful as these. The air held a keenness that made her nose twitch. The harvesting of the corn and cotton, peanuts and squash, made each day a golden surprise that caused excited little tremors to run up her jaws.

Myop carried a short, knobby stick. She struck out at random at chickens she liked, and worked out the beat of a song on the fence around the pigpen. She felt light and good in the warm sun. She was ten, and nothing existed for her but her song, the stick clutched in her dark brown hand, and the tat-de-ta-ta of accompaniment.

Turning her back on the rusty boards of her family's sharecropper cabin, Myop walked along the fence till it ran into the stream made by the spring. Around the spring, where the family got drinking water, silver ferns and wildflowers grew. Along the shallow banks pigs rooted. Myop watched the tiny white bubbles disrupt the thin black scale of soil and the water that silently rose and slid away down the stream.

She had explored the woods behind the house many times. Often, in late autumn, her mother took her to gather nuts among the fallen leaves. Today she made her own path, bouncing this way and that way, vaguely keeping an eye out for snakes. She found, in addition to various common but pretty ferns and leaves, an armful of strange blue flowers with velvety ridges and a sweet suds bush full of the brown, fragrant buds.

By twelve o'clock, her arms laden with sprigs of her findings, she was a mile or more from home. She had often been as far before, but the strangeness of the land made it not as pleasant as her usual haunts. It seemed gloomy in the little cove in which she found herself. The air was damp, the silence close and deep.

Myop began to circle back to the house, back to the peacefulness of the morning. It was then that she stepped smack into his eyes. Her heel became lodged in the broken ridge between brown and nose, and she reached down quickly, unafraid, to free herself. It was only when she saw his naked grin that she gave a little yelp of surprise.

He had been a tall man. From feet to neck covered a long space. His head lay beside him. When she pushed back the leaves and layers of earth and debris Myop saw that he'd had large white teeth, all of them cracked or broken, long fingers, and very big bones. All his clothes had rotted away except some threads of blue denim from his overalls. The buckles of the overalls had turned green. Myop gazed around the spot with interest. Very near where she'd stepped into the head was a wild pink rose. As she picked it to add to her bundle she noticed a raised mound, a ring, around the rose's root. It was the rotted remains of a noose, a bit of shredding plow line, now blending benignly into the soil. Around an overhanging limb of a great spreading oak clung another piece. Frayed, rotted, bleached, and frazzled—barely there—but spinning restlessly in the breeze. Myop laid down her flowers.

And the summer was over.

Response notes

Reread Alice Walker's story. Focus on sensory and action words. Which of the senses is predominant in this story? To find out, make a word chart for the story. Find at least five words for each category. If any words are new to you, try guessing at their sense by the way Walker uses them.

87

Sight Words	Sound Words	Taste Words	Touch Words	Smell Words	Action Words

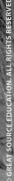

Circle any of Walker's words that are also on your list. Put an asterisk (*) by any that you might like to add to your universe of language.

● ◆ What are some of the concepts that lie behind Alice Walker's story? Select one and explain how Walker uses sensory language and action words to dramatize the meaning of the story.

By looking closely
at a writer's universe of words,
we can better understand what the
writer values and how he or she
sees the world.

No one would mistake a series of football drills (passing, tackling, wind sprints) for the real thing. Looking at the words that you or Alice Walker or anyone else uses might be compared to such exercises. We take the game apart in order to perfect our skills. We look at the words an author uses (the adjectives, the action verbs) to gain insight into the roles that specific words play in the whole piece. But let's not forget that the heart of the matter is much more than individual words. The meaning of a piece grows and changes as words become sentences, poems, stories, or essays. Read the following poem, noting interesting words or ideas as you read.

The Universe
May Swenson

What
    is it about,
  the universe,
    the universe about us stretching out?
We, within our brains,
  within it,
     think
we must unspin
the laws that spin it.
    We think *why*
  because we think
  because.
Because we think,
  we think
    the universe about us.

But does it think,
    the universe?
     Then what about?
       About us?
    If not,
must there be cause
    in the universe?
Must it have laws?
    And what
  if the universe
    is not about us?
  Then what?
    What
     is it about?
  And what
    about *us*?

Response notes

89

Now read the same words set as prose rather than poetry:

What is it about, the universe, the universe about us stretching out? We, within our brains, within it, think we must unspin the laws that spin it. We think *why* because we think *because*. Because we think, we think the universe about us. But does it think, the universe? Then what about? About us? If not, must there be cause in the universe? Must it have laws? And what if the universe is not about us? Then what? What is it about? And what about us?

How does the meaning of any of the key words change for you when you read the poem as prose? Is it easier or harder to understand?

●◆ Look at how the ends of the lines in the poem act as pauses. What differences in meaning arise from reading the lines as Swenson meant them to be read in the poem? Explain.

●◆ Look again at your universe of language. Read back through your lists carefully. Are there any words that you want to drop? Any that you want to add? Make any additions or subtractions to your list. Then explain how the words on your list reflect your world.

Words express our personalities and values. Understanding words and their nuances can help us understand what writers are trying to say.

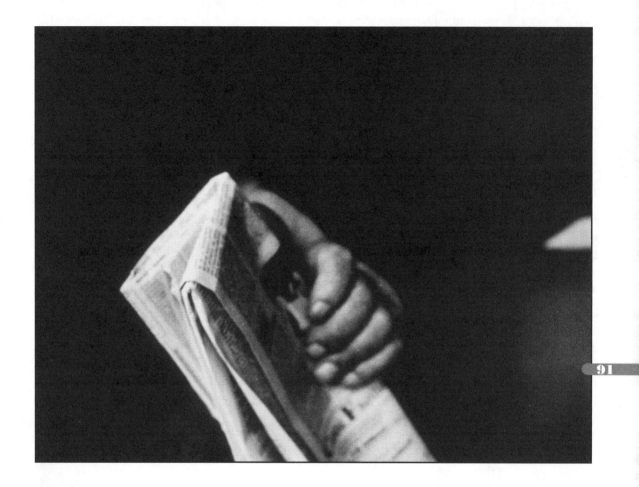

The Power of Language

The next time you are walking down a school corridor, stop talking and listen. What do you hear? Words! Hundreds of words. Happy words. Sad words. Angry words. Writers know that words are their tools. They must use them precisely to create a style.

People also make lots of comparisons as they talk and write. These comparisons are called meta-phors and can make us look at something in a new way. However, when a comparison is used over and over again, it becomes a cliché. One of the marks of a good writer is the ability to make fresh comparisons that let us see old, familiar things with new eyes.

The power of the word is not static. It is constantly being transformed in the feelings, thoughts, and actions that it stimulates in the speaker or the listener, the writer, or the reader. Words link us to the things of this world. They enable us to express our ideas and understand the ideas of others. We can look at how others use language and then try out their ideas in our own speech and writing. Just being aware of the power of language is the first step.

One
Making an Abstraction Concrete

One of the marks of good writing is the use of specific details or concrete images. A concrete image is something that you can see or hear or touch. It is something you know through your five senses. In contrast, an abstraction is an idea or concept that you can think about, but you can't see or hear or touch. Many of the common abstractions have traditional symbols that help make them real to people. For example, the American flag symbolizes the United States of America.

Choose an abstraction that is important to you. Then select a color word to describe the abstraction and three concrete image words that might stand for or symbolize the abstraction. For example, you might choose an abstraction such as peace. What color is peace? You might think of peace as white since white symbolizes a truce or a pause in fighting. Or you might think of peace as blue because it is a cool and calm color. For concrete image words that describe peace, you might choose a dove, the traditional symbol for peace. What other concrete images might you choose?

➥ Choose your words and write them below. Then draw a symbol for your abstraction in the box.

Abstraction	Color word	Three concrete image words
		1.
		2.
		3.

92

➥ Translate your drawing into words. Explain the importance of your abstraction without using the word itself.

> Good writers turn abstract ideas into powerful images by using concrete details to describe them.

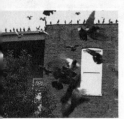

Reading and Making Metaphors

Whenever we speak of one thing in terms of another, we are using a **metaphor.** "Hope is a thing with feathers," wrote Emily Dickinson, "that perches in the soul." The idea of bird is there, but it is unspoken. Her words form a metaphor that is fresh and new. It makes us look at hope in a new way. Making comparisons that aren't overused is the mark of the good writer.

"Metaphors" by Sylvia Plath is a riddle made up of comparisons. Plath doesn't tell us the answer. Read the poem and see whether you can figure out the answer.

Response notes

Metaphors
Sylvia Plath

I'm a riddle in nine syllables,
An elephant, a ponderous house,
A melon strolling on two tendrils.
O red fruit, ivory, fine timbers!
This loaf's big with its yeasty rising.
Money's new-minted in this fat purse.
I'm a means, a stage, a cow in calf.
I've eaten a bag of green apples,
Boarded the train there's no getting off.

93

Once you know the subject of the metaphors is pregnancy it seems obvious, but it is hard to figure it out. What is not so obvious is the craft that Plath uses to construct the riddle. Look, for instance, at the number of lines in the poem. Then count the number of syllables in each line.

➤ Try making up a riddle poem in which you follow these rules:

1. Don't give away the answer in the poem.
2. Use the same number of syllables in each line.
3. Make the number of syllables and the number of lines the same.

A more subtle use of metaphor occurs in Linda Pastan's poem "Camouflage." As you read it, notice how she uses comparison.

Response notes

Camouflage
Linda Pastan

Diffused with the color
of the stone it rests on,
the chameleon turns from simile
to metaphor and back to lizard.
Summer is only camouflage.
Under the thick disguise of leaves
wait last winter's old trees;
the earth is raw clay
under a cowl of topsoil.
And what of us, walking
the spindly boardwalk,
smiles chainlinked across bone?
We say the waves like rosaries,
hour on hour, and later
flat against the sand
turn beach colored ourselves.

Pastan points out the difference between two kinds of comparisons: a *simile* uses the words *like* or *as*, making clear that one thing is not *really* the other but is just *like* it. A *metaphor*, however, states that one thing *is* the other. Explain Pastan's use of the terms *simile* and *metaphor* in the first four lines of the poem.

Reread the whole poem with the title in mind. Now write an explanation of the title of the poem, noting all the ways Pastan uses metaphor to convey her meaning.

95

A metaphor is a thoughtful comparison between two things that writers use to make us look at something in a new way. Old, overused metaphors are clichés that should be avoided.

Three

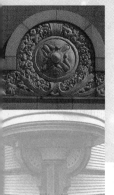

Five-Finger Exercises

While there are many traditional poetic forms, such as the ballad and the sonnet, there are also forms that poets make up just for the fun of it. They often construct elaborate rules, then set out to write practice poems similar to the "five-finger exercises" pianists use to learn dexterity. Try some "five-finger exercises" of your own.

➥ Use your five words from lesson one to write five poems. The stanza patterns (number of lines) are on the left. You may include the words anywhere in the stanza.

#1 ABSTRACT POEM

➥ Introduce abstraction and metaphors. Do not use rhyme.

Line 1   three words

Line 2   two words

Line 3   four words

Line 4   one word

Line 5   five words

#2 DESCRIPTION POEM

➥ Use a color word and a metaphor in each line.

Line 1   five words

Line 2   three words

Line 3   five words

Line 4   three word

Line 5   five words

#3 FULCRUM POEM

This is a fulcrum poem. The *fulcrum* is the center line, like the center of a teeter-totter, with each side balancing the other. Each word must have only one syllable. The word at the center should be abstract.

Line 1   three words

Line 2   one word

Line 3   three words

#4 ALLITERATION POEM

All words should begin with the same consonant sound. Use one metaphor.

One line with five words

#5 WORD WALK POEM

Take a word for a walk. Choose your own magic word. Move this word through the poem so that it appears in each "X" position. There should be six words in each line. Use color, abstraction, and metaphors in your poem.

X

    X

        X

            X

                X

                    X

After you have finished your poems, title the whole set. Then title or number each poem separately.

Writers sometimes use writing exercises to unlock their creativity by forcing theselves to use a particular form or order.

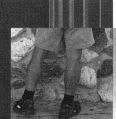

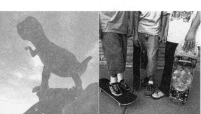

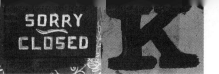

Belief in the power of words continues to influence the way we live our lives. "She is as good as her word," people say, unconsciously reaching back to a time when a person's word was a contract. In many ways, the words we have at our command influence the quality of our lives. Read the following excerpt from the introduction to one of the most widely used "how-to-do-it" books ever published.

Response notes

from *Thirty Days to a More Powerful Vocabulary*
Wilfred Funk and Norman Lewis

The study of words is not merely something that has to do with literature. Words are your tools of thought. *You can't even think at all without them.* Try it. If you are planning to go downtown this afternoon you will find that you are saying to yourself "I think I will go downtown *this afternoon.*" You can't make such a simple decision as this without using words.

Without words you could make no decisions and form no judgments whatsoever. A pianist may have the most beautiful tunes in his head, but if he had only five keys on his piano he would never get *more* than a fraction of these tunes out.

Your words are *your* keys for *your* thoughts. And the more words you have at your command the deeper, clearer and more accurate will be your thinking.

A command of English will not only improve the processes of your mind. It will give you assurance; build your self-confidence; lend color to your personality; and increase your popularity.

Your words are your personality. Your vocabulary is you. Your words are all that we, your friends, have to know and judge you by. You have *no other* medium for telling us your thoughts—for convincing us, persuading us, giving us orders.

●◆ The author uses keys as a metaphor to describe the power of language. Use a metaphor to discuss the role that words play in your own life.

Words are all that we have for expressing our thoughts. Some cultures go even further. In "Magic Words," read about an ancient belief system that has been handed down through generations.

Magic Words
Nalungiaq
translated by Edward Field

In the very earliest time,
when both people and animals lived on earth,
a person could become a human being.
Sometimes they were people
and sometimes animals
and there was no difference.
All spoke the same language.
The human mind had mysterious powers.
A word spoken by chance
might have strange consequences.
It would suddenly come alive
and what people wanted to happen could happen—
all you had to do was say it.
Nobody could explain this:
That's the way it was.

Response notes

99

●◆Compare the two pieces. What does each have to say about the power of words? Which conveys its message more effectively? Explain.

The power of language goes beyond time and culture; our words convey our personal universes.

Octavio Paz, the first Mexican to receive the Nobel Prize for Literature, wrote, "I think the mission of poetry is to create among people the possibility of wonder, admiration, enthusiasm, mystery, the sense that life is marvelous. When you say life is marvelous, you are saying a banality. But to make life a marvel—that is the role of poetry." Read the following poem to learn more about his views of the power of the word.

Response notes

Between What I See and What I Say . . .
for Roman Jakobson
Octavio Paz

1

Between what I see and what I say,
between what I say and what I keep silent,
between what I keep silent and what I dream,
between what I dream and what I forget:
poetry.
          It slips
between yes and no,
                    says
what I keep silent,
                    keeps silent
what I say,
          dreams
what I forget.
              It is not speech:
it is an act.
              It is an act
of speech.
          Poetry
speaks and listens:
                    it is real.
And as soon as I say
                    it is real
it vanishes.
          Is it then more real?

2

Tangible idea,
              intangible
word:
     poetry
comes and goes
              between what is
and what is not.

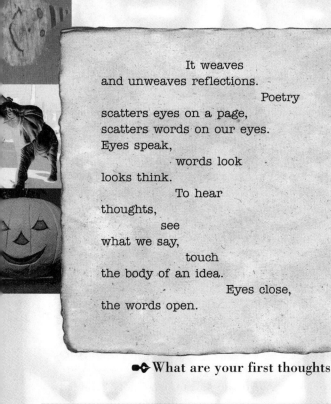

It weaves
and unweaves reflections.
                              Poetry
scatters eyes on a page,
scatters words on our eyes.
Eyes speak,
                words look
looks think.
                To hear
thoughts,
          see
what we say,
                touch
the body of an idea.
                    Eyes close,
the words open.

●◆ **What are your first thoughts about what this poem means?**

....

....

....

Write your ideas about the meaning of the selected phrases. Then select two
additional lines or passages from the poem and write your ideas about them.

Lines from the poem	*My ideas about what they mean*
It is not speech: it is an act. It is an act of speech. Poetry	
scatters eyes on a page, scatters words on our eyes.	

Read this passage in which Octavio Paz expresses his ideas about poetry and poets. As you read, note your responses to his ideas.

I have a great belief in poetry, but not in poets. Poets are the transmitters, the conduits. They are no better than other people. Poets are vain—we have many defects. We must realize that we are human beings, and be humble. Poetry is very important, but poets are not.

Poetry, in the past, was the center of society, but with modernity it has retreated to the outskirts. It has become more and more a marginal art. The situation of poetry in the United States is terrible because poets here are genuinely outside the society. This has been a great loss, especially considering that, in the twentieth century, the United States has given the world some of its greatest poets. It's a sad irony that they are not the center of American society.

I think the exile of poetry is also the exile of the best of humankind. Our society lacks the other dimension, the dimension of light and darkness that is poetry. We live in a kind of electric light—but electric light, the light of industry, is not all the light. Both primordial light and primordial darkness are part of being human, and we have tried to hide these realities.

●◆ What is your idea about the value of poetry or of poets in our society? Refer to Paz's ideas as you either agree or disagree with what he says about the "exile of poetry" in the United States.

The reader of poetry must stay with an image or an idea and read between the lines to experience a poet's deep power of language.

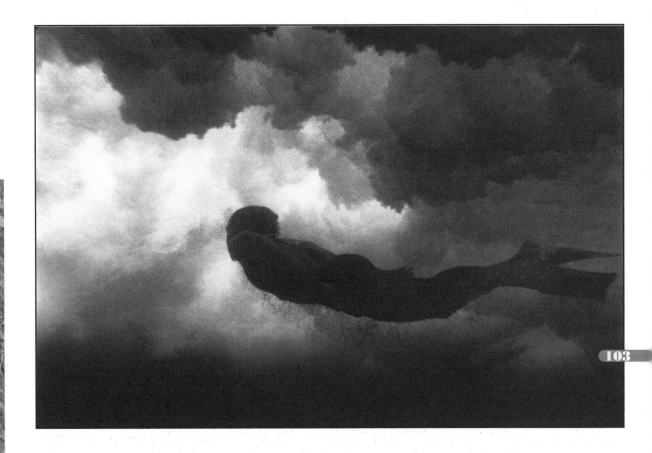

Focus on the Writer: Ursula K. Le Guin

When you read a novel or short story by Ursula K. Le Guin, you are likely to read about life in imaginary worlds such as Gethen or the twin planets of Werel and Yeowe at the far end of our universe. You will find interstellar travelers, starships, and faster-than-light communication in her science fiction. And you will encounter dragons and wizards in the king-dom of Earthsea in her fantasy.

Le Guin has written novels, short stories, books for children, poetry, and essays. She has won numerous literary awards for her out-of-this-world imaginings. Le Guin be-lieves fiction should offer readers the chance to experience new worlds—in the past, in imaginary places, in minds different from theirs. Where do writers such as Le Guin get ideas for the worlds they create? Why do they choose to imagine worlds rather than write about what is in the world around them? What are the challenges for read-ers when they are ex-pected to enter worlds very different from their own? How can an author help readers face the difficulties?

Why are we interested in novels or films that take us into fantasy worlds, the future, or outer space? Why is it that we will believe, temporarily at least, in such worlds? Long before *Star Wars* or *E.T.*, writers invited their readers to journey through galaxies, come face-to-face with aliens, and believe in magical swords, talking animals, and imaginary lands.

Le Guin specializes in these kinds of stories—what she calls thought experiments. For both writer and reader, thought experiment stories require participation in the believing game—a willingness to suspend, temporarily, the rules of the known world. In this way, the reader can play the believing game along with the writer. Look at how Le Guin introduces the world in the opening paragraphs of her novel *The Eye of the Heron*.

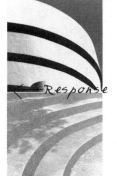

---

from *The Eye of the Heron* by Ursula K. Le Guin

← Response notes →

In the sunlight in the center of a ring of trees Lev sat cross-legged, his head bent above his hands.

A small creature crouched in the warm, shallow cup of his palms. He was not holding it; it had decided or consented to be there. It looked like a little toad with wings. The wings, folded into a peak above its back, were dun-colored with shadowy streaks, and its body was shadow-colored. Three gold eyes like large pinheads adorned its head, one on each side and one in the center of the skull. This upward-looking central eye kept watch on Lev. Lev blinked. The creature changed. Dusty pinkish fronds sprouted out from under its folded wings. For a moment it appeared to be a feathery ball, hard to see clearly, for the fronds or feathers trembled continually, blurring its outlines. Gradually the blur died away. The toad with wings sat there as before, but now it was light blue. It scratched its left eye with the hindmost of its three left feet. Lev smiled. Toad, wings, eyes, legs vanished. A flat moth-like shape crouched on Lev's palm, almost invisible because it was, except for some shadowy patches, exactly the same color and texture as his skin. He sat motionless. Slowly the blue toad with wings reappeared, one golden eye keeping watch on him. It walked across his palm and up the curve of his fingers. The six tiny, warm feet gripped and released, delicate and precise. It paused on the tip of his fingers and cocked its head to look at him with its right eye while its left and central eyes scanned the sky. It gathered itself into an arrow shape, shot out two translucent underwings twice the length of its body, and flew off in a long effortless glide toward a sunlit slope beyond the ring of trees.

"Lev?"

"Entertaining a wotsit." He got up, and joined Andre outside the tree-ring.

"Martin thinks we might get home tonight."

"Hope he's right," Lev said. He picked up his backpack and joined the end of the line of seven men. They set off in single file, not talking from *The Eye of the Heron* by Ursula K. Le Guin

←—Response notes—→

except when one down the line called to indicate to the leader a possible easier way to take, or when the second in line, carrying the compass, told the leader to bear right or left. Their direction was southwestward. The going was not hard, but there was no path and there were no landmarks. The trees of the forest grew in circles, twenty to sixty trees forming a ring around a clear central space. In the valleys of the rolling land the tree-rings grew so close, often interlocking, that the travelers' way was a constant alternation of forcing through undergrowth between dark shaggy trunks, clear going across spongy grass in the sunlit circle, then again shade, foliage, crowded stems and trunks. On the hillsides the rings grew farther apart, and sometimes there was a long view over winding valleys endlessly dappled with the soft rough red circles of the trees.

As the afternoon wore on a haze paled the sun. Clouds thickened from the west. A fine, small rain began to fall. It was mild, windless. The travelers' bare chests and shoulders shone as if oiled. Water drops clung in their hair. They went on, bearing steadily south by west. The light grew grayer. In the valleys, in the circles of the trees, the air was misty and dark.

The lead man, Martin, topping a long stony rise of land, turned and called out. One by one they climbed up and stood beside him on the crest of the ridge. Below a broad river lay shining and colorless between dark beaches.

The eldest of them, Holdfast, got to the top last and stood looking down at the river with an expression of deep satisfaction. "Hullo there," he murmured, as to a friend.

"Which way to the boats?" asked the lad with the compass.

"Upstream," Martin said, tentative.

"Down," Lev proposed. "Isn't that the high point of the ridge, west there?"

They discussed it for a minute and decided to try downstream. For a little longer before they went on they stood in silence on the ridge top, from which they had a greater view of the world than they had had for many days. Across the river the forest rolled on southward in endless interlocking ring patterns under hanging clouds. Eastward, upriver, the land rose steeply; to the west the river wound in gray levels between lower hills. Where it disappeared from sight a faint brightness lay upon it, a hint of sunlight on the open sea. Northward, behind the travelers' backs, the forested hills, the days and miles of their journey, lay darkening into the rain and night.

In all that immense, quiet landscape of hills, forest, river, no thread of smoke; no house; no road.

Circle some of the details that separate this place—the people, animals, or landscape—from ones that you'd expect to find in the world as you know it. In your response notes, explain whether or not these details help you believe in this imaginary place.

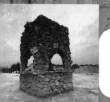

◗◆Imagine that you have been asked to design the cover for this novel. What do you know about Le Guin's world that you would want to include? Draw a cover that emphasizes her world as you imagine it.

In fantasy, or thought experiment, stories, the writer convinces the reader to believe that the fantasy elements of the story are somehow right and reasonable.

Two A Story in Ten Words

Le Guin gives an assignment to her writing workshop students that requires them to invent an artifact and think about how it might be used in a story. In the following story, Le Guin chose to use the artifact that her friend, Roussel Sargent, had created. Sargent named her artifact a "kerastion" and described it as "a musical instrument that cannot be heard." From this, Le Guin imagined a story.

from "The Kerastion" by Ursula K. Le Guin

←—Response notes—→

The small caste of the Tanners was a sacred one. To eat food prepared by a Tanner would entail a year's purification to a Tinker or a Sculptor, and even low-power castes such as the Traders had to be cleansed by a night's ablutions after dealing for leather goods. Chumo had been a Tanner since she was five years old and had heard the willows whisper all night long at the Singing Sands. She had had her proving day, and since then had worn a Tanner's madder-red and blue shirt and doublet, woven of linen on a willow-wood loom. She had made her masterpiece, and since then had worn the Master Tanner's neckband of dried vauti-tuber incised with the double line and double circles. So clothed and so ornamented she stood among the willows by the burying ground, waiting for the funeral procession of her brother, who had broken the law and betrayed his caste. She stood erect and silent, gazing towards the village by the river and listening for the drum.

She did not think; she did not want to think. But she saw her brother Kwatewa in the reeds down by the river, running ahead of her, a little boy too young to have a caste, too young to be polluted by the sacred, a crazy little boy pouncing on her out of the tall reeds shouting, "I'm a mountain lion!"

A serious little boy watching the river run, asking, "Does it ever stop? Why can't it stop running, Chumo?"

A five-year-old coming back from the Singing Sands, coming straight to her, bringing her the joy, the crazy, serious joy that shone in his round face—"Chumo! I heard the sand singing! I heard it! I have to be a Sculptor, Chumo!"

She had stood still. She had not held out her arms. And he had checked his run towards her and stood still, the light going out of his face. She was only his wombsister. He would have truesibs, now. He and she were of different castes. They would not touch again.

Ten years after that day she had come with most of the townsfolk to Kwatewa's proving day, to see the sand-sculpture he had made in the Great Plain Place where the Sculptors performed their art. Not a breath of wind had yet rounded off the keen edges or leveled the lovely curves of the classic form he had executed with such verve and sureness, the Body of Amakumo. She saw admiration and envy in the faces of his truebrothers and truesisters. Standing aside among the sacred castes, she heard the speaker of the Sculptors dedicate Kwatewa's proving piece to Amakumo. As his voice ceased a wind came out of the desert north, Amakumo's wind, the maker hungry for

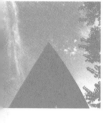

←—Response notes——→

the made—Amakumo the Mother eating her body, eating herself. Even while they watched, the wind destroyed Kwatewa's sculpture. Soon there was only a shapeless lump and a feathering of white sand blown across the proving ground. Beauty had gone back to the Mother. That the sculpture had been destroyed so soon and so utterly was a great honor to the maker.

The funeral procession was approaching. She heard or imagined she heard the drumbeat, soft, no more than a heartbeat. . . .

Le Guin must create a supporting world in which the kerastion develops some significance. List everything that you know about the society and its people. Explain what you think the information reveals about the world that Le Guin has imagined.

	What I Know About	What Is Revealed
Society	caste system by occupation	rules of behavior linked to caste
People		

●◆ Write two to three sentences speculating on how Le Guin will use the kerastion in the story.

_____

_____

_____

_____

_____

_____

_____

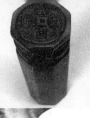

●◆Create a "kerastion" of your own. Decide what your artifact is and its characteristics. Give the artifact a name. Write a ten-word sentence about your artifact in much the same way that Roussel Sargent did: "The kerastion is a musical instrument that cannot be heard." Then write the beginning for your story.

Ten-word Sentence:

Beginning:

109

Writers of fantasy create imaginary objects that add layers of imagining to their work.

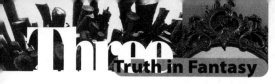

Fantasy invites readers to fasten their seatbelts for a fast-paced journey into a seemingly impossible world. Where do ideas for fantasy come from? Early in her writing career, Le Guin found the subject for one of her fantasy stories in something her daughter said. In her introduction to the following story, Le Guin writes about what sparked the idea:

> When my daughter Caroline was three she came to me with a small wooden box in her small hands and said, "Guess fwat is in this bockus!" I guessed caterpillars, mice, elephants, etc. She shook her head, smiled an unspeakably eldritch smile, opened the box slightly so that I could just see in, and said: "Darkness." Hence, this story.

from **"Darkness Box"** by Ursula K. Le Guin

←— *Response notes* —→

On soft sand by the sea's edge a little boy walked leaving no footprints. Gulls cried in the bright sunless sky, trout leaped from the saltless ocean. Far off on the horizon the sea serpent raised himself a moment in seven enormous arches and then, bellowing, sank. The child whistled but the sea serpent, busy hunting whales, did not surface again. The child walked on casting no shadow, leaving no tracks on the sand between the cliffs and the sea. Ahead of him rose a grassy headland on which stood a four-legged hut. As he climbed a path up the cliff the hut skipped about and rubbed its front legs together like a lawyer or a fly; but the hands of the clock inside, which said ten minutes of ten, never moved.

"What's that you've got there, Dicky?" asked his mother as she added parsley and a pinch of pepper to the rabbit stew simmering in an alembic.

"A box, Mummy."

"Where did you find it?"

Mummy's familiar leaped down from the onion-festooned rafters and, draping itself like a foxfur round her neck, said, "By the sea."

Dicky nodded. "That's right. The sea washed it up."

"And what's inside it?"

The familiar said nothing, but purred. The witch turned round to look into her son's round face. "What's in it?" she repeated.

"Darkness."

"Oh, Let's see."

As she bent down to look the familiar, still purring, shut its eyes. Holding the box against his chest, the little boy very carefully lifted the lid a scant inch.

"So it is," said his mother. "Now put it away, don't let it get knocked about. I wonder where the key got to. Run wash your hands now. Table, lay!" And while the child worked the heavy pump-handle in the yard and splashed his face and hands, the hut resounded with the clatter of plates and forks materializing.

After the meal, while his mother was having her morning nap, Dicky took down the water-bleached, sand-encrusted box from his treasure shelf and set out with it across the dunes, away from the sea. Close at his heels the black familiar followed him, trotting

110

from **"Darkness Box"** by Ursula K. Le Guin

patiently over the sand through the coarse grass, the only shadow he had.

At the summit of the pass Prince Rikard turned in the saddle to look back over the plumes and pennants of his army, over the long falling road, to the towered walls of his father's city. Under the sunless sky it shimmered there on the plain, fragile and shadowless as a pearl. Seeing it so he knew it could never be taken, and his heart sang with pride. He gave his captains the signal for quick march and set spurs to his horse. It reared and broke into a gallop, while his gryphon swooped and screamed overhead. She teased the white horse, diving straight down at it clashing her beak, swerving aside just in time; the horse, bridleless, would snap furiously at her snaky tail or rear to strike out with silver hoofs. The gryphon would cackle and roar, circle back over the dunes and with a screech and swoop play the trick all over. Afraid she might wear herself out before the battle, Rikard finally leashed her, after which she flew along steadily, purring and chirping, by his side.

The sea lay before him; somewhere beneath the cliffs the enemy force his brother led was hidden. The road wound down growing sandier, the sea appearing to right or left always nearer. Abruptly the road fell away; the white horse leaped the ten-foot drop and galloped out over the beach. As he came out from between the dunes Rikard saw a long line of men strung out on the sand, and behind them three black-prowed ships. His own men were scrambling down the drop, swarming over the dunes, blue flags snapping in the sea wind, voices faint against the sound of the sea.

[A battle ensues. After a difficult fight Rikard and his men push the attackers into the sea. Then, Rikard and his army head back toward the city.]

Taking an easier road homeward, Rikard passed not far from the four-legged hut on the headland. The witch stood in the doorway, hailing him. He galloped over, and, drawing rein right at the gate of the little yard, he looked at the young witch. She was bright and dark as coals, her black hair whipped in the sea wind. She looked at him, white-armored on a white horse.

"Prince," she said, "you'll go to battle once too often."

He laughed. "What should I do—let my brother lay siege to the city?"

"Yes, let him. No man can take the city."

"I know. But my father the king exiled him, he must not set foot even on our shore. I'm my father's soldier, I fight as he commands."

The witch looked out to sea, then back at the young man. Her dark face sharpened, nose and chin peaking crone-like, eyes flashing. "Serve and be served," she said, "rule and be ruled. Your brother chose neither to serve nor rule. Listen, prince, take care." Her face warmed again to beauty. "The sea brings presents this morning, the wind blows, the crystals break. Take care."

Gravely he bowed his thanks, then wheeled his horse and was gone, white as a gull over the long curve on the dunes.

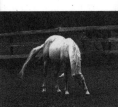

1. The character I identify most with is _____ because

_____

2. The thing that is hardest to believe is

_____

3. I think this story is about

_____

4. This story reminds me of

_____

5. The phrase that gives me the most information about what will happen in the story is

_____

112

6. The story of the battle would be different without the witch because

_____

7. The darkness in the box might represent

_____

8. The characteristics of fantasy that I noticed in the story are

_____

Note how Le Guin uses a familiar, believable scene—a young boy at the beach—and accompanies that with elements of fantasy. For example, the boy leaves no footprints, and the hut skips. Discuss with a partner how the realistic elements help you believe in Le Guin's imaginary world.

Authors often use realistic elements to make their imaginary worlds more believable.

Four: A Tissue of Lies

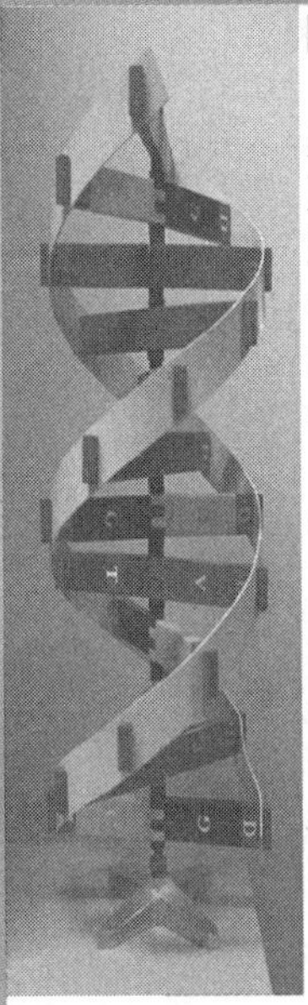

To be an effective writer of fantasy, Le Guin must give enough detail to help her readers believe in her imaginary world. She wrote in her introduction to *The Left Hand of Darkness*, "[writers] may use all kinds of facts to support their tissue of lies." To compose a tissue of lies, the writer needs to include enough information to help the reader understand the society or world that has been created. Writers extrapolate—borrow facts, objects, ideas—from the real world to give a sense of reality to their fantastical worlds. Even the weakest of ties to the known world gives a story some believability.

In what other ways does Le Guin extrapolate in order to ground her readers in the worlds of her imaginings? For example, what characteristics of the "creature" in *The Eye of the Heron* are exaggerations of natural, biological functions of an insect? How effectively does Le Guin exaggerate these natural qualities?

✒ Write a paragraph about the use of extrapolation in one of the stories. First explain how realistic elements are twisted, exaggerated, or extended to work in the more fantastical story that Le Guin creates. End the paragraph with an explanation of whether or not you think the details are effective.

Title of Story:

Writers use familiar concepts and details as a way of grounding readers in reality. That way, the fictional world connects to the world with which readers are familiar.

Dancing at the Edge of the World

What makes one writer choose to write **nonfiction** and another fantasy? Read excerpts from the speech Le Guin made to the "Lost Worlds and Future Worlds" convention to get a better understanding of her reasons for writing about the worlds she imagines.

from **"World-Making"** by Ursula K. Le Guin

← Response notes →

. . . What artists do is make a particularly skillful selection of fragments of cosmos, unusually useful and entertaining bits chosen and arranged to give an illusion of coherence and duration amidst the uncontrollable streaming of events. An artist makes the world her world. An artist makes her world the world. For a little while. For as long as it takes to look at or listen to or watch or read the work of art. Like a crystal, the work of art seems to contain the whole, and to imply eternity. And yet it is an explorer's sketch-map. A chart of shorelines on a foggy coast.

To make something is to invent it, to discover it, to uncover it, like Michelangelo cutting away the marble that hid the statue. Perhaps we think less often of the proposition reversed, thus: To discover something is to make it. As Julius Caesar said, "the existence of Britain was uncertain, until I went there." We can safely assume that the ancient Britons were perfectly certain of the existence of Britain, down to such details as where to go for the best wood. But, as Einstein said, it all depends on how you look at it, and as far as Rome, not Britain, is concerned, Caesar invented (*invenire*, "to come into, to come upon") Britain. He made it be, for the rest of the world.

Alexander the Great sat down and cried, somewhere in the middle of India, I think, because there were no more new worlds to conquer. What a silly man he was. There he sits sniveling, halfway to China! A conqueror. Conquistadores, always running into new worlds, and quickly running out of them. Conquest is not finding, and it is not making our culture, which conquered what is called the New World, and which sees the world of nature as an adversary to be conquered: look at us now. Running out of everything.

The name of our meeting is Lost Worlds and Future Worlds. Whether our ancestors came seeking gold, or freedom, or as slaves, we are the conquerors, we who live here now, in possession, in the New World. We are the inhabitants of a Lost World. It is utterly lost. Even the names are lost. . . .

And one line is left of a dancing song:

Dancing on the brink of the world.

With such fragments I might have shored my ruin, but I didn't know how. Only knowing that we must have a past to make a future with, I took what I could from the European-based cultures of my own forefathers and mothers. I learned, like most of us, to use whatever I could, to filch an idea from China and steal a god from India, and so patch together a world as best I could. But still there is a mystery.

114

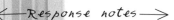

from "World-Making" by Ursula K. Le Guin

This place where I was born and grew up and love beyond all other,
my world, my California, still needs to be made. To make a new world
you start with an old one certainly. To find a world maybe you have to
have lost one. Maybe you have to be lost. The dance of renewal, the
dance that made the world, was always danced here at the edge of
things, on the brink, on the foggy coast.

←Response notes→

●◆ Write a short response to each of the following questions:

• What do you think the connection is between world-making and "dancing on the
brink of the world"?

• What does Le Guin say about why she chooses to write fantasy?

115

• What does she say about why she creates worlds from her imagination rather
than trying to describe the world in which she lives?

• What other points does she make that are particularly interesting to you?

●❖ Write a letter to a friend who is going to read Le Guin in an English class. Tell your friend what you know about Le Guin and give all the advice you can about how to approach the reading of science fiction and fantasy.

Knowing about an author's interests and reasons for writing can help the reader understand the larger meaning behind the stories.

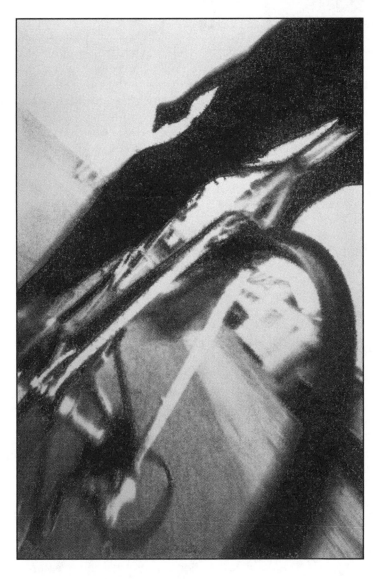

117

Essentials of Reading

There is little room in the popular conception of reading for the apprehension and appreciation of style. I had all along, I would like to think, been responding to style in my earliest attempts to read. I knew that the books I failed to enjoy—Scott's The Black Dwarf *was the worst of these—were texts that remained foggy and indeterminate, like a moving picture experienced through bad eyesight and defective hearing.*

The writer Guy Davenport is describing his own efforts to become an active reader. He recognizes that when a work confused him, it was his failure to get at the essentials of what the author wrote.

Critical readers understand that there are a few essentials to the reading process, including finding the main idea and predicting what will happen next. Among the other essentials are making inferences as you read, rereading and reflecting, and identifying and understanding the author's themes. Equally important is recognizing the author's purpose for writing. In the lessons that follow, you'll examine these and other essentials of reading.

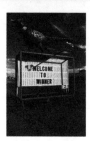

Thinking With the Writer

Active readers constantly ask themselves what will happen next or what might have caused an event or experience to have occurred. Authors encourage readers to make these kinds of predictions and examine the cause and effect of events—to hold a kind of "dialogue" with the words on the page and the person who wrote them.

"A Fable for Tomorrow" was originally published as the first chapter of Rachel Carson's book *A Silent Spring*. As you read the first part, watch for the ways Carson builds suspense and invites readers to examine what's causing the crisis in this town.

"A Fable for Tomorrow" from ***A Silent Spring*** by Rachel Carson

← *Response notes* →

There was once a town in the heart of America where all life seemed to live in harmony with its surroundings. The town lay in the midst of a checkerboard of prosperous farms, with fields of grain and hillsides of orchards where, in spring, white clouds of bloom drifted above the green fields. In autumn, oak and maple and birch set up a blaze of color that flamed and flickered across a backdrop of pines. Then foxes barked in the hills and deer silently crossed the fields, half hidden in the mists of the fall mornings.

Along the roads, laurel, viburnum and alder, great ferns and wildflowers delighted the traveler's eye through much of the year. Even in winter the roadsides were places of beauty, where countless birds came to feed on the berries and on the seed heads of the dried weeds rising above the snow. The countryside was, in fact, famous for the abundance and variety of its bird life, and when the flood of migrants was pouring through in spring and fall people traveled from great distances to observe them. Others came to fish the streams, which flowed clear and cold out of the hills and contained shady pools where trout lay. So it had been from the days many years ago when the first settlers raised their houses, sank their wells, and built their barns.

Then a strange blight crept over the area and everything began to change. Some evil spell had settled on the community: mysterious maladies swept the flocks of chickens; the cattle and sheep sickened and died. Everywhere was a shadow of death. The farmers spoke of much illness among their families. In the town the doctors had become more and more puzzled by new kinds of sickness appearing among their patients. There had been several sudden and unexplained deaths, not only among adults but even among children, who would be stricken suddenly while at play and die within a few hours.

There was a strange stillness. The birds, for example—where had they gone? Many people spoke of them, puzzled and disturbed. The feeding stations in the backyards were deserted. The few birds seen anywhere were moribund; they trembled violently and could not fly. It was a spring without voices. On the mornings that had once throbbed with the dawn chorus of robins, catbirds, doves, jays, wrens, and scores of other bird voices there was now no sound; only silence lay over the fields and woods and marsh.

118

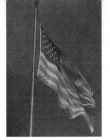

Stop at this point and think about the town Carson describes. Use the cause and effect chart to track the specifics of the crisis facing this town. In the "possible causes" column, make a list of what you think may have caused the problems. In the third column, make some educated guesses about what you think will happen next. After you've finished the chart, move on to the second part of Carson's essay.

problems Carson describes	possible causes for problems	guesses about what may happen
The chickens, cattle, and sheep have all sickened and died.	Has a virus of some sort affected them?	The virus may spread to humans and become a threat to the people in the town.

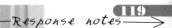

Response notes

119

On the farms the hens brooded, but no chicks hatched. The farmers complained that they were unable to raise any pigs—the litters were small and the young survived only a few days. The apple trees were coming into bloom but no bees droned among the blossoms, so there was no pollination and there would be no fruit.

The roadsides, once so attractive, were now lined with browned and withered vegetation as though swept by fire. These, too, were silent, deserted by all living things. Even the streams were now lifeless. Anglers no longer visited them, for all the fish had died.

In the gutters under the eaves and between the shingle of the roofs, a white granular powder still showed a few patches; some weeks before it had fallen like snow upon the roofs and the lawns, the fields and streams.

No witchcraft, no enemy action had silenced the rebirth of new life in this stricken world. The people had done it themselves.

This town does not actually exist, but it might easily have a thousand counterparts in America or elsewhere in the world. I know of no community that has experienced all the misfortunes I describe. Yet every one of these disasters has actually happened somewhere, and many real communities have already suffered a substantial number of them. A grim specter has crept upon us almost unnoticed, and this imagined tragedy may easily become a stark reality we all shall know.

What has already silenced the voices of spring in countless towns in America? This book is an attempt to explain.

Now that you've finished reading Carson's essay, return to your cause and effect chart and read what you wrote. Which of your guesses proved correct? Which problems remain unsolved at the end of this excerpt? Make some additional notes on the chart. Then explain what you think caused the "silent spring." Be sure you support your explanation with evidence from the text.

Active readers examine the cause and effect of events in stories. Understanding why an event occurred engages them fully in the text.

Two

Discovering the Main Idea

Almost all writing—fiction, nonfiction, or poetry—has a **main idea**. The main idea of a work is its deeper underlying meaning. Sometimes a writer will make direct statements of the main idea. Other times a writer will allow the reader to infer the main idea through **characterization**, **tone**, or **style**.

The simplest way to discover the main idea of a literary work is to first think about the subject of the piece. Then decide what the author is saying about the subject. The author's observations about the subject will often reveal the main idea.

In "Poisoned Water," another excerpt from *A Silent Spring*, Rachel Carson explains the causes for the environmental devastation she described in "A Fable for Tomorrow." As you read "Poisoned Water," keep in mind what you already know about the crisis Carson is describing. Annotate the text by underlining passages you think are significant and noting your questions in the margin.

"Poisoned Water" from *A Silent Spring* by Rachel Carson

If anyone doubts that our waters have become almost universally contaminated with insecticides he should study a small report issued by the United States Fish and Wildlife service in 1960. The Service had carried out studies to discover whether fish, like warm-blooded animals, store insecticides in their tissues. The first samples were taken from forest areas in the West where there had been mass spraying of DDT for the control of the spruce budworm. As might have been expected, all of these fish contained DDT. The really significant findings were made when the investigators turned for comparison to a creek in a remote area about 30 miles from the nearest spraying for budworm control. This creek was upstream from the first and separated from it by a high waterfall. No local spraying was known to have occurred. Yet these fish, too, contained DDT. Had the chemical reached this remote creek by hidden underground streams? Or had it been airborne, drifting down as fallout on the surface of the creek? In still another comparative study, DDT was found in the tissues of fish from a hatchery where the water supply originated in a deep well. Again there was no record of local spraying. The only possible means of contamination seemed to be by means of groundwater.

In the entire water-pollution problem, there is probably nothing more disturbing than the threat of widespread contamination of groundwater. It is not possible to add pesticides to water anywhere without threatening the purity of water everywhere. Seldom if ever does Nature operate in closed and separate compartments, and she has not done so in distributing the earth's water supply. Rain, falling on the land, settles down through pores and cracks in soil and rock, penetrating deeper and deeper until eventually it reaches a zone where all the pores of the rock are filled with water, a dark, subsurface sea, rising under hills, sinking beneath valleys. This groundwater is always on the move, sometimes at a pace so slow that it travels no more than 50 feet a year, sometimes rapidly, by

←— *Response notes* —→

121

←—Response notes—→ comparison, so that it moves nearly a tenth of a mile in a day. It travels by unseen waterways until here and there it comes to the surface as a spring, or perhaps it is tapped to feed a well. But mostly it contributes to streams and so to rivers. Except for what enters streams directly as rain or surface runoff, all the running water of the earth's surface was at one time groundwater. And so, in a very real and frightening sense, pollution of the groundwater is pollution of water everywhere.

What would you say is the main idea of "Poisoned Water"? What is the main idea of "A Fable for Tomorrow"? Use the chart below to make some notes about the subjects and main ideas of the two pieces.

	"Poisoned Water"	"A Fable for Tomorrow"
Subject		
Main Idea		

●◆After you've finished your chart, write a paragraph in which you compare and contrast the main ideas of the two essays. Explain similarities and differences.

_____

_____

_____

_____

_____

_____

_____

_____

The main idea of a work is its underlying meaning. To find the main idea, first find the subject of the piece. The main idea is what the author has to say about the subject.

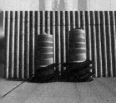

Three
Reading Between the Lines

Another essential of the reading process is the ability to make inferences as you read. (Inferences are the reasonable conclusions a person can form based on the evidence provided.) In literature, readers draw inferences about character and plot from the sometimes limited information presented by the writer. As you read this excerpt from David Guterson's award-winning novel *Snow Falling on Cedars*, underline the words, phrases, or passages that reveal (or hint at) information about the man on trial. What inferences can you make about this man? What inferences can you make about his crime?

from *Snow Falling on Cedars* by David Guterson

← Response notes →

The accused man, Kabuo Miyamoto, sat proudly upright with a rigid grace, his palms placed softly on the defendant's table—the posture of a man who has detached himself insofar as this is possible at his own trial. Some in the gallery would later say that his stillness suggested a disdain for the proceedings; others felt certain it veiled a fear of the verdict that was to come. Whichever it was, Kabuo showed nothing—not even a flicker of the eyes. He was dressed in a white shirt worn buttoned to the throat and gray, neatly pressed trousers. His figure, especially the neck and shoulders, communicated the impression of irrefutable physical strength and of precise, even imperial bearing. Kabuo's features were smooth and angular; his hair had been cropped close to his skull in a manner that made its musculature prominent. In the face of the charge that had been leveled against him he sat with his dark eyes trained straight ahead and did not appear moved at all.

In the public gallery every seat had been taken, yet the courtroom suggested nothing of the carnival atmosphere sometimes found at country murder trials. In fact, the eighty-five citizens gathered there seemed strangely subdued and contemplative. Most of them had known Carl Heine, a salmon gillnetter with a wife and three children, who was buried now in the Lutheran cemetery up on Indian Knob Hill. Most had dressed with the same communal propriety they felt on Sundays before attending church services, and since the courtroom, however stark, mirrored in their hearts the dignity of their prayer houses, they conducted themselves with churchgoing solemnity.

This courtroom, Judge Llewellyn Fielding's, down at the end of a damp, drafty hallway on the third floor of the Island County Courthouse, was run-down and small as courtrooms go. It was a place of gray-hued and bleak simplicity—a cramped gallery, a bench for the judge, a witness stand, a plywood platform for the jurors, and scuffed tables for the defendant and his prosecutor. The jurors sat with studiously impassive faces as they strained to make sense of matters. The men—two truck farmers, a retired crabber, a bookkeeper, a carpenter, a boat builder, a grocer, and a halibut schooner deckhand—were all dressed in coats and neckties. The women all wore Sunday dresses—a retired waitress, a sawmill secretary, two nervous fisher wives. A hairdresser accompanied them as alternate.

The bailiff, Ed Soames, at the request of Judge Fielding, had given a good head of steam to the sluggish radiators, which now and again

123

←—— Response notes ——→

sighed in the four corners of the room. In the heat they produced—a humid, overbearing swelter—the smell of sour mildew seemed to rise from everything.

Snow fell that morning outside the courthouse windows, four tall, narrow arches of leaded glass that yielded a great quantity of weak December light. A wind from the sea lofted snowflakes against the windowpanes, where they melted and ran toward the casements. Beyond the courthouse the town of Amity Harbor spread along the island shoreline. A few wind-whipped and decrepit Victorian mansions, remnants of a lost era of seagoing optimism, loomed out of the snowfall on the town's sporadic hills. Beyond them, cedars wove a steep mat of still green. The snow blurred from vision the clean contours of these cedar hills. The sea wind drove snowflakes steadily inland, hurling them against the fragrant trees, and the snow began to settle on the highest branches with gentle implacability.

The accused man, with one segment of his consciousness, watched the falling snow outside the windows. He had been exiled in the county jail for seventy-seven days—the last part of September, all of October and all of November, the first week of December in jail. There was no window anywhere in his basement cell, no portal through which the autumn light could come to him. He had missed autumn, he realized now—it had passed already, evaporated. The snowfall, which he witnessed out of the corners of his eyes—furious, wind-whipped flakes against the windows—struck him as infinitely beautiful.

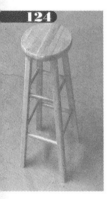

Think about the inferences you made while reading the passage. Notice how Guterson sometimes offers concrete descriptions of Kabuo Miyamoto: "He was dressed in a white shirt worn buttoned to the throat and gray, neatly pressed trousers." At other times, Guterson encourages the reader to infer information about the character: "The snowfall, which he witnessed out of the corners of his eyes—furious, wind-whipped flakes against the windows—struck him as infinitely beautiful." Using the chart below, note other inferences you can make about the character of Kabuo Miyamoto.

What you know about Kabuo	What you can infer about Kabuo

●◆After you complete the chart, take a moment to imagine you are a journalist. Write a piece describing the way Kabuo presents himself to the spectators at the trial.

125

Drawing inferences about what you read will help you understand what the author is really saying. Each inference you make will bring you one step closer to the main idea.

MAIL

Four Doubling Back

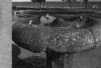

Critical readers know that allowing time for careful reflection is another essential part of reading. Most literary works require a second, and sometimes even a third, reading before they can be fully understood. During the first reading of a text, make notes about any questions you might have and mark any passages you find particularly significant. On your next reading, your notes will help you focus on the various reading essentials: making predictions, inferencing, understanding theme, and so on.

➤ Reread the excerpt from *Snow Falling on Cedars*. What do you notice on the second reading of the text that you didn't notice on the first? Explain.

➤ Now read the text again, knowing that Kabuo Miyamoto is a Japanese-American man whose family has lived for years on a small, remote island just north of the Puget Sound (in western Washington). Miyamoto has been accused of murdering Carl Heine—a salmon fisherman who also has lived for years on the island. The story takes place in 1954, less than ten years after the end of World War II. How does this knowledge change your understanding of the text? Explain.

Returning to a piece of writing for a second— and sometimes a third—reading increases your understanding of the meaning of the piece.

Five
Author's Purpose

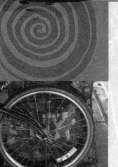

Another essential part of reading is the ability to interpret an author's purpose or intent. Sometimes an author will make a direct statement of purpose: "What has already silenced the voices of spring in countless towns in America? This book is an attempt to explain." Other times readers will need to infer the author's purpose from the language, tone, or theme.

Read this poem by the poet Sylvia Plath. As you read, keep an eye out for the author's purpose. Make sure to take notes.

Sonnet
Sylvia Plath

All right, let's say you could take a skull and break it
The way you'd crack a clock; you'd crush the bone
Between steel palms of inclination, take it,
Observing the wreck of metal and rare stone.

This was a woman: her loves and stratagems
Betrayed in mute geometry of broken
Cogs and disks, inane mechanic whims
And idle coils of jargon yet unspoken.

Not man nor demigod could put together
The scraps of rusted reverie, the wheels
Of notched tin platitudes concerning weather,
Perfume, politics, and fixed ideals.

The idiot bird leaps up and drunken leans
To chirp the hour in lunatic thirteens.

Response notes

127

❧ What would you say is Plath's purpose in this poem? Record it here.

After Plath wrote her sonnet, she sent it to her mother with a quick letter of explanation. Read Plath's letter to her mother. Watch for what she says about her intent in writing the poem.

November 3, 1951

Dear Mother,

. . . . I'm enclosing a sonnet composed when I should have been reading the Mass. It's supposed to be likening the mind to a collection of minute mechanisms, trivial and smooth-functioning when in operation, but absurd and disjointed when taken apart. In other words, the mind as a wastebasket of fragmentary knowledge, things to do, dates to remember, details, and trifling thoughts. The "idiot bird" is to further the analogy of clockwork being the cuckoo in said mechanism. See what you can derive from this chaos . . . .

Love, Sivvy

●◆ According to her letter, what was Plath's intent in writing the poem? Record it here.

_____

_____

●◆ Now think about both the letter and the sonnet. Would you say Plath's sonnet fulfills the intent she describes in her letter? Explain your answer.

_____

_____

_____

_____

_____

_____

Identifying and understanding the writer's purpose adds to your understanding of what you read.

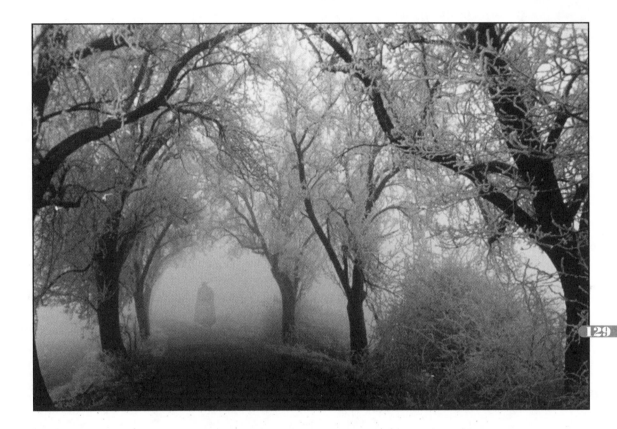

Story Landscapes

Stories may locate you in a variety of landscapes—place, time, season, in a secluded corner, behind a cypress tree, or next to a junkyard. These landscapes are the environments in which the characters of a story live and act. The time of day, sounds, smells, and weather each become a different layer of a story's setting. The various landscapes may each emphasize different aspects—physical, emotional, or spiritual. Together these landscapes constitute the setting of the story. Think, for example, of the differences in what you expect from a story that begins with "It was a dark and stormy night" and one that opens with "A gentle rain had been falling all afternoon." How do writers determine what landscapes they need to include? How do they set the scenes? How do their choices affect you as a reader? These are the types of questions to ask when examining how story landscapes affect meaning.

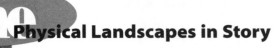

One Physical Landscapes in Story

Stories require a stage of sorts, a setting, for the action. Story landscapes add up to more than places, times, or weather conditions. Story landscapes can help a reader feel, see, and interpret meaning from the story. Pay special attention to setting in the opening paragraphs of a Ray Bradbury story.

from **"There Will Come Soft Rains"** by Ray Bradbury

←— *Response notes* —→

In the living room the voice-clock sang, *Tick-tock, seven o'clock, time to get up, time to get up, seven o'clock!* as if it were afraid that nobody would. The morning house lay empty. The clock ticked on, repeating and repeating its sounds into the emptiness. *Seven-nine, breakfast time, seven-nine!*

In the kitchen the breakfast stove gave a hissing sigh and ejected from its warm interior eight pieces of perfectly browned toast, eight eggs sunnyside up, sixteen slices of bacon, two coffees, and two cool glasses of milk.

"Today is August 4, 2026," said a second voice from the kitchen ceiling, "in the city of Allendale, California." It repeated the date three times for memory's sake. "Today is Mr. Featherstone's birthday. Today is the anniversary of Tilita's marriage. Insurance is payable, as are the water, gas, and light bills."

Somewhere in the walls, relays clicked, memory tapes glided under electric eyes.

Eight-one, tick-tock, eight-one o'clock, off to school, off to work, run, run, eight-one! But no doors slammed, no carpets took the soft tread of rubber heels. It was raining outside. The weather box on the front door sang quietly: "Rain, rain, go away; rubbers, raincoats for today . . ." And the rain tapped on the empty house, echoing.

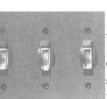

Bradbury demonstrates just how much can be told in a description of setting. What do the details reveal about the subject and meaning of this story?

●✦ Write down two or three questions that you have about what is going on in this story. Circle or highlight five to six phrases that you think give some hints at what the story is about. Talk with a partner about what you think might happen next.

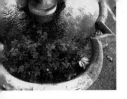

Landscapes may also be used to reveal the personalities or situations of a story's characters. As you read the opening paragraphs of Gabriel García Márquez's story "Tuesday Siesta," notice what you learn about the characters through the way García Márquez sets the scene.

from **"Tuesday Siesta"** by Gabriel García Márquez

The train emerged from the quivering tunnel of sandy rocks, began to cross the symmetrical, interminable banana plantations, and the air became humid and they couldn't feel the sea breeze any more. A stifling blast of smoke came in the car window. On the narrow road parallel to the railway there were oxcarts loaded with green bunches of bananas. Beyond the road, in uncultivated spaces set at odd intervals there were offices with electric fans, red-brick buildings, and residences with chairs and little white tables on the terraces among dusty palm trees and rosebushes. It was eleven in the morning, and the heat had not yet begun.

"You'd better close the window," the woman said. "Your hair will get full of soot."

The girl tried to, but the shade wouldn't move because of the rust. They were the only passengers in the one third-class car. Since the smoke of the locomotive kept coming through the window, the girl left her seat and put down the only things they had with them: a plastic sack with some things to eat and a bouquet of flowers wrapped in newspaper. She sat on the opposite seat, away from the window, facing her mother. They were both in severe and poor mourning clothes.

←— Response notes —→

131

Several landscapes are introduced here: 1) the train's movement and its interior; 2) the countryside; 3) character trappings, that is, the clothes or objects associated with the characters. What do you learn about the characters and their situation from each of these story landscapes?

Descriptions of:	What They Reveal:
Train stifling blast of smoke	unpleasant conditions
Countryside	
Trappings	

●◆ What are the similarities and differences in the ways Bradbury and García Márquez use setting to introduce their stories? Write two paragraphs about setting: one comparing the two settings and one that describes what setting can reveal about a story.

Writers use descriptions and
details of setting to introduce a story's landscapes.
These descriptions will often include information
about the meaning and characters
of the story.

Two Emotional Landscapes in Story

Physical landscapes locate you in a story—they give you a sense of place. A story may also contain landscapes that reflect the emotional life of characters. Emotional landscapes help readers understand what characters are thinking or how they are reacting to the events of the story. It is important to notice what characters see by how they describe what is around them. As you read "The Monkey Garden," keep in mind the various landscapes that the narrator describes.

"The Monkey Garden" from ***The House on Mango Street*** by Sandra Cisneros

←—Response notes —→

The monkey doesn't live there anymore. The monkey moved—to Kentucky—and took his people with him. And I was glad because I couldn't listen anymore to his wild screaming at night, the twangy yakkety-yak of the people who owned him. The green metal cage, the porcelain table top, the family that spoke like guitars. Monkey, family, table. All gone.

And it was then we took over the garden we had been afraid to go into when the monkey screamed and showed its yellow teeth.

There were sunflowers big as flowers on Mars and thick cockscombs bleeding the deep red fringe of theater curtains. There were dizzy bees and bow-tied fruit flies turning somersaults and humming in the air. Sweet, sweet peach trees. Thorn roses and thistle and pears. Weeds like so many squinty-eyed stars and brush that made your ankles itch and itch until you washed with soap and water. There were big green apples hard as knees. And everywhere the sleepy smell of rotting wood, damp earth and dusty hollyhocks thick and perfumy like the blue-blond hair of the dead.

Yellow spiders ran when we turned rocks over and pale worms blind and afraid of light rolled over in their sleep. Poke a stick in the sandy soil and a few blue-skinned beetles would appear, an avenue of ants, so many crusty lady bugs. This was a garden, a wonderful thing to look at in the spring. But bit by bit, after the monkey left, the garden began to take over itself. Flowers stopped obeying the little bricks that kept them from growing beyond their paths. Weeds mixed in. Dead cars appeared overnight like mushrooms. First one and then another and then a pale blue pickup with the front windshield missing. Before you knew it, the monkey garden became filled with sleepy cars.

Things had a way of disappearing in the garden, as if the garden itself ate them, or, as if with its old-man memory, it put them away and forgot them. Nenny found a dollar and a dead mouse between two rocks in the stone wall where the morning glories climbed, and once when we were playing hide and seek, Eddie Vargas laid his head beneath a hibiscus tree and fell asleep there like a Rip Van Winkle until somebody remembered he was in the game and went back to look for him.

This, I suppose, was the reason why we went there. Far away from where our mothers could find us. We and a few old dogs who lived inside the empty cars. We made a club-house once on the back of

133

that old blue pickup. And besides, we liked to jump from the roof of one car to another and pretend they were giant mushrooms.

Somebody started the lie that the monkey garden had been there before anything. We liked to think the garden could hide things for a thousand years. There beneath the roots of soggy flowers were the bones of murdered pirates and dinosaurs, the eye of a unicorn turned to coal.

This is where I wanted to die and where I tried one day but not even the monkey garden would have me. It was the last day I would go there.

Who was it that said I was getting too old to play the games? Who was it I didn't listen to? I only remember that when the others ran, I wanted to run too, up and down and through the monkey garden, fast as the boys, not like Sally who screamed if she got her stockings muddy.

I said, Sally, come on, but she wouldn't. She stayed by the curb talking to Tito and his friends. Play with the kids if you want, she said, I'm staying here. She could be stuck-up like that if she wanted to, so I just left.

It was her own fault too. When I got back Sally was pretending to be mad . . . something about the boys having stolen her keys. Please give them back to me, she said punching the nearest one with a soft fist. They were laughing. She was too. It was a joke I didn't get.

I wanted to go back with the other kids who were still jumping on cars, still chasing each other through the garden, but Sally had her own game.

One of the boys invented the rules. One of Tito's friends said you can't get the keys back unless you kiss us and Sally pretended to be mad at first but she said yes. It was that simple.

I don't know why, but something inside me wanted to throw a stick. Something wanted to say no when I watched Sally going into the garden with Tito's buddies all grinning. It was just a kiss, that's all. A kiss for each one. So what, she said.

Only how come I felt angry inside. Like something wasn't right. Sally went behind that old blue pickup to kiss the boys and get her keys back, and I ran up three flights of stairs to where Tito lived. His mother was ironing shirts. She was sprinkling water on them from an empty pop bottle and smoking a cigarette.

Your son and his friends stole Sally's keys and now they won't give them back unless she kisses them and right now they're making her kiss them, I said all out of breath from the three flights of stairs.

Those kids, she said, not looking up from her ironing.

That's all?

What do you want me to do, she said, call the cops? And kept on ironing.

I looked at her a long time, but couldn't think of anything to say, and ran back down the three flights to the garden where Sally needed to be saved. I took three big sticks and a brick and figured this was enough.

134

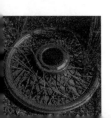

"The Monkey Garden" from ***The House on Mango Street*** by Sandra Cisneros

←— *Response notes* —→

But when I got there Sally said go home. Those boys said, leave us alone. I felt stupid with my brick. They all looked at me and if I was the one that was crazy and made me feel ashamed.

And then I don't know why but I had to run away. I had to hide myself at the other end of the garden, in the jungle part, under a tree that wouldn't mind if I lay down and cried a long time. I closed my eyes like tight stars so that I wouldn't, but I did. My face felt hot. Everything inside hiccupped.

I read somewhere in India there are priests who can will their heart to stop beating. I wanted to will my blood to stop, my heart to quit its pumping. I wanted to be dead, to turn into the rain, my eyes melt into the ground like two black snails. I wished and wished. I closed my eyes and willed it, but when I got up my dress was green and I had a headache.

I looked at my feet in their white socks and ugly round shoes. They seemed far away. They didn't seem to be my feet anymore. And the garden that had been such a good place to play didn't seem mine either.

Esperanza leads us into the garden, walks us around, and helps us discover why this is an important place to her. In order to better understand how Esperanza reveals her feelings through her descriptions of the garden, reread the story, circling the phrases that helped you picture the garden. Underline those phrases that describe Esperanza's attitude toward it.

●❖Sketch a map of the garden. Fill in the physical details first.

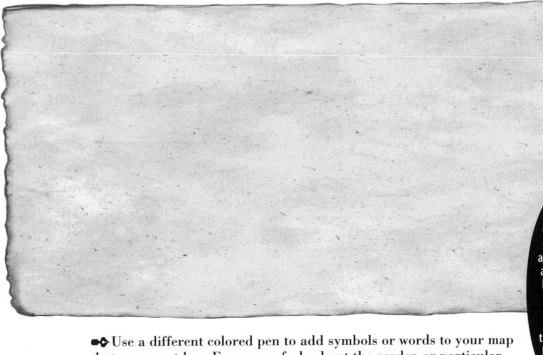

Writers reveal what their characters are thinking and feeling by the way characters see and interpret the physical landscapes around them.

●❖Use a different colored pen to add symbols or words to your map that represent how Esperanza feels about the garden or particular locations in it—that is, the emotional landscape. For example, what word or symbol could be used to represent the sentence: "This was a garden, a wonderful thing to look at in the spring"?

Three
Changing Landscapes

The landscapes within a story seldom stand still. The events that take place often affect how characters think or react to the physical landscapes around them. One way to study the story landscapes is to look for changes in the descriptions of the landscapes. For example, "The Monkey Garden" begins with a description of a change in Esperanza's and her friends' view of the garden. A particular event caused the change: "The monkey doesn't live there anymore."

▰◆ Review how you think Esperanza feels about the garden from the descriptions she gives early in the story. Look over your response notes, your map, and reread pertinent sections to determine what her attitude is as revealed in her descriptions. List three words that describe her attitude.

1.   2.   3.

▰◆ Write a short paragraph explaining how Esperanza feels differently about the garden after the incident with Sally.

●◆ Now, write a new ending for the story. Have Esperanza take the reader back to the garden. How will she describe it a month after the incident with Sally? What details will she describe differently showing her changed feelings towards the garden?

Example beginning: Esperanza (on seeing the old cars again): "I turned toward the skeleton of cars. Rust was eating holes in the roof of the old Chevy.

137

Writers often reveal characters' changing attitudes or reactions to situations by pointing out the differences in the way they describe the landscape around them.

Four
Exploring Your Own Landscapes

R eading Esperanza's remembrances may have reminded you of special places of your own—a certain vacation spot, a secret hideaway, a cool and drafty basement where you've spent time with friends. Reading sometimes works that way. Many writers claim that it is through their constant reading of other writers that they discover ideas for their own work.

➨ Draw a map of a place that is important to you. Sketch in details as if you were above the place looking down—that is, from a bird's-eye view. Include as many specific objects as you can. Label objects, places, or memorable events on the map as you draw it.

Writers often look to places that hold special meaning for inspiration. Through these places, writers can explore their own feelings and ideas.

Share your map with a partner. Take each other on a guided tour of your places. Stop in one particular place and tell each other a story about an incident that occurred there. Give details of both the physical and emotional landscapes of the place.

Five
Writing Your Landscapes

In the opening paragraphs of this short story by Robert Coover, the author offers a reminder that you, as the writer, have license to choose and manipulate the details of landscape to emphasize what you want the reader to notice and experience. Read the opening, paying particular attention to the details of setting that Coover includes.

from "The Magic Poker" by Robert Coover

I wander the island, inventing it. I make a sun for it, and trees—pines and firs—and cause the water to lap the pebbles of its abandoned shores. This, and more: I deposit shadows and dampness, spin webs, and scatter ruins. Yes: ruins. A mansion and guest cabins and boat houses and docks. Terraces, too, and bath houses and even an observation tower. All gutted and window-busted and autographed and shat upon. I impose a hot midday silence, a profound and heavy stillness. But anything can happen.

This small and secretive bay, here just below what was once the caretaker's cabin and not far from the main boat house, probably once possessed its own system of docks, built out to protect boats from the big rocks along the shore. At least the refuse—the long bony planks of gray lumber heaped up at one end of the bay—would suggest that. But aside from the planks, the bay is now only a bay, shallow, floored with rocks and cans and bottles. Schools of silver fish, thin as fingernails, fog the bottom, and dragonflies dart and hover over its placid surface. The harsh snarl of the boat motor—for indeed a boat has been approaching, coming in off the lake into this small bay—breaks off abruptly, as the boat carves a long gentle arc through the bay, and slides, scraping bottom, toward a shallow pebbly corner. There are two girls in the boat.

Bedded deep in the grass, near the path up to the first guest cabin, lies a wrought-iron poker. It is long and slender with an intricately worked handle, and it is orange with rust. It lies shadowed, not by trees, but by the grass that has grown wildly around it. I put it there.

← Response notes →

139

Reread the description and circle the key words that help you visualize the physical and the emotional landscape.

Now choose a place from your map to write about. To get started, think about the place and write down the words that come to mind. List as many physical details as you can, as well as what you like and dislike and the emotions the place brings to mind.

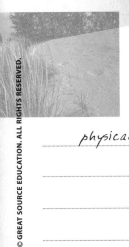

physical details	likes and dislikes	emotions

●◆ Now, write a few paragraphs describing the physical and emotional landscapes of your place. Use Bradbury, García Márquez, Cisneros, and Coover as models to help you organize and craft your piece.

Capture landscapes from your own life stories in the same way that professional writers do. Then use them to help you write descriptions of physical and emotional landscapes, which help reveal your story's meaning.

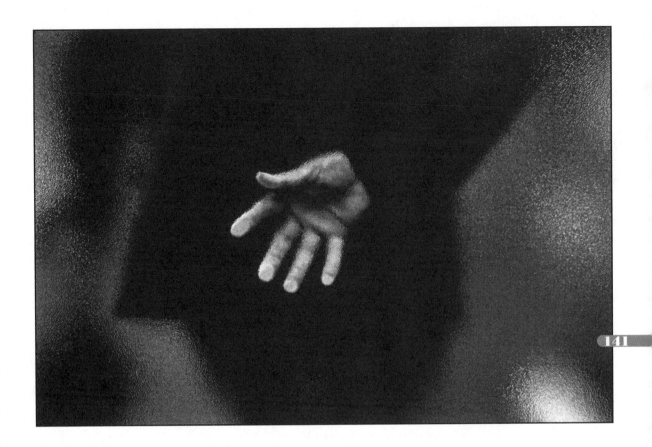

Characters in Stories

The creation of a character presents special demands on a writer. Characters in film, television, or in plays are physically present. They can demonstrate their personalities through gestures, looks, and the way they move their bodies. But the author of a story creates characters through words. Authors give you certain kinds of information from which you form opinions or develop feelings for the characters. Sometimes authors reveal characters by describing what goes on in their minds. Other times they reveal their characters through what the characters say or do and what others say about them. Physical appearances and gestures may also help identify character type.

In what other ways can authors bring their characters to life?

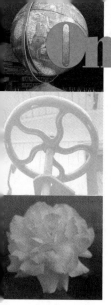

Distinguishing Characteristics

One way to understand a character is to look for distinguishing qualities or features. Once you find them, decide how these are important to the character and the story as a whole. What do you learn about the character of Jamie from the following paragraph?

> Jamie entered the room. She pushed through the door, and the tattoo on her bare arm brushed against Mr. Jameson's blue suit jacket. After sitting down, cross-legged, on the waiting room chair, Jamie leaned toward the woman sitting next to her and tapped her long, blue fingernails on the woman's shoulder. "Could ya quiet your kid down? I'm tryin to concentrate on my lines." Jamie stared hard at the kid who was tugging on his mother's arm and begging for candy.

The descriptions guide you to focus on particular characteristics. Jamie's tattoo suggests that she may be rebellious. Her actions signal that she is assertive. As a reader, you are expected to work with the author's descriptions to determine the qualities of a character.

In Margaret Atwood's novel *Cat's Eye*, Elaine, the narrator, tells about an incident that occurred when she was about ten years old. Note the ways in which the characters come to life through the selection of details used to describe them.

142

---

from ***Cat's Eye*** by Margaret Atwood

← *Response notes* →

It's the middle of March. In the schoolroom windows the Easter tulips are beginning to bloom. There's still snow on the ground, a dirty filigree, though the winter is losing its hardness and glitter. The sky thickens, sinks lower.

We walk home under the low thick sky that is gray and bulging with dampness. Moist soft flakes are falling out of it, piling up on roofs and branches, sliding off now and then to hit with a wet cottony *thunk*. There's no wind and the sound is muffled by the snow.

It isn't cold. I undo the ties on my blue knitted wool hat, let it flap loose on my head. Cordelia takes off her mittens and scoops up snowballs, throwing them at trees, at telephone poles, at random. It's one of her friendly days; she puts her arm through my arm, her other arm through Grace's, and we march along the street, singing *We don't stop for anybody.* I sing this too. Together we hop and slide.

Some of the euphoria I once felt in falling snow comes back to me; I want to open my mouth and let the snow fall into it. I allow myself to laugh, like the others, trying it out. My laughter is a performance, a grab at the ordinary.

Cordelia throws herself backward onto a blank front lawn, spreads her arms out in the snow, raises them above her head, draws them

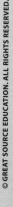

from *Cat's Eye* by Margaret Atwood

← Response notes →

down to her sides, making a snow angel. The flakes fall onto her face, into her laughing mouth, melting, clinging to her eyebrows. She blinks, closing her eyes against the snow. For a moment she looks like someone I don't know, a stranger, shining with unknown, good possibilities. Or else a victim of a traffic accident, flung onto the snow.

She opens her eyes and reaches up her hands, which are damp and reddened, and we pull her upward so she won't disturb the image she's made. The snow angel has feathery wings and a tiny pin head. Where her hands stopped, down near her sides, are the imprints of her fingers, like little claws.

We've forgotten the time, it's getting dark. We run along the street that leads to the wooden footbridge. Even Grace runs, lumpily, calling, "Wait up!" For once she is the one left behind.

Cordelia reaches the hill first and runs down it. She tries to slide but the snow is too soft, not icy enough, and there are cinders and pieces of gravel in it. She falls down and rolls. We think she's done it on purpose, the way she made the snow angel. We rush down upon her, exhilarated, breathless, laughing, just as she's picking herself up.

We stop laughing, because now we can see that her fall was an accident, she didn't do it on purpose. She likes everything she does to be done on purpose.

Carol says, "Did you hurt yourself?" Her voice is quavery, she's frightened, already she can tell that this is serious. Cordelia doesn't answer. Her face is hard again, her eyes baleful.

Grace moves so that she's beside Cordelia, slightly behind her. From there she smiles at me, her tight smile.

Cordelia says, to me, "Were you laughing?" I think she means, was I laughing at her because she fell down.

"No," I say.

"She was," says Grace neutrally. Carol shifts to the side of the path, away from me.

"I'm going to give you one more chance," says Cordelia. "Were you laughing?"

"Yes," I say, "but . . ."

"Just yes or no," says Cordelia.

I say nothing. Cordelia glances over at Grace, as if looking for approval. She sighs, an exaggerated sigh, like a grown-up's. "Lying again," she says. "What are we going to do with you?"

We seem to have been standing there for a long time. It's colder now. Cordelia reaches out and pulls off my knitted hat. She marches the rest of the way down the hill and onto the bridge and hesitates for a moment. Then she walks over to the railing and throws my hat down into the ravine. Then the white oval of her face turns up toward me. "Come here," she says.

Nothing has changed, then. Time will go on, in the same way, endlessly. My laughter was unreal after all, merely a gasp for air.

I walk down to where Cordelia stands by the railing, the snow not crunching but giving way under my feet like cotton wool packing. It

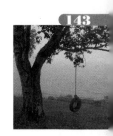

143

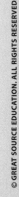

← Response notes →

sounds like a cavity being filled, in a tooth, inside my head. Usually I'm afraid to go so near the edge of the bridge, but this time I'm not. I don't feel anything as positive as fear.

"There's your stupid hat," says Cordelia; and there it is, far down, still blue against the white snow, even in the dimming light. "Why don't you go down and get it?"

I look at her. She wants me to go down into the ravine where the bad men are, where we're never supposed to go. It occurs to me that I may not. What will she do then?

I can see this idea gathering in Cordelia as well. Maybe she's gone too far, hit, finally, some core of resistance in me. If I refuse to do what she says this time, who knows where my defiance will end? The two others have come down the hill and are watching, safely in the middle of the bridge.

"Go on then," she says, more gently, as if she's encouraging me, not ordering. "Then you'll be forgiven."

I don't want to go down there. It's forbidden and dangerous; also it's dark and the hillside will be slippery, I might have trouble climbing up again. But there is my hat. If I go home without it, I'll have to explain, I'll have to tell. And if I refuse to go, what will Cordelia do next? She might get angry, she might never speak to me again. She might push me off the bridge. She's never done anything like that before, never hit or pinched, but now that she's thrown my hat over there's no telling what she might do.

I walk along to the end of the bridge. "When you've got it, count to a hundred," says Cordelia. "Before coming up." She doesn't sound angry any more. She sounds like someone giving instructions for a game.

I start down the steep hillside, holding on to branches and tree trunks. The path isn't even a real path, it's just a place worn by whoever goes up and down here: boys, men. Not girls.

When I'm among the bare trees at the bottom I look up. The bridge railings are silhouetted against the sky. I can see the dark outlines of three heads, watching me.

My blue hat is out on the ice of the creek. I stand in the snow, looking at it. Cordelia is right, it's a stupid hat. I look at it and feel resentment, because this stupid-looking hat is mine, and deserving of ridicule. I don't want to wear it ever again.

I can hear water running somewhere, down under the ice. I step out onto the creek, reach for the hat, pick it up, go through. I'm up to my waist in the creek, slabs of broken ice upended around me.

Cold shoots through me. My overshoes are filling, and the shoes inside them; water drenches my snowpants. Probably I've screamed, or some noise has come out of me, but I can't remember hearing anything. I clutch the hat and look up at the bridge. Nobody is there. They must have walked away, run away. That's why the counting to a hundred: so they could run away.

144

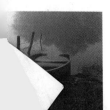

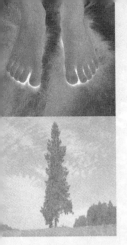

What distinguishes each of these girls—Elaine, Cordelia, Grace, and Carol—from one another? In order to answer this question, go back into the text of the story.

- Circle places that reveal particular qualities of each girl. Then write a statement in your response notes about the distinguishing characteristics you identify. For example, the sentence "It's one of her friendly days" describes Cordelia.

"It's one of her friendly days."

Response notes
moody or not friendly all the time

- Write about a person you know who reminds you of a character in the story. First, create a cluster of characteristics (physical traits, actions, qualities of character, etc.) of the person.

qualities of character

physical traits

Name

actions

145

◆❖ Use the cluster to create a character sketch describing the person you've chosen. Include enough details to show how he or she is similar to a character in the story.

....

....

....

....

....

....

....

....

When you read, try to determine the qualities that define a character, distinguish one character from another, and explain how each character contributes to the whole of the story.

Two Character Motivation

If you speak of a character's motives—what pushes or drives a person to do something—then you're trying to get at what causes certain behaviors and reactions. But motivations are complicated and not easy to portray. Many times a character's motivation is not stated directly. You, as the reader, must make guesses based on what you know motivates people's actions.

What motivates Cordelia to act as she does? What about Elaine or the other girls? Reread the excerpt, looking for hints from Atwood about what motivates characters.

●◆ Write a brief statement about each character's motivations.

Cordelia: ....

....

Elaine: ....

....

Grace: ....

....

Carol: ....

....

One way to explore what you understand about characters' motivations is to think about how they would explain their behavior.

●◆ Write an imagined monologue, the thoughts going through one character's mind, that justifies Cordelia's or Grace's actions during the incident with Elaine. Think about how you can best show that character's motivations through the way she explains the situation and her part in the incident.

....

....

....

....

....

....

....

Knowing what motivates characters helps you explain why they act as they do.

Three
Character Development

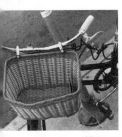

Authors have a responsibility to show how characters evolve and change, how they respond to the action of the story. For example, how will the incident between Elaine and the other girls change their relationship with one another?

As the next scene begins, Elaine has just managed to reach the top of the hill. Before this, she had fallen through the ice on the creek while trying to retrieve her hat. She made her way back to the bank, lay down, exhausted and numb. During this moment she believed someone had come to help her. First, she thought it was Cordelia. Then, she realized that it was an image of a woman, one she later believed was the Virgin Mary. As she came to the top of the hill, she saw her mother. As you read, look for changes in Elaine's character.

from ***Cat's Eye*** by Margaret Atwood

"I fell in," I say. "I was getting my hat." My voice sounds thick, the words mumbled. Something is wrong with my tongue.

My mother does not say, *Where have you been?* or *Why are you so late?* She says, "Where are your overshoes?" They are down in the ravine, covering over with snow. I have forgotten them, and my hat as well.

"It fell over the bridge," I say. I need to get this lie over with as soon as possible. Telling the truth about Cordelia is still unthinkable for me.

My mother takes off her coat and wraps it around me. Her mouth is tight, her face is frightened and angry at the same time. It's the look she used to have when we would cut ourselves, a long time ago, up north. She puts her arm under my armpit and hurries me along. My feet hurt at every step. I wonder if I will be punished for going down into the ravine.

When we reach the house my mother peels off my soggy half-frozen clothes and puts me into a lukewarm bath. She looks carefully at my fingers and toes, my nose, my ear lobes. "Where were Grace and Cordelia?" she asks me. "Did they see you fall in?"

"No," I say. "They weren't there."

I can tell she's thinking about phoning their mothers no matter what I do, but I am too tired to care. "A lady helped me," I say. "What lady?" says my mother, but I know better than to tell her. If I say who it really was I won't be believed. "Just a lady," I say.

My mother says I'm lucky I don't have severe frostbite. I know about frostbite: your fingers and toes fall off, as punishment for drink. She feeds me a cup of milky tea and puts me into bed with a hot water bottle and flannelette sheets, and spreads two extra blankets on top. I am still shivering. My father has come home and I hear them talking in low, anxious voices out in the hallway. Then my father comes in and puts his hand on my forehead, and fades to a shadow.

I dream I'm running along the street outside the school. I've done something wrong. It's autumn, the leaves are burning. A lot of people are chasing after me. They're shouting.

←— *Response notes* —→

147

←—Response notes—→

An invisible hand takes mine, pulls upward. There are steps into the air and I go up them. No one else can see where the steps are. Now I'm standing in the air, out of reach above the upturned faces. They're still shouting but I can no longer hear them. Their mouths close and open silently, like the mouths of fish.

I am kept home from school for two days. The first day I lie in bed, floating in the glassy delicate clarity of fever. By the second day I am thinking about what happened. I can remember Cordelia throwing my blue knitted hat over the bridge, I remember falling through the ice and then my mother running toward me with her sleety hair. All these things are certain, but in between them there's a hazy space. The dead people and the woman in the cloak are there, but in the same way dreams are. I'm not sure, now, that it really was the Virgin Mary. I believe it but I no longer know it.

I'm given a get-well card with violets on it from Carol, shoved through the letter slot. On the weekend Cordelia calls me on the telephone. "We didn't know you fell in," she says. "We're sorry we didn't wait. We thought you were right behind us." Her voice is careful, precise, rehearsed, unrepentant.

I know she's told some story that conceals what really happened, as I have. I know that this apology has been exacted from her, and that I will be made to pay for it later. But she has never apologized to me before. This apology, however fake, makes me feel not stronger but weaker. I don't know what to say. "It's okay," is what I manage. I think I mean it.

When I go back to school, Cordelia and Grace are polite but distant. Carol is more obviously frightened, or interested. "My mother says you almost froze to death," she whispers as we stand in line, two by two, waiting for the bell. "I got a spanking, with the hairbrush. I really *got* it."

The snow is melting from the lawns; mud reappears on the floors, at school, in the kitchen at home. Cordelia circles me warily. I catch her eyes on me, considering, as we walk home from school. Conversation is artificially normal. We stop at the store for licorice whips, which Carol buys. As we stroll along, sucking in licorice, Cordelia says, "I think Elaine should be punished for telling on us, don't you?"

"I didn't tell," I say. I no longer feel the sinking in my gut, the held-back tearfulness that such a false accusation would once have produced. My voice is flat, calm, reasonable.

"Don't contradict me," Cordelia says. "Then how come your mother phoned our mothers?"

"Yeah, how come?" says Carol.

"I don't know and I don't care," I say. I'm amazed at myself.

"You're being insolent," says Cordelia. "Wipe that smirk off your face."

I am still a coward, still fearful; none of that has changed. But I turn and walk away from her. It's like stepping off a cliff, believing the air will hold you up. And it does. I see that I don't have to do

from **Cat's Eye** by Margaret Atwood

what she says, and, worse and better, I've never had to do what she says. I can do what I like.

"Don't you dare walk away on us," Cordelia says behind me. "You get back here right now!" I can hear this for what it is. It's an imitation, it's acting. It's an impersonation, of someone much older. It's a game. There was never anything about me that needed to be improved. It was always a game, and I have been fooled. I have been stupid. My anger is as much at myself as at them.

"Ten stacks of plates," says Grace. This would once have reduced me. Now I find it silly. I keep walking. I feel daring, light-headed. They are not my best friends or even my friends. Nothing binds me to them. I am free.

They follow along behind me, making comments on the way I walk, on how I look from behind. If I were to turn I would see them imitating me. "Stuck up! Stuck up!" they cry. I can hear the hatred, but also the need. They need me for this, and I no longer need them. I am indifferent to them. There's something hard in me, crystalline, a kernel of glass. I cross the street and continue along, eating my licorice.

I stop going to Sunday school. I refuse to play with Grace or Cordelia or even Carol after school. I no longer walk home over the bridge, but the long way around, past the cemetery. When they come in a group to the back door to collect me I tell them I'm busy. They try kindness, to lure me back, but I am no longer susceptible to it. I can see the greed in their eyes. It's as if I can see right into them. Why was I unable to do this before?

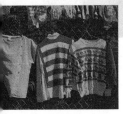

Make a "before and after" chart that shows how Elaine changed after the ravine incident.

Elaine Before	Elaine After

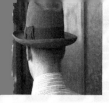

➡️ Use the chart to write three paragraphs about Elaine's character development. Structure your paragraphs to:

1. explain how Elaine changed
2. explain the reasons you think she changed
3. discuss what she gained or lost as a result of what happened

....

....

....

....

....

....

....

....

150

....

....

....

....

....

....

....

....

....

Authors use various methods to show character development because in fiction, as in life, people are affected or changed by their experiences.

Four
Point of View

In Atwood's novel *Cat's Eye*, Elaine tells the story from a first-person point of view. You learn how she interprets the events and other characters' actions. You learn about everything through her perspective and what she chooses to tell.

Skim both excerpts again. Decide what each of the other girls might say about the events that have taken place. List a few words that tell how each girl might have viewed the situation based on what you know about them.

Incident:	Cordelia	Carol	Grace
Cordelia's Fall			
Retrieving the Hat			
Elaine's Rebellion			

151

◗◆Rewrite one of the incidents, shifting the point of view to one of the other girls. For example, you might describe Cordelia's perspective on Elaine's decision to walk away.

152

Share your version of the incident with a partner. Discuss how the story changed.

Point of view affects what is included and how a story is told.

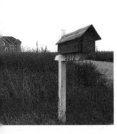

Five

Dialogue Reveals Character

The way characters talk and what they say help reveal who they are:

> "It's too dark. I can't see the way out," said Jacob.
> "Shhh," Lauren said. "I'm sure he's following. Move faster."
> "It's hopeless," he told her.
> "It's up to us to outsmart them," she whispered.

What do you learn about Jacob and Lauren in these four sentences? Write one or two words to describe each character based on what they have said (for example, you might describe Jacob as timid or assertive). Note how dialogue alone can tell you something about the characters.

As you read an excerpt from Tobias Wolff's **autobiography**, *This Boy's Life*, make notes in the margins about how the **dialogue** reveals character.

153

from ***This Boy's Life*** by Tobias Wolff

⟵ Response notes ⟶

I stood and left the confessional. Sister James came toward me from where she'd been standing against the wall. "That wasn't so bad now, was it?" she asked.

"I'm supposed to wait," I told her.

She looked at me. I could see she was curious, but she didn't ask any questions.

The priest came out soon after. He was old and very tall and walked with a limp. He stood close beside me, and when I looked up at him I saw the white hair in his nostrils. He smelled strongly of tobacco. "We had a little trouble getting started," he said.

"Yes, Father?"

"He's just a bit nervous is all," the priest said. "Needs to relax. Nothing like a glass of milk for that."

She nodded.

"Why don't we try again a little later. Say twenty minutes?"

"We'll be here, Father."

Sister James and I went to the rectory kitchen. I sat at a steel cutting table while she poured me a glass of milk. "You want some cookies?" she asked.

"That's all right, Sister."

"Sure you do." She put a package of Oreos on a plate and brought it to me. Then she sat down. With her arms crossed, hands hidden in her sleeves, she watched me eat and drink. Finally she said, "What

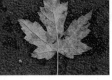

happened, then? Cat get your tongue?"

"Yes, Sister."

"There's nothing to be afraid of."

"I know."

"Maybe you're just thinking of it wrong," she said.

I stared at my hands on the tabletop.

"I forgot to give you a napkin," she said. "Go on and lick them. Don't be shy."

She waited until I looked up, and when I did I saw that she was younger than I'd thought her to be. Not that I'd given much thought to her age. Except for the really old nuns with canes or facial hair they all seemed outside of time, without past or future. But now — forced to look at Sister James across the narrow space of this gleaming table — I saw her differently. I saw an anxious woman of about my mother's age who wanted to help me without knowing what kind of help I needed. Her good will worked strongly on me. My eyes burned and my throat swelled up. I would have surrendered to her if only I'd known how.

"It probably isn't as bad as you think it is," Sister James said. "Whatever it is, someday you'll look back and you'll see that it was natural. But you've got to bring it to the light. Keeping it in the dark is what makes it feel so bad." She added, "I'm not asking you to tell me, understand. That's not my place. I'm just saying that we all go through these things."

Sister James leaned forward over the table. "When I was your age," she said, "maybe even a little older, I used to go through my father's wallet while he was taking his bath at night. I didn't take bills, just pennies and nickels, maybe a dime. Nothing he'd miss. My father would've given me the money if I'd asked for it. But I preferred to steal it. Stealing from him made me feel awful, but I did it all the same."

She looked down at the tabletop. "I was a backbiter, too. Whenever I was with one friend I would say terrible things about my other friends, and then turn around and do the same thing to the one I had just been with. I knew what I was doing, too. I hated myself for it, I really did, but that didn't stop me. I used to wish that my mother and my brothers would die in a car crash so I could grow up with just my father and have everyone feel sorry for me."

Sister James shook her head. "I had all these bad thoughts I didn't want to let go of. Know what I mean?"

I nodded, and presented her with an expression that was meant to register dawning comprehension.

"Good!" she said. She slapped her palms down on the table. "Ready to try again?"

I said that I was.

Sister James led me back to the confessional. I knelt and began again: "Bless me Father, for —"

"All right," he said. "We've been here before. Just talk plain."

"Yes Father."

from ***This Boy's Life*** by Tobias Wolff

Again I closed my eyes over my folded hands. "Come come," he said, with a certain sharpness. "Yes, Father." I bent close to the screen and whispered, "Father, I steal."

He was silent for a moment. Then he said, "What do you steal?"

"I steal money, Father. From my mother's purse when she's in the shower."

"How long have you been doing this?"

I didn't answer.

"Well?" he said. "A week? A year? Two years?"

I chose the one in the middle. "A year."

"A year," he repeated. "That won't do. You have to stop. Do you intend to stop?"

"Yes, Father."

"Honestly, now."

"Honestly, Father."

"All right. Good. What else?"

"I'm a backbiter."

"A backbiter?"

"I say things about my friends when they're not around."

"That won't do either," he said.

"No, Father."

"That certainly won't do. Your friends will desert you if you persist in this and let me tell you, a life without friends is no life at all."

"Yes, Father."

"Do you sincerely intend to stop?"

"Yes, Father."

"Good. Be sure that you do. I tell you this in all seriousness. Anything else?"

← Response notes →

155

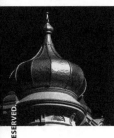

What do you learn about Sister James, the priest, and Wolff from the way each speaks? Circle or highlight with a marker places that reveal particular qualities of each character. Explain in your response notes what is revealed about each. For example, what is implied when Sister James says:

"That wasn't so bad now."

Response notes
helpful, reassuring, concerned

- Examine the speech tags for additional information. Through speech tags, "he said" and "she said," we get information from the author about characters. Speech tags shouldn't intrude but can help you visualize what the character is doing while speaking—she leans forward, fidgets, averts her eyes, uncrosses her legs. Sometimes the speech tag helps you keep track of who is talking. How does Wolff use speech tags? Underline tags that you think are particularly effective in providing information about the characters.

●◆ Write a segment of dialogue that involves three characters you create. You might choose to model the characters after people you know or ones you imagine. To begin, create lists of distinguishing traits that you want to emphasize for each character.

	Name	*Name*	*Name*
qualities of character			
physical traits			
actions			

Now, write the dialogue among your three characters. Include speech tags. Think about how your characters' speech will reveal something about their character.

The dialogue in a story reveals information about characters and can help you understand characters' motivations, values, and why and how they act as they do.

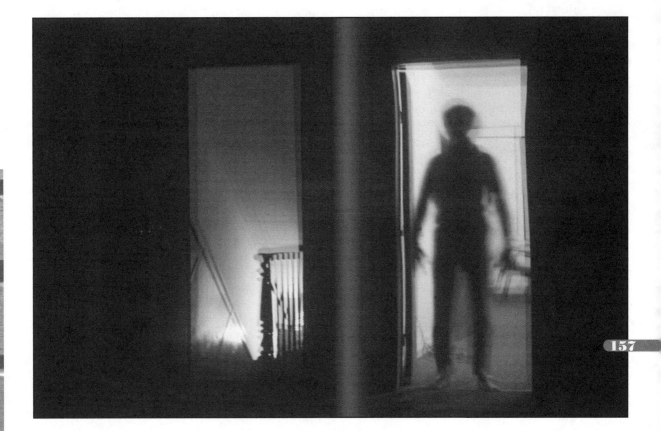

Shifting Forms: Nonfiction and Poetry

The form of a work must fit the writer's audience, purpose, and intended effect. Writers usually choose from among the many conventional genres—poetry, fiction, essay, drama. But within these broad genres, a writer must choose a form: short story or novel, sonnet or ballad, comedy or tragedy, and so on.

Critical readers know that the form of a text influences their expectations about the content of a poem or a novel. We may read about the same idea or event in both prose and poetry. But we can expect to find differences in word choice and selection of details. Ultimately, a different effect or impression is created in each genre.

In autobiography, one kind of nonfiction, we read about incidents and details from the writer's life. But the writer does not merely report them. He or she interprets them for the reader by selecting key incidents and details. In poetry, incidents and details are distilled to their essence, often leaving the reader to determine their importance.

Readers expect nonfiction to be true. And, it mostly is. But some **forms** are more **objective** than others. Newspaper articles generally report **facts** without interpreting them. **Editorials** give **opinions** supported by facts. Producers of television **documentaries** select and arrange facts to make the information interesting to a viewer. Producers of **docudramas** may add incidents and characters that were not in the original event to make a better story.

Objectivity and subjectivity are determined, in part, by the writer's involvement in the events and by the details he or she chooses. Read the opening four paragraphs of a story from the August 27, 1997, *New York Times*.

Response notes

from **Many Smokers Who Can't Quit Are Mentally Ill**
Jane E. Brody

People who have been smoking for years and have been unable to quit may have more health problems than either they or their physicians realize. A University of Michigan researcher has gathered evidence that many if not most hard-core smokers are suffering from an underlying psychiatric problem that nicotine may help to ameliorate.

This not-too-surprising conclusion was drawn by Dr. Cynthia S. Pomerleau, who cited "mounting evidence that smoking is becoming increasingly concentrated in people at risk for major depressive disorders, adult attention deficit hyperactivity disorder, anxiety disorders and bulimia or binge-eating."

The idea that many smokers may be medicating themselves is not new. For example, several researchers have linked smoking to an attempt to counter depression and have shown that various antidepressants can often help a hard-core depressed smoker quit.

But the extent of the relationship between various psychological disorders and self-medication with nicotine has not been widely recognized or well documented.

158

In the article, circle the conclusions that Brody is drawing. In the response notes, write down the support for each conclusion.

Discuss with a partner the objectivity of this story.
- How objective is it?
- Is the writer a participant in the events or just reporting them?
- What details does she present to support her own opinions?
- How would the story be different if it were more subjective?

➥ Explore the last question by rewriting the article as a letter trying to persuade a friend not to smoke. Then compare your letter with the original article. How are the two similar? How are they different?

159

Critical reading of nonfiction requires evaluating the objectivity of the selection.

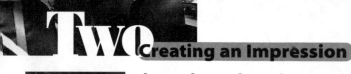

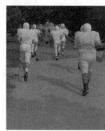

An **autobiography** is often considered to be more **subjective** than a **biography**. The writer selects incidents and presents them in such a way that the reader is left with an impression of the writer's personality and the significance of the events. As critical readers, we need to be alert to the impression the writer wants us to have.

The following excerpt is from *Always Running*, Luis Rodriguez's autobiography about growing up with gangs, poverty, and prejudice in Los Angeles. In the excerpt, Rodriguez talks about his relationship with the brother who was three years older than he.

from ***Always Running*** by Luis J. Rodriguez

←—Response notes—→

Although we moved around the Watts area, the house on 105th Street near McKinley Avenue held my earliest memories, my earliest fears and questions. It was a small matchbox of a place. Next to it stood a tiny garage with holes through the walls and an unpainted barnlike quality. The weather battered it into a leaning shed. The backyard was a jungle. Vegetation appeared to grow down from the sky. There were banana trees, huge "sperm" weeds (named that because they stank like semen when you cut them), foxtails and yellowed grass. An avocado tree grew in the middle of the yard and its roots covered every bit of ground, tearing up cement walks while its branches scraped the bedroom windows. A sway of clothes on some lines filled the little bit of grassy area just behind the house.

My brother and I played often in our jungle, even pretending to be Tarzan (Rano mastered the Tarzan yell from the movies). The problem, however, was I usually ended up being the monkey who got thrown off the trees. In fact, I remember my brother as the most dangerous person alive. He seemed to be wracked with a scream which never let out. His face was dark with meanness, what my mother called *maldad*. He also took delight in seeing me writhe in pain, cry or cower, vulnerable to his own inflated sense of power. This hunger for cruelty included his ability to take my mom's most wicked whippings—without crying or wincing. He'd just sit there and stare at a wall, forcing Mama to resort to other implements of pain—but Rano would not show any emotion.

Yet in the streets, neighborhood kids often chased Rano from play or jumped him. Many times he came home mangled, his face swollen. Once somebody threw a rock at him which cut a gash across his forehead, leaving a scar Rano has to this day.

Another time a neighbor's kid smashed a metal bucket over Rano's head, slicing the skin over his skull and creating a horrifying scene with blood everywhere. My mother in her broken English could remedy few of the injustices, but she tried. When this one happened, she ran next door to confront that kid's mother. The woman had been sitting on her porch and saw everything.

"¿Qué pasó aquí?" Mama asked.

"I don't know what you want," the woman said. "All I know is your

160

from *Always Running* by Luis J. Rodriguez

boy picked up that bucket and hit himself over the head—that's all I know."

In school, they placed Rano in classes with retarded children because he didn't speak much English. They even held him back a year in the second grade.

For all this, Rano took his rage out on me. I recall hiding from him when he came around looking for a playmate. My mother actually forced me out of closets with a belt in her hand and made me play with him.

One day we were playing on the rooftop of our house.

"Grillo, come over here," he said from the roof's edge. "Man, look at this on the ground."

I should have known better, but I leaned over to see. Rano then pushed me and I struck the ground on my back with a loud thump and lost my breath, laying deathly still in suffocating agony, until I slowly gained it back.

Another time he made me the Indian to his cowboy, tossed a rope around my neck and pulled me around the yard. He stopped barely before it choked the life out of me. I had rope burns around my neck for a week.

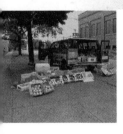

Rodriguez says that Rano had a "hunger for cruelty." Circle specific words or phrases that describe Rano's cruelty. Notice how the author reinforces his point through repeated incidents and details.

161

●◆ What are your impressions of Luis and Rano? Why do you think they act the ways they do? How do you think the incidents would change if they were included in Rano's autobiography? Explain.

Authors often use repeated details and a series of similar events to create a strong impression in the reader's mind.

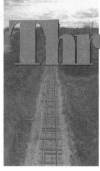

Shifting Emphasis

Good writers show more than one side of important characters. Rodriguez shifts his emphasis when he describes a significant incident in detail. Notice how he shows another side of Rano.

from ***Always Running*** by Luis J. Rodriguez

←—Response notes—→

One day, my mother asked Rano and me to go to the grocery store. We decided to go across the railroad tracks into South Gate. In those days, South Gate was an Anglo neighborhood, filled with the families of workers from the auto plant and other nearby industry. Like Lynwood or Huntington Park, it was forbidden territory for the people of Watts.

My brother insisted we go. I don't know what possessed him, but then I never did. It was useless to argue; he'd force me anyway. He was nine then, I was six. So without ceremony, we started over the tracks, climbing over discarded market carts and torn-up sofas, across Alameda Street, into South Gate: all-white, all-American.

We entered the first small corner grocery store we found. Everything was cool at first. We bought some bread, milk, soup cans and candy. We each walked out with a bag filled with food. We barely got a few feet, though, when five teenagers on bikes approached. We tried not to pay attention and proceeded to our side of the tracks. But the youths pulled up in front of us. While two of them stood nearby on their bikes, three of them jumped off theirs and walked over to us.

"What do we got here?" one of the boys said. . . .

He pushed me to the ground; the groceries splattered onto the asphalt. I felt melted gum and chips of broken beer bottle on my lips and cheek. Then somebody picked me up and held me while the others seized my brother, tossed his groceries out, and pounded on him. They punched him in the face, in the stomach, then his face again, cutting his lip, causing him to vomit.

I remember the shrill, maddening laughter of one of the kids on a bike, this laughing like a raven's wail, a harsh wind's shriek, a laugh that I would hear in countless beatings thereafter. I watched the others take turns on my brother, this terror of a brother, and he doubled over, had blood and spew on his shirt, and tears down his face. I wanted to do something, but they held me and I just looked on, as every strike against Rano opened me up inside.

They finally let my brother go and he slid to the ground, like a rotten banana squeezed out of its peeling. They threw us back over the tracks. In the sunset I could see the Watts Towers, shimmers of seventy thousand pieces of broken bottles, sea shells, ceramic and metal on spiraling points puncturing the heavens, which reflected back the rays of a falling sun. My brother and I then picked ourselves up, saw the teenagers take off, still laughing, still talking about those stupid greasers who dared to cross over to South Gate.

162

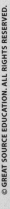

from **Always Running** by Luis J. Rodriguez

←—Response notes —→

Up until then my brother had never shown any emotion to me other than disdain. He had never asked me anything, unless it was a demand, an expectation, an obligation to be his throwaway boy-doll. But for this once he looked at me, tears welled in his eyes, blood streamed from several cuts—lips and cheeks swollen.

"Swear—you got to swear—you'll never tell anybody how I cried," he said.

I suppose I did promise. It was his one last thing to hang onto, his rep as someone who could take a belt whipping, who could take a beating in the neighborhood and still go back risking more—it was this pathetic plea from the pavement I remember. I must have promised.

Luis writes, "every strike against Rano opened me up inside." Circle in the text other details that show Luis was sympathetic toward Rano.

●◆ What are your impressions of Luis and Rano now? Have your impressions changed? What is your opinion of Rano's cruelty now?

Authors can change the reader's impressions of people and events through the details they choose to present.

Four

In "'Race' Politics" Luis Rodriguez shifts genres. He presents the incident where his brother was beaten in a different form—with a different focus. Read the poem twice: once to get an initial overall impression and a second time to annotate it with your questions, impressions, and responses.

Response notes

"Race" Politics
Luis J. Rodriguez

My brother and I—shopping for *la jefita*—
decided to get the "good food"
over on the other side of the tracks.

We dared each other.
Laughed a little.
Thought about it.
Said, what's the big deal.
Thought about that.
Decided we were men,
not boys.
Decided we should go wherever
we damn wanted to.

Oh, my brother—now he was bad.
Tough dude. Afraid of nothing.
I was afraid of him.

So there we go,
climbing over
the iron and wood ties,
over discarded sofas and bent-up market carts,
over a weed-and-dirt road,
into a place called South Gate
—all white. All-American.

We entered the forbidden
narrow line of hate,
imposed,
transposed,
supposed,
a line of power/powerlessness
full of meaning,
meaning nothing—
those lines that crisscross
the abdomen of this land,
that strangle you
in your days, in your nights.
When you dream.

There we were, two Mexicans,
six and nine—from Watts, no less.
Oh, this was plenty reason
to hate us.

164

Plenty reason to run up behind us.
Five teenagers on bikes.
Plenty reason to knock
the groceries out from our arms—
    a splattering heap of soup
    cans, bread and candy.

Plenty reason to hold me down
on the hot asphalt; melted gum
    and chips of broken
    beer bottle on my lips and cheek.

Plenty reason to get my brother
by the throat, taking turns
    punching him in the face,
    cutting his lower lip,
    punching, him vomiting.

Punching until swollen and dark blue
he slid from their grasp
like a rotten banana from its peeling.
When they had enough, they threw us back,
dirty and lacerated,
back to Watts, its towers shiny
across the orange-red sky.

My brother then forced me
to promise not to tell anybody
how he cried.
He forced me to swear to God,
to Jesus Christ, to our long-dead
Indian Grandmother—
keepers of our meddling souls.

Create a cluster to illustrate your main impression of Rano in the poem. Identify one word or phrase that represents the central impression. Put that word or phrase in the center oval on the next page, then add the details that support that word or idea. For example, a cluster for the autobiographical excerpt in lesson one might focus on Rano's cruelty and look like this:

His face was "dark with meanness."

He pushed Luis off the roof.

Rano was incredibly cruel.

He never showed emotion.

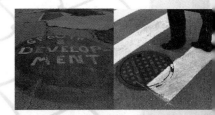

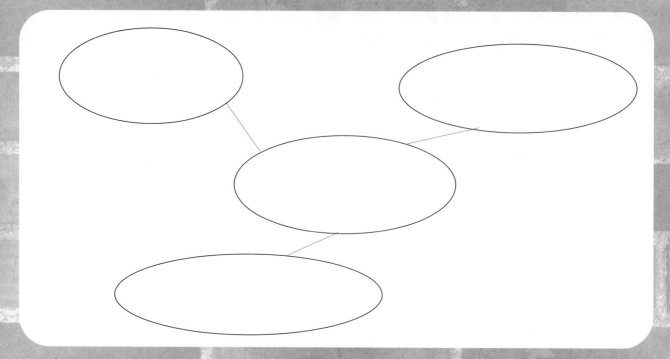

●◆Describe your reaction to the beating incident. What difference, if any, did reading it as a poem make?

Different genres can provide a different focus for an event.

Five — Comparing Genres

Compare the details in the two tellings of the beating incident. Return to the poem and the autobiographical excerpt about the beating and underline all details that are similar. Use the chart below to compare the prose excerpt and the poem, filling in the blanks with details from the pieces.

IMPRESSION OR FOCUS	PROSE	POEM
The relationship between Rano and Luis is complex.		
Luis feels sympathy for his brother.		
There is a focus on the issue of race relations.		
The reader can empathize with the feelings of both boys.		
The contrast between what the boys want and what they have is vivid.		
Rodriguez implies that they should not have tried to "cross the tracks."		
Does Rodriguez use more subjective details or objective details?		

167

●◆The autobiography excerpt and the poem leave different impressions. Create a different impression of your own by turning the excerpt in lesson two into a poem. Determine the impression you want to create, either about Rano or the relationship between the brothers, then find words and phrases that you can arrange into a poem of about five to eight lines. Share your poem with a partner and discuss the changes from the autobiography.

Details often assume different meanings in different forms. They may be subjective or objective, depending on the writer's involvement in the events and the impression he or she wants to create.

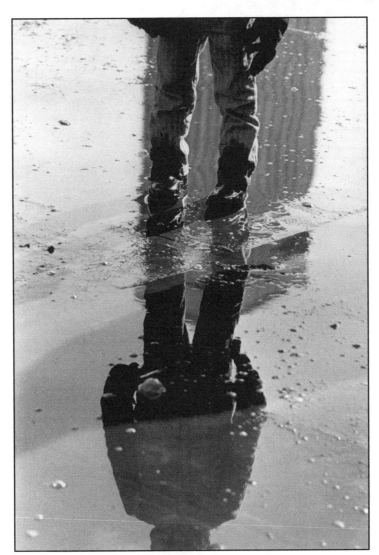

Interpretations: A New Look at Poems

Poems can be exciting to read and write about, provided we understand them. Sometimes poems seem too much like riddles or puzzles that we are never able to solve. Looking at poems by using interpretive strategies can provide a better perspective for understanding them. An interpretive strategy such as asking questions is a way to explain the poem and to understand it.

Active readers learn a variety of ways to make sense of poems. They may first read just to get a sense of the whole poem. They may ask questions or collaborate with others. Or they may compare two or more poems. Poems do not need to be puzzles when you have strategies for understanding them.

The various perspectives you use, and your ability to shift those perspectives, will help you take a new look at poems.

One

Getting a Sense of a Poem

One strategy for understanding and interpreting a poem is to listen to it and read it over a few times, letting images and impressions sink in. When you first look at this poem by E. E. Cummings, you may think you will never be able to make sense of it. However, pay attention to the clues that Cummings gives you and to the punctuation that he does use. He also structures the stanzas to give you clues to meaning. At this point, don't worry about analyzing the form of the poem; just try to get a sense of it.

- First, listen while someone reads the poem aloud. Write or draw your impressions and observations in the response notes.
- Next, listen while a second person reads the poem aloud. Add words or drawings to your initial impressions.
- Then, read the poem to yourself twice. Each time, add words or drawings.

Response notes

170

if everything happens that can't be done
E. E. Cummings

if everything happens that can't be done
(and anything's righter
than books
could plan)
the stupidest teacher will almost guess
(with a run
skip
around we go yes)
there's nothing as something as one

one hasn't a why or because or although
(and buds know better
than books
don't grow)
one's anything old being everything new
(with a what
which
around we come who)
one's everyanything so

so world is a leaf so tree is a bough
(and birds sing sweeter
than books
tell how)
so here is away and so your is a my
(with a down
up
around again fly)
forever was never till now

now i love you and you love me
(and books are shuter
than books
can be)
and deep in the high that does nothing but fall
(with a shout
each
around we go all)
there's somebody calling who's we

we're anything brighter than even the sun
(we're everything greater
than books
might mean)
we're everyanything more than believe
(with a spin
leap
alive we're alive)
we're wonderful one times one

Response notes

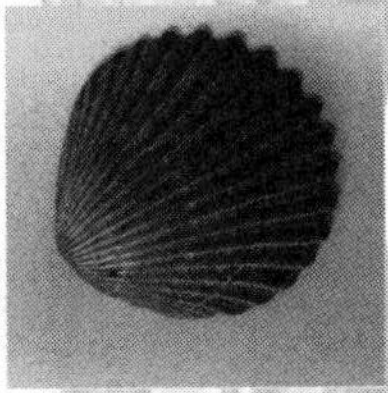

Look back over the poem and your notes. Write down four statements that represent certainties you have about the poem, such as "There are five stanzas," or "He uses parentheses." Also, write down one question that you have about the poem. We will return to these in the next lesson.

Certainties:

1.

2.

3.

4.

Question:

Get an impression of what a poem means before trying to interpret it.

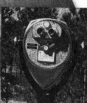

Questioning and commenting are two good ways to make sense of a poem. Discuss "if everything happens that can't be done" with three or four other people to share your notes from lesson one. Commenting on the observations of others is a way to continue making sense of the poem. Read the notes that other students made when reading Cummings' poem. In the right-hand column, write your comments about their observations.

E. E. Cummings	other student	you
one hasn't a why or because or		
although		
(and buds know better	he seems to be saying	
than books	that flowers are better	
don't grow)	than books	
one's anything old being		
everything new		
(with a what		
which		
around we come who)		
one's everyanything so	"everyanything" combines	
• • •	two ideas, kind of like the	
we're anything brighter than	poem does	
even the sun	This time "everyanything" is	
(we're everything greater	with "we." Before it was	
than books	with "one." I wonder if	
might mean)	that means anything?	
we're everyanything more than		
believe		
(with a spin		
leap		
alive we're alive)	the first stanza and the	
we're wonderful one times one	last stanza both end with	
	"one"	

172

●◆In one or two sentences, write down the sense you have made of this poem. What do you think is the subject, and why do you think so?

Respond to the questions and comments of others to help make sense of a poem.

Three

Juxtaposing Texts

Another way to understand a poem better is to see how it relates to other poems. As you juxtapose texts, or read them together, you examine elements of the poems side by side to construct meaning.

Have someone read aloud "When I Heard the Learn'd Astronomer" and "Have You Ever Hurt About Baskets?" Write or draw your initial impressions of the poems together and separately.

When I Heard the Learn'd Astronomer
Walt Whitman

When I heard the learn'd astronomer,
When the proofs, the figures, were ranged in column
    before me,
When I was shown the charts and diagrams, to add, divide
    and measure them,
When I sitting heard the astronomer where he lectured
    with much applause in the lecture room,
How soon unaccountable I became tired and sick,
Till rising and gliding out I wander'd off by myself,
In the mystical moist night-air, and from time to time,
Look'd up in perfect silence at the stars.

173

Have You Ever Hurt About Baskets?
Marylita Altaha

Have you ever hurt about baskets?
I have, seeing my grandmother weaving for a long time.
Have you ever hurt about work?
I have, because my father works too hard and he tells
    how he works.
Have you ever hurt about cattle?
I have, because my grandfather has been working on the
    cattle for a long time.
Have you ever hurt about school?
I have, because I learned a lot of words from school,
And they are not my words.

Discuss your reactions with at least two other people. Add to your response notes after hearing what others thought.

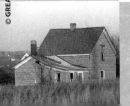

Reread the two poems silently. Note the connections that the poems have. What seems to be the subject of each poem? How does the speaker in each poem feel about the subject? How else can you relate the poems to each other? What connections can you make to "if everything happens that can't be done"? Write your notes below.

Juxtaposing texts gives you different perspectives on a topic. Use those perspectives to interpret each poem.

Four
Using Venn Diagrams

Extend your understanding of poems by comparing and contrasting them. Use a Venn diagram, a graphic organizer with overlapping circles, to chart information and ideas about the poems by Whitman, Cummings, and Altaha. Write what the poems have in common in the areas where the circles overlap. Write what is distinct about each poem in the area where there is no overlap.

WHITMAN

Cummings

ALTAHA

➥ What do you know about the three poems now that you did not know when you first read them? Write down your ideas about the perspective each poet gives on the subject and how the structure and voice of the poem reflect the perspective. In several sentences, speculate on why each author might have made the decisions that he or she did. (Speculating is merely informed guessing, not necessarily having correct answers.)

Comparing
and contrasting help you
determine a poet's point of
view toward the topic.

Five
Selecting Strategies

As you read poems, you will need to select one or more interpretive strategies that work best for you. If the poem seems difficult at first, you may want to begin by getting a sense of it. Asking questions and drawing conclusions are good ways to make sense of poems. Juxtaposing the texts and using Venn diagrams can help you shift perspectives on individual poems. Writing about your understandings will help you keep track of your thinking about the poem or poems. You may not use all of these strategies all of the time and you may not use them in this order, but you need to be aware of how you read poems and why you read the way you do.

Read the following poems, conscious of the strategies that you are using to understand them. Record your observations in the margins as you read or immediately after you have read each poem.

Response notes

R-P-O-P-H-E-S-S-A-G-R
E. E. Cummings

                    r-p-o-p-h-e-s-s-a-g-r
            who
a)s w(e loo)k
upnowgath
            PPEGORHRASS
                            eringint(o-'
aThe):l
        eA
            !p:
S   a
                (r
rIvInG   .gRrEaPsPhOs)
                            to
rea(be)rran(com)gi(e)ngly
,grasshopper;

The Negro Speaks of Rivers
Langston Hughes

I've known rivers:
I've known rivers ancient as the world and older than the
    flow of human blood in human veins.

My soul has grown deep like the rivers.

I bathed in the Euphrates when dawns were young. I built
my hut near the Congo and it lulled me to sleep.
I looked upon the Nile and raised the pyramids above it.
I heard the singing of the Mississippi when Abe Lincoln
        went down to New Orleans, and I've seen its muddy
    bosom turn all golden in the sunset.

I've known rivers:
Ancient, dusky rivers.

My soul has grown deep like the rivers.

●◆ Write an interpretive summary of one of the poems. Tell what you think the poem is about and why you think so.

....

....

....

....

....

....

....

....

●◆ Now describe what strategies you used to understand the poem. How did you decide what strategies to select? What else did you do to understand the poem?

....

....

....

....

....

....

Being aware of how you read poems and of the various interpretive strategies available to you will help you read poetry.

The Use of Questions

Why is the sky blue? Where does the sun go at night? How do birds fly? Questions come naturally to us when we're children and the world is new. As we grow older, however, we often replace questions with assumptions. We think we know; we assume that we know when we really need to ask in order to learn.

Questions are at the heart of learning. We need to learn how to ask them, where they lead, and what they provoke. Sometimes writers pose questions when they are trying to get readers to participate in their own explorations. Sentences written as statements are closed. They may provoke thoughts, but they already tell us what the speaker or writer thinks. Sentences written as questions are open; they invite us to see possibilities that we hadn't thought of before.

Questions and Answers

The game "Twenty Questions" is based on asking *yes* or *no* questions to identify what the object is. By learning to ask the right kind of question, narrowing the object down by such attributes as size and use, a player can get quite good at solving the riddle. Read the poem below in which Donald Justice plays a different kind of "Twenty Questions."

Response notes

Twenty Questions
Donald Justice

Is it raining out?
Is it raining in?
Are you a public fountain?
Are you an antique musical instrument?
Are you a famous resort, perhaps?
What is your occupation?
Are you by chance a body of water?
Do you often travel alone?
What is your native language, then?
Do you recall the word for carnation?

Are you sorry?
Will you be sorry?
Is this your handkerchief?
What is your destination?
Are you Aquarius?
Are you the watermelon flower?
Will you please take off your glasses?
Is this a holiday for you?
Is that a scar, or a birthmark?
Is there no word for calyx in your tongue?

●◆ Make up your own "Twenty Questions" poem. Use these guidelines:

• Make the first ten of your twenty questions apply directly to some aspect of your object.

• Make the last ten questions less obvious.

180

181

Trade poems with a partner and discuss each other's riddles.

Writers sometimes use questions as a way of making remarks or statements. Writing your own question poem helps you understand this technique.

Two

Simple Questions, Complex Answers

Sometimes writers use questions to get their readers to think about complex issues. Read the three poems by Pablo Neruda below, concentrating on where the questions lead. Neruda was a Chilean poet famous for his love poems as well as for his political involvement in Chile. Can you spot any hints of Neruda's political struggles?

Response notes

182

from **The Book of Questions**
Pablo Neruda

VII

Is peace the peace of the dove?
Does the leopard wage war?

Why does the professor teach
the geography of death?

What happens to swallows
who are late for school?

Is it true they scatter
transparent letters across the sky?

XVI

Do salt and sugar work
to build a white tower?

Is it true that in an anthill
dreams are a duty?

Do you know what the earth
meditates upon in autumn?

(Why not give a medal
to the first golden leaf?)

XXIV

Is 4 the same 4 for everybody?
Are all sevens equal?

When the convict ponders the light
is it the same light that shines on you?

For the diseased, what color
do you think April is?

Which occidental monarchy
will fly flags of poppies?

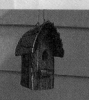

Reread the poems carefully, looking at the kinds of questions in each poem. The chart below lists several kinds of questions, each with an example. Find more examples of these types of questions.

Playful question: What happens to swallows who are late for school?

Your examples

_____

_____

_____

_____

Questions about nature: Is it true that in an anthill dreams are a duty?

Your examples

_____

183

_____

_____

_____

Questions about perception or ways of understanding:
Is 4 the same 4 for everybody? / Are all sevens equal?

Your examples

_____

_____

_____

_____

_____

●◆ Think about an issue that is important to you, such as the value of friendship or the controversy over animal rights. Write a question poem of your own. Include at least one question for each of the three categories in the chart. The questions should force your reader to reflect on the subject.

Writers often use questions to explore their own ideas. Even simple or childlike questions can be extremely deep or even unanswerable.

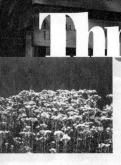

Three

Questions and Antecedents

The connections in poems are often subtle, resting on your understanding of a pronoun. The word *pronoun* literally means "a word standing for a noun." In order to understand the meanings of the pronouns, you need to identify the antecedents, the words the pronouns stand for.

Read two more of Neruda's question poems and pay attention to what the pronouns stand for.

---

from ***The Book of Questions***
Pablo Neruda

XXII

Love, love, his and hers,
if they've gone, where did they go?

Yesterday, yesterday I asked my eyes
when will we see each other again?

And when you change the landscape
is it with bare hands or with gloves?

How does rumor of the sky smell
when the blue of water sings?

XLIV

Where is the child I was,
still inside me or gone?

Does he know that I never loved him
and that he never loved me?

Why did we spend so much time
growing up only to separate?

Why did we both not die
when my childhood died?

And why does my skeleton pursue me
if my soul has fallen away?

Response notes

185

Locate the antecedents for the following pronouns in poem XXII; the first one is done for you.

PRONOUNS	ANTECEDENTS
line 2: "they've" and "they"	*the loves his and hers*
line 4: "we"	
line 5: "you"	

●◆ Now that you've analyzed the antecedents, what do you think the third stanza means?

Now locate the antecedents for the pronouns listed from poem XLIV.

PRONOUNS	ANTECEDENTS
Line 3: "he" and "him"	
line 4: "he"	
line 5: "we"	
line 7: "we"	

●◆ Select one of the first four stanzas in XLIV. Write about what you think it means. Then tell what you think the last stanza in this poem means.

Good readers analyze a poem word-by-word and sentence-by-sentence in order to understand the meaning of the whole.

Four
Questions and Similes

One of the ways poets deal with abstract concepts such as love and death and the soul is to make comparisons between what we know and what we don't know. In "Some Questions You Might Ask," Mary Oliver uses a sequence of similes (direct comparisons using the words *like* or *as*) to get to her basic question: what is the soul? First read the poem for the pictures it creates in your mind.

Some Questions You Might Ask
Mary Oliver

Is the soul solid, like iron?
Or is it tender and breakable, like
the wings of a moth in the beak of the owl?
Who has it, and who doesn't?
I keep looking around me,
The face of the moose is as sad
as the face of Jesus.
The swan opens her white wings slowly.
In the fall, the black bear carries leaves into the darkness.
One question leads to another.
Does it have a shape? Like an iceberg?
Like the eye of a hummingbird?
Does it have one lung, like the snake and the scallop?
Why should I have it, and not the anteater
who loves her children?
Why should I have it, and not the camel?
Come to think of it, what about the maple trees?
What about the blue iris?
What about all the little stones, sitting alone in the moonlight?
What about roses, and lemons, and their shining leaves?
What about the grass?

Response notes

187

Reread the poem, this time looking carefully at the comparisons Oliver makes between the soul and some aspects of nature. Add your comments or observations to your response notes.

Fill out the following chart, listing five similes you find in the poem. In the second column, explain what quality of the soul Oliver is referring to in the simile.

The soul is like . . .	What quality forms the basis for the comparison?
line 1: iron	solid
line	
line	
line	
line	
line	

●◆ Extend Oliver's poem by writing more questions. Include similes in your extension. Remember to use some aspect of nature in your similes so they will be compatible with Oliver's questions.

Writers often use metaphors and similes to reflect on questions about large, abstract ideas. The images in the comparisons allow a reader to see and feel the ideas more clearly.

Five Questions and Paradoxes

A paradox is a statement that appears to contradict itself. Questions can sometimes be seen as paradoxes as well. Read this poem and see what you can make of it. Write your questions and notes about its meaning in the response notes.

What Is It?
Mary Oliver

Who can say,
is it a snowy egret
or a white flower
standing

at the glossy edge
of the lily-
and frog-filled pond?
Hours ago the orange sun

opened the cups of the lilies
and the leopard frogs
began kicking
their long muscles,

breast-stroking
like little green dwarves
under the roof of the rich,
iron-colored water.

Now the soft
eggs of the salamander
in their wrappings of jelly
begin to shiver.

They're tired of sleep.
They have a new idea.
They want to swim away
into the world.

Who could stop them?
Who could tell them
to go cautiously, to flow slowly
under the lily pads?

Off they go,
hundreds of them,
like the black
fingerprints of the rain.

The frogs freeze
into perfect five-fingered
shadows, but suddenly the flower
has fire-colored eyes

Response notes

Response notes

and one of the shadows vanishes.
Clearly, now, the flower is a bird.
It lifts its head,
it lifts the hinges

of its snowy wings,
tossing a moment of light
in every direction
like a chandelier,

and then once more is still.
The salamanders,
like tiny birds, locked into formation,
fly down into the endless mysteries

of the transforming water,
and how could anyone believe
that anything in this world
is only what it appears to be—

that anything is ever final—
that anything, in spite of its absence,
ever dies
a perfect death?

190

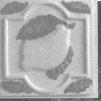

●◆ This poem can be visualized in three parts: the opening description, the action, and the closing commentary. Draw a sketch of each scene in the boxes below. (Don't worry about your drawing; the goal is to try to visualize what the words depict.)

the description

the action

the commentary

●◆Now write a paraphrase of Mary Oliver's poem.

●◆How did reading the poem as prose or seeing it as sketches affect your understanding? Which was more useful in helping you understand the poem?

●❖ Write your ideas about the paradox Oliver poses at the end of the poem: "how could anyone believe / that anything in this world / is only what it appears to be"?

192

Writers use questions to present and explore paradoxes. In this way, they can expand their search or their understanding of the apparent contradiction.

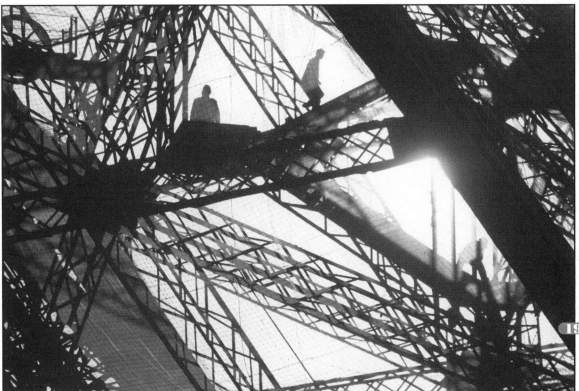

Writing from Models

I once wrote endless imitations, though I never thought them to be imitations, but, rather, wonderfully original things, like eggs laid by tigers.

Dylan Thomas

Painters have long known that they could learn two things from imitating other artists. One, they could learn about the artist's style as they imitated the brushstrokes and mixed colors to match the original. Two, they could extend their own ability to paint as they practiced different styles. Writers, too, imitate other writers, often, like Dylan Thomas, without being aware of it.

Writing from models requires close reading. It lets you get inside the author's mind. As you work with a poem, you imitate the author's intent, point of view, and sentence structure. At the same time, you practice ways of writing that will give you additional options in creating your own structure and style.

When writers find a poem they like, they often write their own version of it. Sometimes, it is in the form of a spinoff poem, which keeps the first line of the original. The poem "The Unloved" by Kathleen Raine is the kind of poem that is easy to model. You will see why when you read it.

Response notes

The Unloved
Kathleen Raine

I am pure loneliness
I am empty air
I am drifting cloud.

I have no form
I am boundless
I have no rest.

I have no house
I pass through places
I am indifferent wind.

I am the white bird
Flying away from land
I am the horizon.

I am a wave
That will never reach the shore.

I am an empty shell
Cast up on the sand.

I am the moonlight
On the cottage with no roof.

I am the forgotten dead
In the broken vault on the hill.

I am the old man
Carrying his water in a pail.

I am light
Travelling in empty space.

I am a diminishing star
Speeding away
Out of the universe.

194

Look closely at Raine's poem. To get a quick insight into it, make a series of sketches, one beside each stanza. Note which lines have images, which you can draw realistically, and which deal with abstractions, which can only be drawn as symbols.

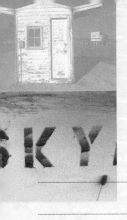

Now write a spinoff poem. Select a stanza that you like and "borrow" it for your poem. Use it as your first stanza, then go on from there, making up a series of metaphors beginning "I am…" Make each of your stanzas two or three lines until you get to the end. Finish with a metaphor of three lines, the way Raine does. When you have finished, give your poem an original title. Under the title, write "after a poem by Kathleen Raine." That is how you designate that you have borrowed her form and some of her lines.

195

Writing a spinoff poem allows you the freedom of writing your own poem and the discipline of following someone else's model.

Good writers use specific, vivid details to add richness to their work. Read "Where I'm From" by George Ella Lyon, poet, novelist, and children's book writer. Note her use of details to bring her childhood to life.

Response notes

Where I'm From
George Ella Lyon

I am from clothespins,
from Clorox and carbon-tetrachloride.
I am from the dirt under the back porch.
(Black, glistening
it tasted like beets.)
I am from the forsythia bush,
the Dutch elm
whose long gone limbs I remember
as if they were my own.

I'm from fudge and eyeglasses,
        from Imogene and Alafair.
I'm from the know-it-alls
        and the pass-it-ons,
from perk up and pipe down.
I'm from He restoreth my soul
        with a cottonball lamb
        and ten verses I can say myself.

I'm from Artemus and Billie's Branch,
fried corn and strong coffee.
From the finger my grandfather lost
        to the auger
the eye my father shut to keep his sight.
Under my bed was a dress box
spilling old pictures,
a sift of lost faces
to drift beneath my dreams.
I am from those moments—
snapped before I budded—
leaf-fall from the family tree.

Reread the poem, looking this time for the kinds of things that the poet says she is "from." Use the margin to make notes. Decide on four categories that things seem to fit into. Name the categories, then list all the things that fit into each category in the chart on the next page.

196

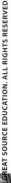

Category: Category: Category: Category:

●◆ Now, use the poem as a take-off point for one of your own. Begin by making the same categories as you did for the items in Lyon's poem. Then, brainstorm all the things that characterize where you are from. Use the chart to help you write your own "Where I'm From" poem.

Category: Category: Category: Category:

197

"Where I'm From"

Creating categories for the images in a writer's work helps you focus on the details.

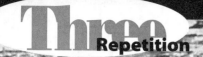

Repetition

nother, more subtle, technique writers use to add richness and vividness to their
work is **repetition**. Read "My Father After Work" by Gary Gildner. Note his use
of repetition. What is its effect?

Response notes

My Father After Work
Gary Gildner

Putting out the candles
I think of my father asleep
on the floor beside the heat,
his work shoes side by side
on the step, his cap
capping his coat on a nail,
his socks slipping down,
and the gray hair over his ear
marked black by his pencil.

Putting out the candles
I think of winter, that quick dark time
    before dinner
when he came upstairs after
shaking the furnace alive,
his cheek patched with soot,
his overalls flecked with
sawdust and snow,
and called for his pillow,
saying to wake him
when everything was ready.

Putting out the candles
I think of going away
and leaving him there,
his tanned face turning
white around his mouth,
and his left hand under his head
hiding a blue nail,
the other slightly curled
at his hip, as if
the hammer had just fallen out of it
and vanished.

●◆ Reread the poem, one **stanza** at a time. Think of a picture or **symbol** for each
of the three stanzas. Draw what you see in the boxes on the next page. Then draw
one image or symbol for the father.

Stanza 1

Stanza 2

Stanza 3

Image/Symbol for the Father

Now make notes for your own poem:
- Choose a person who is important to you for the subject of your poem.

- Think of a typical time of day or a specific place where you often see this person.

- Think of a dominant image or symbol for each stanza.

- Jot down or draw a symbol you might use to characterize this person.

Symbol

- Choose an opening line for your poem. It should be an action that you take, one that happens frequently. It might be something as simple as "Opening the door…" or "Listening to their conversation…" Follow that line with something else that you do, like "I think…" or "I wonder…" Use these lines as the beginning of each stanza. Remember to make each stanza a separate scene.

199

Title: _____

_____

_____

_____

_____

_____

_____

_____

_____

_____

_____

_____

_____

_____

_____

Writers repeat words or phrases on purpose. It helps them make a point and reinforce it.

Four Extended Metaphor

Read "Marshall" by George Macbeth. The first time through read just to get a sense of the poem. Note your responses as you read.

Marshall
George Macbeth

It occurred to Marshall
that if he were a vegetable, he'd
be a bean. Not
one of your thin, stringy
green beans, or your

dry, marbly
Burlotti beans. No, he'd be
a broad bean,
a rich, nutritious,
meaningful bean,

alert for advantages,
inquisitive with potatoes,
mixing with every kind
and condition of vegetable,
and a good friend

to meat and lager. Yes, he'd
leap from his huge
rough pod with a loud
popping sound
into the pot: always

in hot water
and out of it with a soft
heart inside
his horny carapace. He'd
carry the whole

world's hunger on
his broad shoulders, green
with best butter
or brown with gravy. And if
some starving Indian saw his

flesh bleeding
when the gas was turned on
or the knife went in
he'd accept the homage and prayers,
and become a god, and die like a man,

which, as things were, wasn't so easy.

Response notes

201

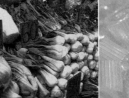

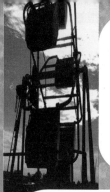

Notice that the entire poem is based on a single comparison, that of Marshall, the character of the poem, to a bean. This is an example of an extended **metaphor**. Macbeth develops the metaphor by first saying what kind of bean Marshall is not, then describing the kind of bean that he is. About halfway through, he moves from an extended description of character qualities to the kinds of action Marshall would take. Draw an arrow by the line in the poem where this transition occurs.

Make a list of vegetables and write down some of their characteristics. What kind of people would they be? What would they look like? How would they act?

Vegetable	Characteristics	What kind of person would it be?	How would it act?

Choose one of your vegetables for your poem. Give the vegetable a name. Then, following the general format of "Marshall," draft your poem.

> An extended metaphor is a comparison carried on for much if not an entire piece of writing. Writers may use the metaphor to highlight both serious and silly aspects of the comparison.

Five
Word-for-Word Modeling

R ead "Acquainted with the Night" by Robert Frost. The first time through read just to get a sense of the poem.

Acquainted with the Night
Robert Frost

Response notes

I have been one acquainted with the night.
I have walked out in rain—and back in rain.
I have outwalked the furthest city light.

I have looked down the saddest city lane.
I have passed by the watchman on his beat
And dropped my eyes, unwilling to explain.

I have stood still and stopped the sound of feet
When far away an interrupted cry
Came over houses from another street,

But not to call me back or say good-by;
And further still at an unearthly height,
One luminary clock against the sky

Proclaimed the time was neither wrong nor right.
I have been one acquainted with the night.

203

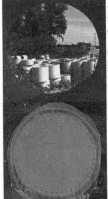

Now read the poem again, looking carefully for meaning. As you reread, **annotate** the poem with observations about Frost's use of **repetition**, **rhythm**, and **rhyme**. To get a better understanding of Frost's technique, imitate or, more precisely, emulate, Frost's style by writing a word-for-word model. **Emulation** lets you get inside the author's head and see how the words form sentences and sentences form lines that end up making a poem.

•❖Choose a topic to write about. (Your topic does not need to have anything to do with the subject of Frost's poem.)

GUIDELINES FOR WRITING AN EMULATION

1. Replace every word of the original with a word of your own that serves the same grammatical purpose. (In other words, replace a noun with a noun, verb with a verb, adjective with an adjective, and so on.)
2. There are places where you can simply use the words of the original. Words such as *and, but, or* may be kept; prepositions (words such as *in, out, above, through, with*) may be kept or replaced; and any form of the verb to be (*am, is, was, were*, etc.) may be used as in the original.
3. Where entire lines are repeated in the original, you should repeat lines as well. (Notice that the first and last lines of the Frost poem are the same.)

I have been one acquainted with the night.

I have walked out in rain—and back in rain.

I have outwalked the furthest city light.

I have looked down the saddest city lane.

I have passed by the watchman on his beat

And dropped my eyes, unwilling to explain.

I have stood still and stopped the sound of feet

When far away an interrupted cry

Came over houses from another street,

But not to call me back or say good-by;

And further still at an unearthly height,

One luminary clock against the sky

Proclaimed the time was neither wrong nor right.

I have been one acquainted with the night.

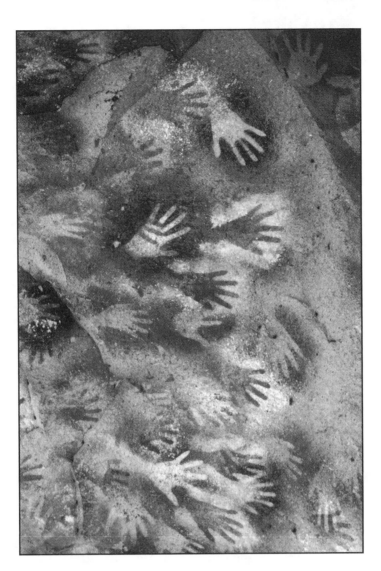

Focus on the Writer: Rudolfo Anaya

Reading several works by one writer is an important way to deepen your understanding of his or her ideas. You will begin to see how a writer has developed and recognize the writer's key concerns. By reading a variety of works, you will grow to recognize an author's style and its distinctive elements. You gain important insights, at a deeper, more intimate level, into the craft of writing. Biographical information will also help you understand the author's beliefs and ideas.

Rudolfo Anaya's first novel, *Bless Me, Ultima* (1972), was awarded the Premio Quinto Sol national Chicano literary award. His novels, short stories, essays, poems, and plays have further established his reputation. César A. González writes that Anaya is "acknowledged as the *padrino*, the godfather, of the rapidly developing canon of Chicano letters. He is a major voice in exploring the meeting of cultures in the New World persons of Chicanos and Chicana, and in our evolving self-definition through our writings. Anaya is, moreover, a leading figure in the field of Latino letters in this country."

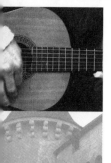

One Finding a Voice

Rudolfo Anaya wanted to write, but he was confronted with a problem many writers have—finding an authentic way to express ideas. Each writer's way is necessarily a little different because it grows out of life experiences, background, culture, education, and reading.

In a speech entitled "An American Chicano in King Arthur's Court," Anaya discussed the initial difficulty he had in finding a voice. His title is a reference to Mark Twain's *A Connecticut Yankee in King Arthur's Court*, a novel in which American and British ideas and values conflict.

← Response notes →

from **"An American Chicano in King Arthur's Court"** by Rudolfo Anaya

I remember when I started writing as a young man, fresh out of the university, my mind teeming with the great works I had read as a student. I was affected, as were most of my generation, by the poetry of Dylan Thomas, Eliot, Pound, Wallace Stevens. I had devoured the works of world authors, as well as the more contemporary Hemingway, Faulkner, Steinbeck, and Thomas Wolfe, and I felt I had learned a little about style and technique. I tried to imitate the work of those great writers, but that was not effective for the stories I had to tell. I made a simple discovery. I found I needed to write in *my* voice, of *my* characters, using *my* indigenous symbols. I needed to write about my culture, my history, and the collective experience of my cultural group. But I had not been prepared to explore *my* indigenous, American experience; all my education from first grade through a graduate degree had prepared me to understand King Arthur's Court. I discovered that the underlying worldview of King Arthur's Court could not serve to tell the stories about my communal group.

I suppose Ultima saved me. That strong, old curandera of my first novel, *Bless Me, Ultima*, came to me one night and pointed the way. Was she the anima, a woman of wisdom, the collective mothers of the past, or a reflection of the real curanderas I had seen do their work? I know she became a guide and mentor who was to lead me into the world of my native American experience. Write what you know, she said. Do not fear to explore the workings of your soul, your dreams, your memory. Dive deep into the lake of your subconsciousness, your memory! Find the symbols, unlock the secrets! Learn who you really are! You can't be a writer of any merit if you don't know who you are!

I took her kind and wise advice. I dove into the common memory, into the dark and hidden past which was a lake full of treasure. The symbols I discovered had very little to do with the symbols I knew from King Arthur's Court—they were new symbols, symbols I did not fully understand, but symbols that I was sure spoke of the indigenous American experience. The symbols and patterns I found connected me to the past, and that past was not only my Hispanic, Catholic heritage; that past was also Indian Mexico. I did what I had never been taught to do at the university. I explored myself and began to learn the workings of my soul. I was a reflection of that totality of the past which had worked for eons to produce me.

206

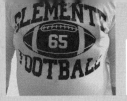

What forces contributed to Anaya's voice? List them in the chart. Then, show their relative importance to him by creating a pie chart. (The narrower the wedge of the circle, the less importance that force has.)

FORCES	IMPORTANCE

207

POUNDS PER SQUARE INCH

KILOGRAMS PER SQUARE CENTIMETER

A writer's voice develops from a series of influences. You must know who you are to write well.

In much of Rudolfo Anaya's work, the past is a potent force. He stresses the importance of respect for values passed on from generation to generation. He values learning from those he calls the "old ones." Think about what he learned from his grandfather as you read part one of his essay "A Celebration of Grandfathers."

---

from "A Celebration of Grandfathers" by Rudolfo Anaya

← Response notes →

"Buenos días le de Dios, abuelo." God give you a good day, grandfather. This is how I was taught as a child to greet my grandfather, or any grown person. It was a greeting of respect, a cultural value to be passed on from generation to generation, this respect for the old ones.

The old people I remember from my childhood were strong in their beliefs, and as we lived daily with them, we learned a wise path of life to follow. They had something important to share with the young, and when they spoke, the young listened. These old *abuelos* and *abuelitas* had worked the earth all their lives, and so they knew the value of nurturing, they knew the sensitivity of the earth. . . . They knew the rhythms and cycles of time, from the preparation of the earth in the spring to the digging of the *acequias* that brought the water to the dance of harvest in the fall. They shared good times and hard times. They helped each other through the epidemics and the personal tragedies, and they shared what little they had when the hot winds burned the land and no rain came. They learned that to survive one had to share in the process of life. . . .

My grandfather was a plain man, a farmer from the valley called Puerto de Luna on the Pecos River. He was probably a descendant of those people who spilled over the mountain from Taos, following the Pecos River in search of farmland. There in that river valley he settled and raised a large family.

Bearded and walrus-mustached, he stood five feet tall, but to me as a child he was a giant. I remember him most for his silence. In the summers my parents sent me to live with him on his farm, for I was to learn the ways of a farmer. My uncles also lived in that valley, there where only the flow of the river and the whispering of the wind marked time. For me it was a magical place.

I remember once, while out hoeing the fields, I came upon an anthill, and before I knew it I was badly bitten. After he had covered my welts with the cool mud from the irrigation ditch, my grandfather calmly said: "Know where you stand." That is the way he spoke, in short phrases, to the point.

One very dry summer, the river dried to a trickle; there was no water for the fields. The young plants withered and died. In my sadness and with the impulse of youth I said, "I wish it would rain!" My grandfather touched me, looked up into the sky and whispered, "Pray for rain." In his language there was a difference. He felt connected to the cycles that brought the rain or kept it from us. His prayer was a meaningful action, because he was a participant with the forces that filled our world; he was not a bystander.

A young man died at the village one summer. A very tragic death.

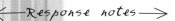

from **"A Celebration of Grandfathers"** by Rudolfo Anaya

He was dragged by his horse. When he was found, I cried, for the boy   ⟵ *Response notes* ⟶
was my friend. I did not understand why death had come to one so
young. My grandfather took me aside and said: "Think of the death of
the trees and the fields in the fall. The leaves fall, and everything
rests, as if dead. But they bloom again in the spring. Death is only
this small transformation in life."

Anaya says of his grandfather, "I remember him most for his silence." When
he did speak, he spoke "in short phrases, to the point." Look again at the
lessons Anaya learned and complete the chart.

EVENT	WHAT GRANDFATHER SAID	IMPLIED LESSON
Anaya stood on an anthill and was severely bitten.	"Know where you stand."	
The year it did not rain.		
A young man died.		

●◆ What do you think is Anaya's conclusion about the importance of learning
from the "old ones"?

●◆ What have you learned from the "old ones," either those in your family or others you know about? How did they teach the lessons you learned?

210

Writing about the past can give meaning to the present.

The Importance of Values

Cultural values are extremely important in Anaya's writing. On the seventy-fifth anniversary of New Mexico statehood, Rudolfo Anaya wrote an essay entitled, "At a Crossroads," about the changes to the Hispanic community since 1912. He said, "*Respeto* is a key value in our culture. Respect for the elders. We were bred on it as we are bred on tortillas and beans. It's a very important element in the family. Now we see signs of that respect and concern for the *viejitos* breaking down. That quality of respect for the elders in the culture is like the faith in the earth, and like honor in the family, pride in community, and awe in the beauty and mystery of the universe. It's those important ingredients in our culture the family has to safeguard."

●◆ Think for a few minutes about the "important ingredients" in your culture. Then, write about what those ingredients are and whether, like Anaya, you see them breaking down.

211

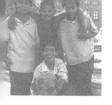

**Now read the conclusion of "A Celebration of Grandfathers" where Anaya
focuses on the importance of safeguarding the ingredients of the culture.**

from **"A Celebration of Grandfathers"** by Rudolfo Anaya

←—Response notes —→

I grew up speaking Spanish, and oh! how difficult it was to learn
English. Sometimes I would give up and cry out that I couldn't learn.
Then he would say, "*Ten paciencia*." Have patience. *Paciencia*, a word
with the strength of centuries, a word that said that someday we
would overcome . . . . "You have to learn the language of the
Americanos," he said. "Me, I will live my last days in my valley. You
will live in a new time."

A new time did come; a new time is here. How will we form it so it
is fruitful? We need to know where we stand. We need to speak softly
and respect others, and to share what we have. We need to pray not
for material gain, but for rain for the fields, for the sun to nurture
growth, for nights in which we can sleep in peace, and for a harvest in
which everyone can share. Simple lessons from a simple man. These
lessons he learned from his past, which was as deep and strong as the
currents of the river of life.

He was a man; he died. Not in his valley but nevertheless cared for
by his sons and daughters and flocks of grandchildren. At the end, I
would enter his room, which carried the smell of medications and
Vicks. Gone were the aroma of the fields, the strength of his young
manhood. Gone also was his patience in the face of crippling old age.
Small things bothered him; he shouted or turned sour when his
expectations were not met. It was because he could not care for
himself, because he was returning to that state of childhood, and all
those wishes and desires were now wrapped in a crumbling, old body.

"*Ten paciencia*," I once said to him, and he smiled. "I didn't know I
would grow this old," he said . . . .

I would sit and look at him and remember what was said of him
when he was a young man. He could mount a wild horse and break it,
and he could ride as far as any man. He could dance all night at a
dance, then work the *acequia* the following day. He helped the
neighbors; they helped him. He married, raised children. Small
legends, the kind that make up every man's life. . . .

I returned to Puerto de Luna last summer to join the community in a
celebration of the founding of the church. I drove by my grandfather's
home, my uncles' ranches, the neglected adobe washing down into the
earth from whence it came. And I wondered, how might the values of
my grandfather's generation live in our own? What can we retain to
see us through these hard times? I was to become a farmer, and I
became a writer. As I plow and plant my words, do I nurture as my
grandfather did in his fields and orchards? The answers are not
simple.

"They don't make men like that anymore," is a phrase we hear
when one does honor to a man. I am glad I knew my grandfather. I
am glad there are still times when I can see him in my dreams, hear

212

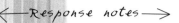

from **"A Celebration of Grandfathers"** by Rudolfo Anaya

him in my reverie. Sometimes I think I catch a whiff of that earthy
aroma that was his smell. Then I smile. How strong these people were
to leave such a lasting impression.

So, as I would greet my *abuelo* long ago, it would help us all to
greet the old ones we know with this kind and respectful greeting:
"*Buenos días le de Dios.*"

←—Response notes—→

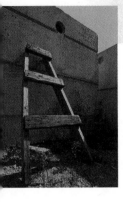

●❖Anaya asks two important questions that show his concern for
safeguarding the ingredients of the culture. "How might the values of
my grandfather's generation live in our own?" "What can we retain to
see us through these hard times?" He answers the questions indirectly.
Unless you are a careful reader, you might think that he does not
answer them at all. Select one of the two questions. Write what his
answer would be if he stated it directly, then quote phrases from the
essay that support your conclusion.

QUESTION: ....

213

ANSWER: ....

....

....

....

....

QUOTES: ....

....

....

....

....

....

....

....

An
author's
ideas
about
important
values are
often
implied
rather than
stated
explicitly.

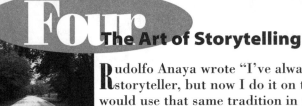

Four

The Art of Storytelling

Rudolfo Anaya wrote "I've always used the technique of the *cuento*. I am an oral storyteller, but now I do it on the printed page. I think if we were very wise we would use that same tradition in videocassettes, in movies, and on radio." In an excerpt from *Bless Me, Ultima*, Antonio (nicknamed Tony) hears a story that makes him question everything he has ever believed. Tony has stopped by the river to fish with Samuel on his way home from the last day of school. He is excited because he has been promoted two grades—from first to third—and will be in Samuel's class next year. He admires Samuel's knowledge of the world.

---

from *Bless Me, Ultima* by Rudolfo Anaya

←—Response notes—→

The afternoon sun was warm on the sand. The muddy waters after-the-flood churned listlessly south, and out of the deep hole by the rock in front of us the catfish came. They were biting good for the first fishing of summer. We caught plenty of channel catfish and a few small yellow-bellies.

"Have you ever fished for the carp of the river?"

The river was full of big, brown carp. It was called the River of the Carp. Everybody knew it was bad luck to fish for the big carp that the summer floods washed downstream. After every flood, when the swirling angry waters of the river subsided, the big fish could be seen fighting their way back upstream. It had always been so.

The waters would subside very fast and in places the water would be so low that, as the carp swam back upstream, the backs of the fish would raise a furrow in the water. Sometimes the townspeople came to stand on the bridge and watch the struggle as the carp splashed their way back to the pools from which the flood had uprooted them. Some of the town kids, not knowing it was bad luck to catch the carp, would scoop them out of the low waters and toss the fish upon the sand bars. There the poor carp would flop until they dried out and died, then later the crows would swoop down and eat them.

Some people in town would even buy the carp for a nickel and eat the fish! That was very bad. Why, I did not know.

It was a beautiful sight to behold, the struggle of the carp to regain his abode before the river dried to a trickle and trapped him in strange pools of water. What was beautiful about it was that you knew that against all the odds some of the carp made it back and raised their families, because every year the drama was repeated.

"No," I answered, "I do not fish for carp. It is bad luck."

"Do you know why?" he asked and raised an eyebrow.

"No," I said and held my breath. I felt I sat on the banks of an undiscovered river whose churning, muddied waters carried many secrets.

"I will tell you a story," Samuel said after a long silence, "a story that was told to my father by Jasón's Indian—"

I listened breathlessly. The lapping of the water was like the tide of time sounding on my soul.

"A long time ago, when the earth was young and only wandering tribes touched the virgin grasslands and drank from the pure streams,

214

from *Bless Me, Ultima* by Rudolfo Anaya

a strange people came to this land. They were sent to this valley by their gods. They had wandered lost for many years but never had they given up faith in their gods, and so they were finally rewarded. This fertile valley was to be their home. There were plenty of animals to eat, strange trees that bore sweet fruit, sweet water to drink and for their fields of maíz—"

"Were they Indians?" I asked when he paused.

"They were *the people*," he answered simply and went on. "There was only one thing that was withheld from them, and that was the fish called the carp. This fish made his home in the waters of the river, and he was sacred to the gods. For a long time the people were happy. Then came the forty years of the sun-without-rain, and crops withered and died, the game was killed, and the people went hungry. To stay alive they finally caught the carp of the river and ate them.

I shivered. I had never heard a story like this one. It was getting late and I thought of my mother.

"The gods were very angry. They were going to kill all of the people for their sin. But one kind god who truly loved the people argued against it, and the other gods were so moved by his love that they relented from killing the people. Instead, they turned the people into carp and made them live forever in the waters of the river—"

The setting sun glistened on the brown waters of the river and turned them to bronze.

"It is a sin to catch them," Samuel said, "it is a worse offense to eat them. They are a part of *the people*." He pointed towards the middle of the river where two huge back fins rose out of the water and splashed upstream.

"And if you eat one," I whispered, "you might be punished like they were punished."

"I don't know," Samuel said. He rose and took my fishing line.

"Is that all the story?" I asked.

He divided the catfish we had caught and gave me my share on a small string. "No, there is more," he said. He glanced around as if to make sure we were alone. "Do you know about the golden carp?" he asked in a whisper.

"No," I shook my head.

"When the gods had turned the people into carp, the one kind god who loved the people grew very sad. The river was full of dangers to the new fish. So he went to the other gods and told them that he chose to be turned into a carp and swim in the river where he could take care of his people. The gods agreed. But because he was a god they made him very big and colored him the color of gold. And they made him the lord of all the waters of the valley."

"The golden carp," I said to myself, "a new god?" I could not believe this strange story, and yet I could not disbelieve Samuel. "Is the golden carp still here?"

"Yes," Samuel answered. His voice was strong with faith. It made me shiver, not because it was cold but because the roots of everything I had ever believed in seemed shaken. If the golden carp was a god, who was the man on the cross? The Virgin? Was my mother praying to the wrong God?

Where does Anaya use some of the content and techniques of an oral storyteller? Number the places in the text, where he has the speaker, Samuel:

1. prepare the listener to hear a story

2. establish a sense of mystery

3. refer to superstition or luck

4. use more formal language than one would use in conversation (for example, "This fish made his home in the waters of the river," rather than "The carp lived in the river.")

5. represents in print the way we connect ideas in talking with "and," "but," and "so."

✎ Write a paragraph about what you think are the strengths and weaknesses of writing like an oral storyteller. Use examples from the text.

216

Stories often connect listeners with traditions and give them a sense of the connections between human beings.

Five Finding a Style

Anaya's ideas invite the reader to share in the "common memory." He stresses the importance of learning from traditional cultures and finding your roots. Look at how he presents his ideas by filling out the following topic chart.

Topic	"An American Chicano . . ."	"Celebration of Grandfathers"	Bless Me, Ultima
Meeting of cultures			the religion Tony was raised in conflicts with the story of the golden carp
Importance of respect			
Importance of the past			
Awe in the beauty and mystery of the universe		Grandfather said "Pray for rain."	

217

●◆ Write a letter describing Anaya's writing style to someone who has never read any of his work. Draw in ideas from all three pieces and explain Anaya's sense of tradition and its importance to him.

Writers' experiences and values influence all facets of their writing style.

Texts

10 "Early in the Morning" from *Rose* by Li-Young Lee. Copyright © 1986 by Li-Young Lee. Reprinted with the permission of Boa Editions, Ltd., 260 East Ave., Rochester, NY 14604.

11 "The Gift" from *Rose* by Li-Young Lee. Copyright © 1986 by Li-Young Lee. Reprinted with the permission of Boa Editions, Ltd., 260 East Ave., Rochester, NY 14604.

14 "Eating Together" from *Rose* by Li-Young Lee. Copyright © 1986 by Li-Young Lee. Reprinted with the permission of Boa Editions, Ltd., 260 East Ave., Rochester, NY 14604.

17 "Mnemonic" from *Rose* by Li-Young Lee. Copyright © 1986 by Li-Young Lee. Reprinted with the permission of Boa Editions, Ltd., 260 East Ave., Rochester, NY 14604.

20 Excerpt from *The Winged Seed* by Li-Young Lee. Copyright © 1995 by Li-Young Lee. Reprinted by permission of Simon and Schuster.

22 "Sunday in the Park" by Bel Kaufman. Copyright © by Bel Kaufman. Reprinted with permission.

27 "We Bad" by Salazar Arrué. Copyright © 1988 by Thomas Christenson. Reprinted by permission of City Lights Books.

30 "Why Tortise's Shell Is Not Smooth" from *Things Fall Apart* by Chinua Achebe. Copyright © 1958 by Chinua Achebe. First published by William Heinemann Ltd. 1958. First published in African Writers Series 1962. Reproduced by permission of REPP. Reprinted by permission of Heinemann Educational Publishers, a division of Reed Educational & Professional Publishing Limited, London, England.

34 Excerpt from "Gambling: Remembrances and Assertions," from *Walking Light: Essays and Memoirs* by Stephen Dunn. Copyright © 1993 by Stephen Dunn. Reprinted by permission of W. W. Norton & Company, Inc.

34 Excerpt from "The War Between Men and Women," from *Running in the Family* by Michael Ondaatje. Copyright © 1982 by Michael Ondaatje. Reprinted by permission of W. W. Norton & Company, Inc.

34 Excerpt from "The Circus" by Tibor Déry. Reprinted by permission of Exile Editions, Ltd.

36 Excerpt from *Paula* by Isabel Allende. Copyright © 1994 by Isabel Allende. Translation copyright © 1995 by HarperCollins Publishers. Reprinted by permission of HarperCollins Publishers, Inc. For additional rights/territory, contact Agencia Literaria Carmen Balcells, Diagonal 580, 08021 Barcelona, Spain.

41 Excerpt from *Annie John* by Jamaica Kincaid. Copyright © 1985 by Jamaica Kincaid. Reprinted by permission of Farrar, Straus & Giroux. Inc.

46 Excerpt from "I Get Born" from *Dust Tracks on the Road* by Zora Neale Hurston. Copyright © 1942 by Zora Neale Hurston. Copyright renewed 1970 by John C. Hurston. Reprinted by permission of HarperCollins Publishers, Inc.

49 Excerpt from *Long, Quiet Highway* by Natalie Goldberg. Copyright © 1993 by Bantam March.

52 "The Last Wolf" by Mary TallMountain. Copyright © Mary TallMountain from *No Word For Goodbye: The Blue Mountain Quarterly*, Vol. 27, No. 1. Reprinted with permission.

54 Excerpt from *Brave Men* by Ernie Pyle. Reprinted by permission of Scripps Howard Foundation.

58 Excerpt from *Woodsong* by Gary Paulsen. Text copyright © 1990 Gary Paulsen. Reprinted with the permission of Simon & Schuster Books for Young Readers, an imprint of Simon & Schuster Children's Publishing Division.

61 "A Poem for 'Magic' " by Quincy Troupe. Reprinted from *Avalanche*, a volume of poems published by Coffee House Press, 1996.

67 Excerpt from *Raising Demons* by Shirley Jackson. Reprinted by permission of Academy Chicago Publishers.

68 Excerpt from pages 99–100 of *An American Childhood* by Annie Dillard. Copyright © 1987 by Annie Dillard. Reprinted by permission of HarperCollins Publishers, Inc.

70 "Hall of Famer Still on Cloud 9" by Sam Lacy, published by Dutton of the Penguin Group in 1997. Reprinted by permission of the Afro-American Newspapers Archives and Research Center.

74 "Memoir" by Ann Hood. Copyright © 1993 by Ann Hood. Reprinted by permission of Brandt & Brandt Literary Agents, Inc. All rights reserved.

77 Excerpt from "Celebration" by Roger Angell from *Once More Around the Park*. Copyright © 1991 by Roger Angell Reprinted by permission of Ballantine Books, a Division of Random House Inc.

80 "Thumbprint" by Eve Merriam from *It Doesn't Always Have to Rhyme*. Copyright © 1964, 1992 by Eve Merriam. Reprinted by permission of Marian Reiner.

86 "The Flowers" by Alice Walker from *In Love & Trouble: Stories of Black Women*. Copyright © 1973 by Alice Walker, reprinted by permission of Harcourt Brace & Company.

89 "The Universe" by May Swenson. Used with permission of the Literary Estate of May Swenson.

93 All lines from "Metaphors" by Sylvia Plath from *Crossing the Water*. Copyright © 1960 by Ted Hughes. Copyright Renewed. Reprinted by permission of HarperCollins Publishers, Inc.

94 "Camouflage" by Linda Pastan. Copyright © by Linda Pastan. Reprinted with permission.

98 Excerpt from *Thirty Days To a More Powerful Vocabulary* by Wilfred Funk and Norman Lewis. Copyright © 1942 by Harper & Row, Publishers, Inc. Copyright renewed. Reprinted by permission of HarperCollins Publishers, Inc.

99 "Magic Words" by Nalungiaq from *Magic Words*. Copyright © 1968, 1967 by Edward Field, reprinted by permission of Harcourt Brace & Company.

100 "Between What I See and What I Say…" by Octavio Paz from *Collected Poems 1957–1987*. Copyright © 1986 by Octavio Paz and Eliot Weinberger. Reprinted by permission of New Directions Publishing Corp.

102 From *The Language Of Life: A Festival of Poets* by Bill Moyers. Copyright © 1995 by Public Affairs Television, Inc. and David Grubin Productions, Inc. Used by permission of Doubleday, a division of Bantam Doubleday Dell Publishing Group, Inc.

104 Excerpt from "The Eye of the Heron" by Ursula K. Le Guin. Copyright © 1978 by Ursula K. Le Guin; first appeared in *Millenial Women*. Reprinted by permission of the author and the author's agent, Virginia Kidd.

107 Excerpt from "The Kerastion" by Ursula K. Le Guin. Copyright © 1990 by Ursula K. Le Guin; first appeared in the *Westercon 1990 Program Book*. Reprinted by permission of the author and the author's agent, Virginia Kidd.

110 Excerpt from "The Darkness Box" by Ursula K. Le Guin. Copyright © 1963, 1991 by Ursula K. Le Guin; first appeared in *Fantastic*. Reprinted by permission of the author and the author's agent, Virginia Kidd.

114 Excerpt from "World-Making" by Ursula K. Le Guin. Copyright © 1981 by Ursula K. Le Guin.

118, 121 Excerpts from *A Silent Spring* by Rachel Carson. Copyright © 1962 by Rachel L. Carson, © renewed 1990 by Roger Christie. Reprinted by permission of Houghton Mifflin Company. All rights reserved.

123 Excerpt from *Snow Falling on Cedars* by David Guterson. Copyright © 1994 by David Guterson. Reprinted by permission of Harcourt Brace & Company.

127, 128 "Sonnet" and November 3, 1951, Postcard from *Letters Home By Sylvia Plath: Correspondence 1950–1963* by Aurelia Schober Plath. Copyright © 1975 by Aurelia Schober Plath. Reprinted by permission of HarperCollins Publishers, Inc.

130 Excerpt from "There Will Come Soft Rains" by Ray Bradbury. Reprinted by permission of Don Congdon Associates, Inc. Copyright © 1950 by the Crowell-Collier Publishing Co., renewed 1977 by Ray Bradbury.

131 All pages from "Tuesday Siesta" from *No One Writes to the Colonel* by Gabriel García Márquez. Copyright © 1968 in the English translation by Harper & Row, Publishers, Inc. Reprinted by permission of HarperCollins Publishers, Inc.

133 Excerpt from *The House on Mango Street* by Sandra Cisneros. Copyright © 1991 by Sandra Cisneros. Published by Vintage Books, a division of Random House, Inc. and in hardcover by Alfred A. Knopf. Reprinted by permission of Susan Bergholz Literary Services, New York. All Rights Reserved.

139 Excerpt from "The Magic Poker" by Robert Coover, from *Pricksongs & Descants*. Copyright © 1969 by Robert Coover. Used by permission of Dutton Signet, a division of Penguin Books USA Inc.

142, 147 Excerpts from *Cat's Eye* by Margaret Atwood. Copyright © 1988 by O. W. Toad, Ltd. Used by permission of Doubleday, a division of Bantam Doubleday Dell Publishing Group, Inc.

153 Excerpt from *This Boy's Life* by Tobias Wolff. Copyright © 1989 by Tobias Wolff. Used by permission of Grove/Atlantic Inc.

158 Excerpt from "Many Smokers Who Can't Quit Are Mentally Ill" by Jane E. Brody. Copyright © 1997 by The New York Times Co. Reprinted by permission.

160, 162 Excerpts from *Always Running* by Luis J. Rodriguez. Copyright © 1993 by Luis J. Rodriguez. Reprinted with permission of Curbstone Press.

164 " 'Race' Politics" by Luis J. Rodriguez from *Poems Across the Pavement*. Copyright © 1989 by Tia Chucha Press. Reprinted with permission.

170 "if everything happens that can't be done" by e. e. cummings. Copyright 1944, © 1972, 1991 by the Trustees for the E. E. Cummings Trust from *Complete Poems: 1904–1962* by E. E. Cummings, edited by George J. Firmage. Reprinted by permission of Liveright Publishing Corporation.

173 "Have You Ever Hurt About Baskets" by Marylita Altaha. Reprinted from *Classroom Discourse: The Language of Teaching and Learning* by permission of Courtney B. Cazden and Heinemann, a division of Greenwood Publishing Group, Portsmouth, NH.

177 "r-p-o-p-h-e-s-s-a-g-r" by E. E. Cummings. Copyright 1935, © 1963, 1991 by the Trustees for the E. E. Cummings Trust. Copyright © 1978 by George James Firmage. From *Complete Poems: 1904–1962* by E. E. Cummings, edited by George J. Firmage. Reprinted by permission of Liveright Publishing Corporation.

177 "The Negro Speaks of Rivers" by Langston Hughes from *Collected Poems*. Copyright © 1994 by the Estate of Langston Hughes. Reprinted by permission of Alfred A. Knopf, Inc.

180 "Twenty Questions" by Donald Justice. Copyright © by Donald Justice. Reprinted with permission.

182, 185 Poems VII, XVI, XXII, XXIV, XLIV from *The Book of Questions* by Pablo Neruda. Copyright © 1991 by Pablo Neruda, translated by William O'Daly. Reprinted by permission of Copper Canyon Press, P. O. Box 271, Port Townsend, WA 98368.

187, 189 "Some Questions You Might Ask" and "What Is It?" by Mary Oliver from *House of Light*. Copyright © 1990 by Mary Oliver. Reprinted by permission of Beacon Press, Boston.

194 "The Unloved" by Kathleen Raine from *The Collected Poems* (London: Hamish Hamilton, 1981).

196 "Where I'm From" by George Ella Lyon. Copyright © by George Ella Lyon. Reprinted with permission.

198 "My Father After Work" by Gary Gildner from *Blue Like the Heavens: New and Selected Poems*. Copyright © 1984. Reprinted by permission of the University of Pittsburgh Press.

201 "Marshall" by George Macbeth. Reprinted with permission of Sheil Land Associates.

203 "Acquainted with the Night" by Robert Frost from *The Poetry of Robert Frost* edited by Edward Connery Lathem. Copyright © 1956 by Robert Frost, Copyright © 1928 by Henry Holt and Company, Inc. Reprinted by permission of Henry Holt and Company, Inc.

206 Excerpt from "An American Chicano in King Arthur's Court" by Rudolfo Anaya from *The Anaya Reader*. Copyright © 1995 by Rudolfo Anaya. Published by Warner Books. First published in *Old Southwest / New Southwest: Essays on a Region and its Literature*, ed. Indy Nolte Lengink, the Tucson-Pima Public Library (1987).

208, 212 Excerpts from "A Celebration of Grandfathers." Copyright © 1983 by Rudolfo Anaya. First published in *New Mexico Magazine*, March 1983.

214 Excerpt from *Bless Me, Ultima* by Rudolfo Anaya. Copyright © 1974 by Rudolfo Anaya. Published in hardcover and mass market paperback by Warner Books Inc. 1994; originally published by TQS Publications.

Design: Christine Ronan Design

Picture Research: Feldman and Associates

Front and Back Cover Photographs: Mel Hill

Interior Photographs: Unless otherwise noted below, all photographs are the copyrighted work of Mel Hill.

9 Copyright © Michael Bank/Tony Stone Images

21 Copyright © Jerry Gay/Tony Stone Images

35 Copyright © Russell Hart/Photonica

51 Copyright © Rob Bodreau/Tony Stone Images

65 Copyright © Anne-Marie Weber/FPG International

79 Copyright © Telegraph Color Library/FPG International

91 Copyright © Masao Muka/Photonica

103 Copyright © Wayne Levin/FPG International

117 Copyright © Jonathan Morgan/Tony Stone Images

129 SuperStock International

141 SuperStock International

157 Copyright © Frank Sarangesa/FPG International

169 Copyright © Gene Tahoff/FPG International

179 Copyright © John Brown/Tony Stone Images

193 Copyright © Stephen Simpson/FPG International

205 Copyright © Philip and Karen Smith/Tony Stone Images

220

Glossary

alliteration, the repetition of the same initial sound in two or more nearby words in poetry or prose. "When to the sessions of sweet silent thought." (William Shakespeare, Sonnet 30) (See ASSONANCE and CONSONANCE.)

annotation, a note or comment added to a text to question, explain, or critique the text.

antecedent, the noun that a pronoun refers to or replaces. All pronouns must have an antecedent, and they must agree in number, person, and gender.

antithesis, a FIGURE OF SPEECH that uses an opposition, or contrast, of ideas for effect. "It was the best of times, it was the worst of times...." (Dickens, *A Tale of Two Cities*)

assonance, the repetition of the same vowel sounds in two or more nearby words in poetry or prose. Assonance is similar to ALLITERATION, but not confined to the initial sound in a word. "That dolphin-torn, that gong-tormented sea." (W. B. Yeats, "Byzantium") (See CONSONANCE.)

audience, those people who read or hear what a writer has written.

autobiography, an author's account of his or her own life. (See BIOGRAPHY and MEMOIR.)

biography, the story of a person's life written by another person. (See AUTOBIOGRAPHY.)

canon, body of books accepted as being of the highest quality.

characterization, the method an author uses to reveal or describe characters and their various personalities.

consonance, the repetition of the same consonant sound before or after different vowels in two or more nearby words in poetry or prose. It is similar to ALLITERATION, but not confined to the initial sound in a word. "Courage was mine, and I had mystery / Wisdom was mine, and I had mastery." (Wilfred Owen, "Strange Meeting") (See ASSONANCE.)

cuento, an oral storyteller who recites and preserves the folk traditions and stories of New Mexico and Central America. The name comes from *cuentos*, the Spanish word for the old folk legends of these areas.

description, writing that paints a colorful picture of a person, place, thing, or idea using concrete, vivid DETAILS.

detail, words from a DESCRIPTION that paint a picture for the AUDIENCE, explain a process, or in some way support the MAIN IDEA. Details are generally vivid, colorful, and appeal to the senses.

dialogue, the conversation carried on by the characters in a literary work.

docudrama, a television program that combines elements of a factual DOCUMENTARY with fictional dramatic sequences.

documentary, a movie or television program presenting factual information in an artistic manner. (See DOCUDRAMA.)

drama, a genre or form of literature meant to be performed by actors before an audience. Drama tells its story through action and dialogue. Dramas are also known as plays. (See GENRE.)

editorial, a brief persuasive article in a newspaper expressing an opinion about a timely issue.

emulation, a copy or IMITATION of a piece of literature, done to practice and study the style of the original author.

essay, a type of NONFICTION in which ideas on a single topic are explained, argued, described, and explored. The essay is an immensely varied form.

fiction, PROSE writing that tells an imaginary story. (See NOVEL and SHORT STORY.)

figurative language, language used to create a special effect or feeling. It is characterized by FIGURES OF SPEECH or language that compares, exaggerates, or means something other than what it first appears to mean.

221

figures of speech, literary devices used to create special effects or feelings by making comparisons. The most common types are ALLITERATION, ANTITHESIS, HYPERBOLE, METAPHOR, METONYMY, PERSONIFICATION, REPETITION, SIMILE, and UNDERSTATEMENT.

first-person, See POINT OF VIEW.

form, the structure or organization a writer uses for a literary work. There are a large number of possible forms: fable, parable, romance, satire, farce, slapstick, etc.

genre, a category or type of literature based on its style, form, and content. The major genres are DRAMA, FICTION, NONFICTION, and POETRY.

hyperbole, a FIGURE OF SPEECH that uses exaggeration, or overstatement, for effect. "I have seen this river so wide it had only one bank." (Mark Twain, *Life on the Mississippi*)

imagery, the words or phrases a writer uses to represent objects, feelings, actions, ideas, etc. Imagery is usually based on sensory DETAILS.

222 **imitation**, a piece of literature consciously modeled after an earlier piece. Imitations can be copies done for practice or a serious homage to a writer. (See EMULATION.)

journal, a daily record of thoughts, impressions, and autobiographical information. A journal can be a source for ideas about writing.

main idea, the central point or purpose in a work of literature. It is often stated in a thesis statement or topic sentence. Main idea is more commonly employed in discussing NONFICTION than the other GENRES.

memoir, a type of AUTOBIOGRAPHY that generally focuses on a specific subject or period rather than the complete story of the author's life.

metaphor, a FIGURE OF SPEECH in which one thing is described in terms of another. The comparison is usually indirect, unlike a SIMILE in which it is direct. "My thoughts are sheep, which I both guide and serve." (Sir Philip Sidney, *Arcadia*)

metonymy, a FIGURE OF SPEECH that substitutes one word for another that is closely related. "The White House has decided to provide a million more public service jobs" is an example. *White House* is substituting for *president*.

monologue, a literary work (or part of one) in which a character is speaking as if another person were present. The speaker's words reveal something important about his or her character or comments on the action.

narrative, writing or speaking that tells a story or recounts an event.

nonfiction, prose writing that tells a real story. There are many categories of nonfiction, including AUTOBIOGRAPHY, BIOGRAPHY, and ESSAY. (See GENRE.)

novel, a lengthy fictional story with a plot that is revealed by the speech, action, and thoughts of the characters. Novels differ from SHORT STORIES in being developed in much greater depth and detail. (See FICTION and GENRE.)

objective, refers to NONFICTION writing that relates information in an impersonal manner; without feelings or opinions. (See SUBJECTIVE.)

oral literature, stories (most often POETRY) composed orally or made up as the author goes along. This is the oldest form of literature and is characterized by REPETITION, patterns, and fluidity. Many poetic forms, such as the ballad and the epic, originated as oral literature.

personification, a FIGURE OF SPEECH in which an author embodies an inanimate object with human characteristics. "The rock stubbornly refused to move" is an example.

perspective, See POINT OF VIEW.

plot, the action or sequence of events in a story. It is usually a series of related incidents that build upon one another as the story develops.

poetry, a GENRE of writing that is an imaginative response to experience reflecting a keen awareness of language. Poetry is generally characterized by rhythm and, often, rhyme.

point of view, the perspective from which a story is told. In the first-person point of view, the story is told by one of the characters: "I don't know what I'm doing tonight. What about you?" In the third-person point of view, the story is told by someone outside the story: "The simple fact is that he lacked confidence. He would rather do something he wasn't that crazy about doing than risk looking foolish."

prose, writing or speaking in the usual or ordinary form. Prose is any form of writing that is not POETRY.

repetition, a FIGURE OF SPEECH in which a word, phrase, or idea is repeated for emphasis and rhythmic effect in a piece of literature. "Bavarian gentians, big and dark, only dark / darkening the day-time, torch-like with the smoking blueness of Pluto's gloom." (D. H. Lawrence, "Bavarian Gentians")

rhyme, the similarity or likeness of sound existing between two words. *Sat* and *cat* are a perfect rhyme because the vowel sounds and final consonant of each word exactly match. Rhyme is a characteristic of POETRY.

rhythm, the ordered occurrence of sound in POETRY. Regular rhythm is called meter. Poetry without regular rhythm is called free verse.

riddle, an ancient FORM of literature that is generally a puzzle or question. "Brothers and sisters have I none. / This man's father is my father's son. / Who am I?"

scene, See SETTING.

setting, the time and place in which the action of a literary work occurs.

short story, a brief fictional story. It usually contains one major theme and one major character. (See FICTION, GENRE, and NOVEL.)

simile, a FIGURE OF SPEECH in which one thing is likened to another. It is a direct comparison employing the word *like* or *as*. Cicero's "A room without books is a like a body without a soul" is an example. (See METAPHOR.)

stanza, a group of lines that are set off to form a division in POETRY. A two-line stanza is call a couplet. A four-line stanza is a quatrain.

structure, See FORM.

style, how an author uses words, phrases, and sentences to form his or her ideas. Style is also thought of as the qualities and characteristics that distinguish one writer's work from another's.

subjective, refers to NONFICTION writing that includes personal feelings, attitudes, or opinions. (See OBJECTIVE.)

symbol, a person, place, thing, or event used to represent something else. The dove is a symbol of peace. Characters in literature are often symbolic of an idea.

theme, the statement that a writer is trying to get across in a piece of writing. Lengthy pieces may have several themes. In stories written for children, the theme is generally spelled out at the end. In more complex literature, the theme is implied.

third-person, See POINT OF VIEW.

tone, a writer's attitude toward the subject. A writer's tone can be serious, sarcastic, solemn, OBJECTIVE, etc.

tradition, the inherited past that is available to an author to study and learn from. This generally includes language, the body of literature, FORMS, and conventions.

understatement, a FIGURE OF SPEECH that states an idea with restraint to emphasize what is being written about. The common usage of "Not bad" to mean *good* is an example of understatement.

voice, an author's distinctive STYLE and unique way of expressing ideas.

223